Osteoporosis Treatment

Elaine Dennison
Editor

Osteoporosis Treatment

A Clinical Overview

Springer

Editor
Elaine Dennison
MRC Lifecourse Epidemiology Centre
University of Southampton
Southampton
UK

ISBN 978-3-030-78127-9 ISBN 978-3-030-78128-6 (eBook)
https://doi.org/10.1007/978-3-030-78128-6

This Springer imprint is published by the registered company Springer Nature Switzerland AG
The registered company address is: Gewerbestrasse 11, 6330 Cham, Switzerland

Foreword

Osteoporosis is a disorder whose time has come (Fig. 1). Recognised since antiquity, the impact of the condition through its association with age-related fractures; an understanding of its cellular and molecular pathology; development of risk assessment algorithms; and the discovery of a wide range of effective therapeutic interventions which attenuate bone loss and prevent fracture; have led over three decades to a conceptual transformation of our understanding of this disorder. The term *osteoporosis* was coined by pathologists in France and Germany during the middle decade of the nineteenth century. The description was morphologic, based upon reductions in cortical thickness and trabecular architecture. It was paralleled by observations on the patterns of occurrence of fractures in older people, made by orthopaedic surgeons in France and the United Kingdom. These pointed out the increasing frequency of fracture with advancing age; the greater predilection of osteoporosis in women; and early observations on seasonal variation in fracture incidence. Although these observations postulated a potential role for impaired bone strength in the aetiology of fracture, it remained for Fuller Albright, senior endocrinologist at Massachusetts General Hospital in the mid twentieth century, to link oestrogen deficiency in postmenopausal women with reduced bone mineral density and elevated fracture risk. The subsequent demonstration that postmenopausal oestrogen replacement reduced fracture risk, and that this effect might be mediated by an inhibitory influence on osteoclastic bone resorption, led to a resurgent interest in the non-invasive assessment of bone density, which culminated in the launch of dual-energy X-ray absorptiometry (DXA) in 1987.

The provision of this intermediary biomarker of fracture risk permitted the World Health Organization to define osteoporosis according to the population bone mineral density distribution (2.5 standard deviations below the young normal mean) in 1994. This heralded a quarter century of intensive pharmacologic innovation with release of a variety of antiresorptive and formation stimulating agents now available. The last decade has witnessed the delineation of national and international strategies to target these agents most effectively and thereby reduce the fracture burden in increasingly older populations. This volume attempts to integrate these innovations and to contextualise them within broad international attempts to combat musculoskeletal ageing and preserve physical function. These are entirely commensurate with the recently launched WHO Decade of Health Ageing.

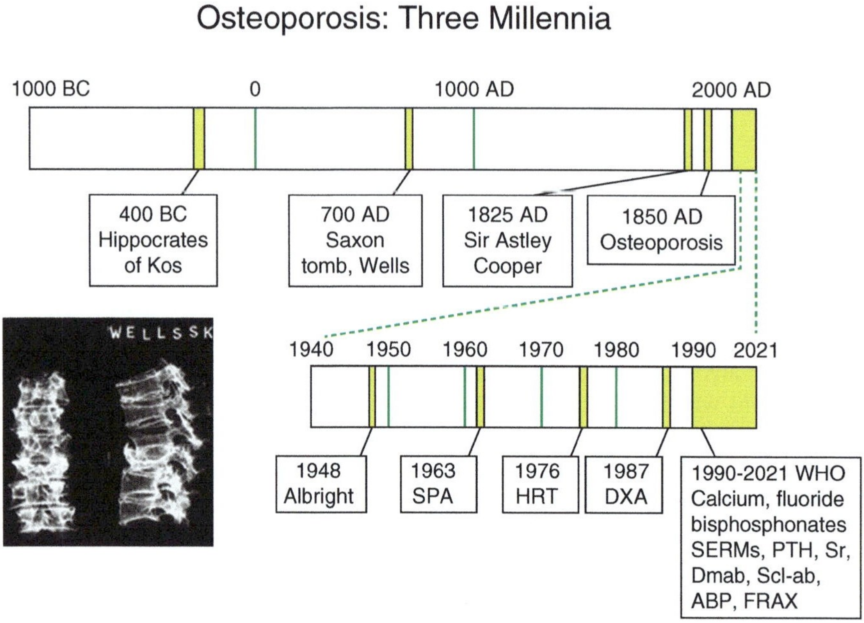

Fig. 1 Osteoporosis through the ages

Cyrus Cooper
MRC Lifecourse Epidemiology Centre
University of Southampton, Southampton General Hospital
Southampton, UK

Rheumatology Department
University Hospitals Southampton NHS Foundation Trust
Southampton, UK

NIHR Southampton Biomedical Research Centre
University of Southampton and University Hospitals Southampton NHS Foundation Trust
Southampton, UK

NIHR Oxford Biomedical Research Unit
University of Oxford
Oxford, UK

Contents

Chapter 1
The Epidemiology of Fracture: Why Treatment Matters

Elaine Dennison and Cyrus Cooper

Introduction

Osteoporosis is a skeletal disorder characterised by low bone mass and microarchitectural deterioration of bone tissue with a consequent increase in the fragility of bone and consequent susceptibility to fracture [1]. Historically, the term 'osteoporosis' first entered medial terminology in France and Germany in the nineteenth century, as a descriptive term emphasizing the porosity of the histological appearances of aged human bone. Prior to this however, work published by Sir Astley Cooper suggested that certain types of fracture may occur due to age-related reduction in bone mass or quality [2]. He described the original classical epidemiological hallmarks of these fractures: incidence rates that increase with age; rates which are higher among women than men; and fractures which are associated with only moderate trauma at sites containing large amounts of trabecular bone. These features are typified by fractures of the proximal femur, distal radius and vertebra, but fractures at other sites such as the pelvis, proximal humerus, and proximal tibia, also show similar patterns. These fractures are the serious and important outcomes of the condition and lead to severe mortality and morbidity, a significant burden on society in general and a huge impact economically. Osteoporotic fractures alone cost the United States around \$17.9 billion per annum and the United Kingdom around £1.7 billion [3]. A recent systematic review considered both direct and indirect costs associated with fragility fracture, since an additional burden to the initial costs of

E. Dennison (✉)
MRC Lifecourse Epidemiology Centre,
University of Southampton, Southampton, UK
e-mail: emd@mrc.soton.ac.uk

C. Cooper
MRC Lifecourse Epidemiology Centre, University of Southampton,
Southampton General Hospital, Southampton, UK
e-mail: cc@mrc.soton.ac.uk

E. Dennison (ed.), *Osteoporosis Treatment*, https://doi.org/10.1007/978-3-030-78128-6_1

managing fractures they are also associated with loss in quality of life, increased dependency and higher costs due to loss of productivity [4]. Although the literature was relative sparce, the authors concluded that the direct costs associated with fragility fracture generally far outweigh the indirect costs, although the changing role of women in coming generations may increase indirect costs as they play an increasing role in the workplace.

This chapter will review the epidemiology of fragility fractures, and highlight the importance of fracture at a personal and societal level.

Definition of Osteoporosis

The definition of osteoporosis has been difficult. A definition based solely on bone mineral density (BMD) does not encompass all the risk factors for fracture, whereas a fracture-based definition will not enable identification of at risk population An expert panel convened by the World Health Organisation (WHO) in 1994 tried to resolve this issue resulting in the current, most widely used definition that encompasses both BMD and previous fracture [5]; osteoporosis is defined when BMD measurements in women fall more than 2.5 standard deviations (SD) below the young mean. However this definition only takes into account the deterioration in bone mineralization and does not consider any of the micro-architectural changes that may weaken bone independently of any effect on BMD [5]. Recently there has been a move towards assessing an individual's 5- or 10- year absolute risk of osteoporotic fracture [6], a topic discussed further in Chap. 4.

Prevalence and Incidence of Osteoporosis

It has been estimated that 10 million Americans >50 years old have osteoporosis and a further 34 million are at risk of the disease [7]. There are an estimated 1.5 million fragility fractures each year. While most American women under the age of 50 have normal BMD, 27% are osteopenic and 70% are osteoporotic at the hip, lumbar spine or forearm by the age of 80 years [7]. Epidemiological studies from North America have estimated the remaining lifetime risk of common fragility fractures to be 17.5% for hip fracture, 15.6% for clinically diagnosed vertebral fracture and 16% for distal forearm fracture among white women aged 50 years. Corresponding risks among men are 6%, 5% and 2.5%. Data from the General Practice Research Database in the United Kingdom (which includes 6% of the UK population) [8] has indicated that the risk is similar in the UK. The lifetime risk of any fracture was found to be 53.2% at age 50 years among women, and 20.7% at the same age among men. Thus, one in two women and one in five men that are 50 years of age will have an osteoporotic fracture in their remaining lifetime [8].

Health Impact of Osteoporotic Fracture

All osteoporotic fractures are associated with significant morbidity, but both hip and vertebral fractures are also associated with excess mortality. In the year 2000 there were an estimated 9 million new osteoporotic fractures of which 1.6 million were at the hip, 1.7 million at the forearm and 1.4 million were clinical vertebral fractures [9].

It has been estimated that there are around 740,000 deaths per year associated with hip fracture [10]. Worldwide, osteoporotic fractures account for 0.83% of the global burden of non-communicable disease and 1.75% in Europe, where osteoporotic fractures account for more disability adjusted life years (DALYs) than many other chronic non-communicable diseases [10]. A recent Spanish study went further, and attempted to relate DALYs to level of bone density, achieving this in a sample size of 2782 (67%) out of 4157 postmenopausal women, with a mean age of 61.0 years [11]. Overall individual undiscounted DALYs per woman were significantly higher in women with severe osteoporosis with prior bone fracture compared to women with less severe osteoporosis or those with treated osteoporosis receiving anti-osteoporosis medication. AOM. Overall, however, DALY losses were considerable amongst postmenopausal women with osteoporosis but not having a prior bone fracture, being older, using a SERM and having fewer osteoporotic risk factors were all associated with less marked DALY losses.

Mortality

For fractures of the femur/hip and vertebral body, previous studies have shown clear evidence of excess mortality up to 5 years following fracture in both sexes, although fractures of the radius/ulna were only associated with slight excess mortality amongst men [12]. While this may represent complications of the fracture, such as infection and thrombo-embolism and subsequent surgery for hip fractures, it is likely to reflect coexisting co-morbidity in individuals sustaining a vertebral fracture. It has been estimated that 8% of men and 3% of women over 50 years die whilst hospitalised for their hip fracture. These mortality rates continue to rise over the subsequent months and at 1 year, mortality is 36% for men (higher for the very elderly) and 21% for women [13]. By 2 years after hip fracture mortality rates tend to decline back to baseline except in elderly patients and amongst men. The four main predictors for higher mortality appear to be: male sex, increasing age, coexisting illness and poor pre-fracture functional status.

In individuals following a vertebral fracture, the excess mortality appears to increase progressively after diagnosis of the fracture [14]. This has been observed in studies using both clinically diagnosed vertebral deformities and in those using radiological morphometric approaches to classify vertebral deformity. Impaired survival is more pronounced for vertebral fractures that follow moderate trauma, rather than severe trauma, of which only 8% are actually attributable to osteoporosis. Five-year survival appears to be worse for men (72% 5 year survival) than for women (84% 5 year survival). In women, an excess risk of death from cardiovascular and pulmonary disease that rises with increasing number of vertebral fractures has been observed [15].

Morbidity

In 2004 a study weighted osteoporotic fracture according to their morbidity—loss in utilities—in relation to hip fractures, to try and obtain a definition of the true burden of osteoporotic fracture [16]. To obtain the true morbidity of hip fractures in men between the ages of 50–54 years, the incidence of hip fractures should be multiplied by 4.48. Thus for men between 50–54 years, the disability caused by osteoporotic fractures is 4.48 times that accounted for by hip fracture alone. Four vertebral fractures appear to have the same morbidity as one hip fracture. For women of the same age, the incidence of hip fractures should be multiplied by a factor of 6.07 to obtain the true morbidity. Thus for women 50–54 years, the disability caused is 6.07 times that accounted for by fracture alone.

In the United States about 7% of survivors of all types of fragility fractures have a degree of permanent disability and 8% end up requiring long term nursing home care. Overall, after any type of fracture, a 50 year old US white woman has a 13% chance of experiencing attributable functional decline [17]. Hip fracture invariably requires hospitalisation and patients are prone to developing acute complications such as pressure sores, bronchopneumonia and urinary tract infections. The degree of functional recovery after hip fracture is age-dependent. Data published in 1996 from the US suggested that 14% of hip fracture patients in the 50–55 age group were discharged to nursing homes versus 55% of those aged over 90 years [17]. The length of hospital stay is also age related.

Pre-morbid status is also a strong predictor of outcome. In the US 25% of formerly independent people became at least partially dependent, 50% of those who were dependent pre-fracture were admitted to nursing homes, and those who were already in nursing homes remained there [18]. Results appear to be similar in France [19].

Hip fracture has a significant effect on an individual's ability to walk; 40% of individuals are still unable to walk independently 1 year after fracture, with 60% requiring assistance with at least one essential activity of daily living (e.g. dressing, bathing). Eighty percent are unable to perform at least one instrumental activity of daily living such as driving or shopping [13].

Despite only a minority of vertebral fractures coming to clinical attention, they account for around 52,000 hospital admissions in the US and 2188 in England and Wales each year in patients aged 45 years or over. The impact of a single vertebral fracture can often be low but multiple fractures lead to a progressive loss of height and kyphosis and severe back pain in both the acute and chronic stages [15]. The resultant loss of mobility can further exacerbate underlying osteoporosis leading to increased risk of further fractures [20]. The psychological impact of functional loss can lead to depression and social isolation as well as loss of self-esteem. Participants in the European Prospective Osteoporosis Study (EPOS) with radiologically identified vertebral fracture at baseline had repeat radiographs performed 3 years later. Women who had suffered a further fracture during this period experienced substantial levels of disability with impairment in key physical functions of independent living [21].

Wrist fractures do not seem to increase mortality [7]. They may impact on some activities such as writing or meal preparation, but few patients are completely disabled, even though over 50% report only fair to poor function at 6 months. This is often due to complications such as reflex sympathetic dystrophy, neuropathies and post-traumatic arthritis [7].

Fracture Epidemiology

Osteoporotic fractures characteristically occur in those areas of the skeleton with high amounts of trabecular bone after low or moderate trauma. The frequency of fracture increases with age in both sexes (Fig. 1.1), reflecting a combination of lower bone density and the increased tendency to fall in the elderly. Racial variation exists, with lower fracture rates observed in black than in Caucasian or Asian populations. Geographic variations in fracture rates have been demonstrated (see Fig. 1.2) even within countries, suggesting that environmental factors (including dietary factors and vitamin D levels) are important in the pathogenesis of hip fracture.

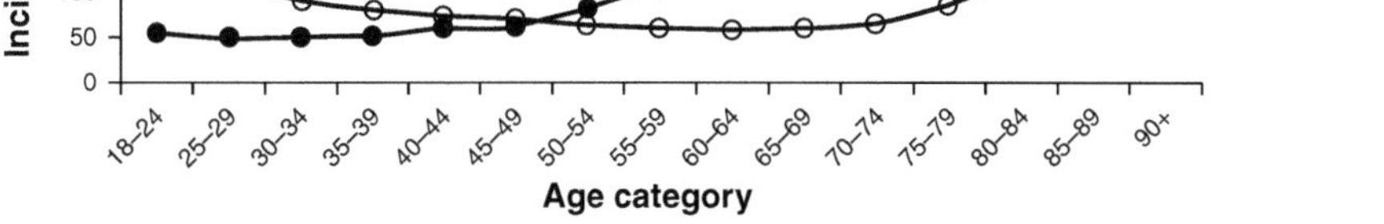

Fig. 1.1 Age- and sex-specific fracture incidence rate at any site among adults, 1988–2012, UK. (Reproduced with permission from Elizabeth M. Curtis, Robert van der Velde, Rebecca J. Moon, Joop P.W. van den Bergh, Piet Geusens, Frank de Vries, Tjeerd P. van Staa, Cyrus Cooper, Nicholas C. Harvey, Epidemiology of fractures in the United Kingdom 1988–2012: Variation with age, sex, geography, ethnicity and socioeconomic status, Bone, Volume 87, 2016, Pages 19–26)

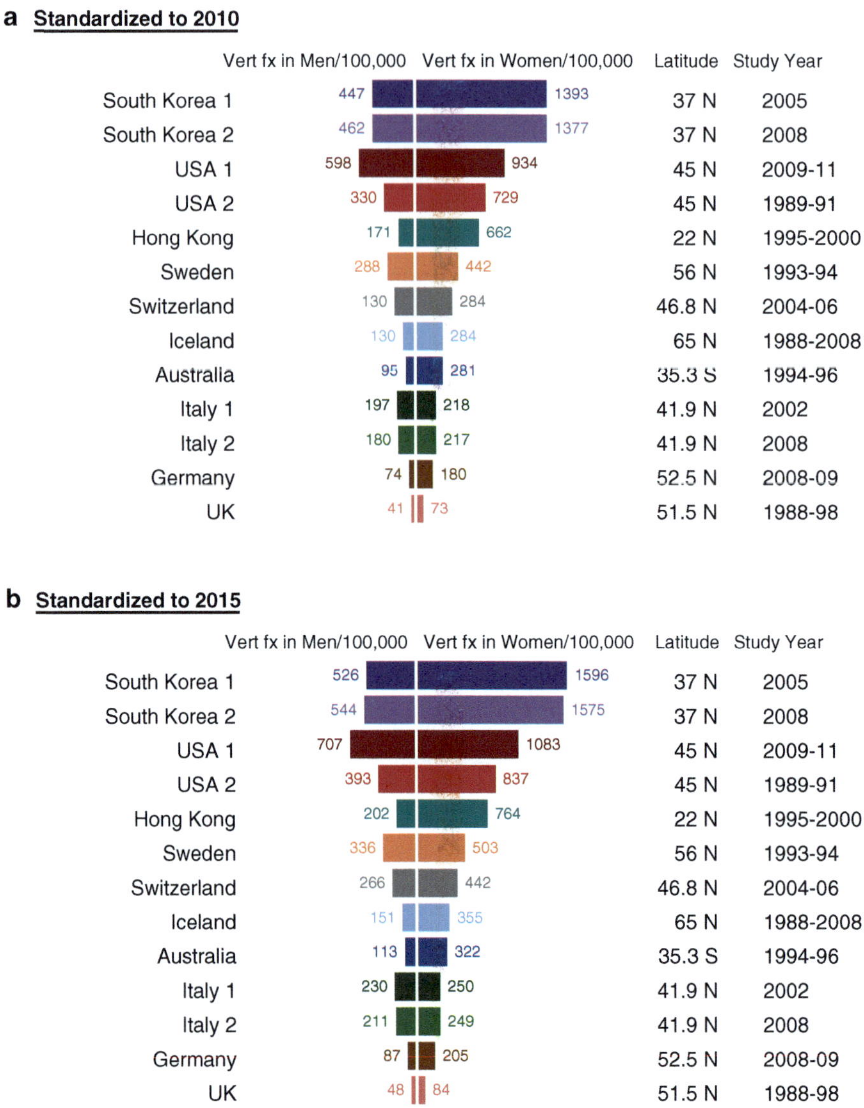

Fig. 1.2 Age-standardized incidence rates in women worldwide, combining hospitalized and ambulatory vertebral fractures, ranked by descending incidence. Standardization to 2010 UN population (**a**) and 2015 UN population (**b**). (Reproduced with permission from Ballane G, Cauley JA, Luckey MM, El-Hajj Fuleihan G. Worldwide prevalence and incidence of osteoporotic vertebral fractures. *Osteoporos Int*. 2017;28(5):1531–1542. https://doi.org/10.1007/s00198-017-3909-3 (Fig. 1.1))

Hip Fracture

Hip fractures represent the most devastating consequence of osteoporosis as they necessitate hospital admission and cause both excess mortality and significant morbidity. In most populations, hip fracture incidence increases exponentially with age. Most hip fractures occur following a fall from standing height. It has been estimated that worldwide there were 1.66 million hip fractures in 1990, representing 1,197,000 fractures in females and 463,000 among males, and that this figure will rise to 6.3 million by 2050 due to an increasing number of elderly people in the population [22]. In Western populations, among individuals above 50 years of age, there is a female preponderance of hip fracture with a female to male incidence ratio of approximately two to one. Overall 98% of hip fractures occur among people >35 years of age, and 80% occur in women. Hip fractures are seasonal, with an increase in winter in temperate countries, but occur mainly indoors, suggesting that rather than slipping on icy pavements being the primary aetiological cause, but rather the seasonal winter higher rates may be related to slowed neuromuscular reflexes and lower sunlight (and hence vitamin D levels) in winter weather.

Incidence rates vary considerably according to geographic area and race, and may vary widely within the same country and within populations of a given sex and race. In Europe, hip fracture rates vary seven-fold between countries [19]. In general people who live in latitudes further from the equator seem to have a higher incidence of fracture [23]. The highest rates of hip fracture are seen in Caucasians living in northern Europe, especially Scandinavians [24]. The rates are intermediate in Asians [25], China [26], Kuwait [27] and lowest in black populations [28]. Genetic factors may play an important role in the aetiology of hip fracture, as well as environmental factors.

Vertebral Fracture

The advent of description of morphometric and semi-quantitative visual techniques has now enabled a number of studies to report on the prevalence of vertebral fracture. Only about a third of all vertebral deformities noted on radiographs come to medical attention, and less than 10% necessitate admission to hospital [29]. In Rochester, Minnesota the prevalence of any vertebral deformity was estimated at 25.3% per 100 women aged 50 years and above, whilst the incidence of a new deformity in this group was estimated at 17.8 per 1000 person-years [30]. By contrast, in the European Vertebral Osteoporosis Study, one in eight women and men aged 50 years and over had evidence of vertebral deformity [31]. Prevalence of vertebral deformity increased steadily with age in both sexes although the gradient was steeper for women. There was a three-fold variation in occurrence of deformity across Europe and up to a two-fold variation in centres within individual countries, perhaps reflecting a combination of environmental and genetic factors. The risk of vertebral deformity among men was significantly elevated in those with high levels of physical activity suggesting the aetiological importance of trauma. By contrast, women with higher levels of customary physical activity have a reduced risk of deformity [32].

In instances where comparable methods and definitions have been used in studies, the prevalence of vertebral fractures has been more similar across regions than seen for hip fractures [33]. Recent data from the EPIDOS study have yielded estimates of prevalence of vertebral fractures of 19% among women aged 75–79 years to 21.9% among 80–84 years to 41.4% among those aged 85 years and older, and are broadly in accord with estimates from other populations [34]. Only a quarter of vertebral fractures result from falls, and most are precipitated by routine daily activities such as bending or lifting light objects, reflecting the compressive load of such acts.

Wrist Fracture

Distal forearm fracture almost always results as a consequence of a fall onto an outstretched hand. These fractures show a steep rise in incidence during the perimenopausal period among women, but tend to plateau thereafter. In men there is no apparent increase in incidence of wrist fracture with age. In white women, the incidence increases linearly between the ages of 40 and 65 and then stabilises, while in men the incidence remains constant between 20 and 80 years. A much stronger sex ratio exists for this fracture than for most others and this has been estimated to be 4:1 in favour of women. Recent data from Dorset, UK showed that among women, the incidence of distal radius fracture rose from a pre-menopausal baseline of 10 per 10,000 of the population per year to a peak of 120 per 10,000 of the population per year over 85 years [35]. Although geographic variation exists, a partial explanation may be methodological considerations of case ascertainment, as less than 20% of forearm fracture patients are hospitalised. A winter peak is again demonstrated, but unlike hip fractures, this probably is due to falls outside on icy surfaces. The plateau with age in women may be due to mode of falls; later in life a woman is more likely to fall onto a hip than an outstretched hand as her neuromuscular co-ordination deteriorates.

Other Fractures

The incidence rates of proximal humeral, pelvic, and proximal tibial fractures also rise steeply with age, and are greater in women than men. These are often termed frailty fractures, as they typically occur in women who are losing weight involuntarily [36]. Furthermore, there is some direct evidence that these fractures are associated with low bone mineral density [37]. Three quarters of all proximal humeral fractures are due to moderate trauma, typically a fall from standing height or less, and tend to be more common in women with poor neuromuscular function [38].

A recent analysis centred in the GLOW study evaluated healthcare utilization associated with treating fracture types in >51,000 women aged ≥55 years [39]. Over the course of 1 year, there were five times more non-hip, non-spine fractures than hip or spine fractures, resulting in twice as many days of hospitalization and rehabilitation/nursing home care for non-hip, non-spine fractures. Using imformation collected via self-administered patient questionnaires at baseline and year 1 in over 50,000 participants, researchers identified that during 1-year follow-up, there were 195 spine, 134 hip, and 1654 non-hip, non-spine fractures. Clinical vertebral fractures resulted in 617 days of hospitalization and 512 days of rehabilitation/nursing home care; hip fractures accounted for 1306 days of hospitalization and 1650 days of rehabilitation/nursing home care. Non-hip, non-spine fractures resulted in 3805 days in hospital and 5186 days of rehabilitation/nursing home care.

Clustering of Fractures

There is evidence from several epidemiological studies that patients with different types of fragility fractures are at an increased risk of developing further osteoporotic fractures, both at the same site and at other site. In general, the presence of previous vertebral deformities has been shown to increase the risk of subsequent vertebral deformities by seven- to ten-fold [40]. This is comparable to the increase in risk of second hip fracture observed amongst those who have already sustained their first hip fracture. In Rochester, Minnesota residents aged 70 years or less with radiologically diagnosed vertebral deformities were followed up to assess the development of subsequent limb fractures [41]. Among residents who experienced their first distal forearm fracture aged 35 years or older, and excluding fractures that occurred on the same day as the index forearm fracture, hip fracture risk was increased 1.4-fold in women (95% CI 1.1–1.8) and 2.7-fold in men (95% CI 0.98–5.8). Excess risk in women was confined to those individuals who sustained their first forearm fracture at age 70 years or greater. By contrast, vertebral fracture was increased at all ages, with a 5.2-fold (95% CI 4.5–5.9) increase in risk among women and a 10.7-fold (95% CI 6.7–16.3) increased risk among men. This increased risk was more marked in subjects with vertebral deformities associated with moderate or minimal trauma than with severe trauma.

Data from the European Prospective Osteoporosis Study (EPOS) indicates that prevalent vertebral deformity predicts incident hip fracture with a rare ratio of 2.8–4.5, and this increases with the number of vertebral deformities [42]. In the US, data from the Study of Osteoporotic Fractures (a prospective study of 9704 US women aged 65 years or older,) has demonstrated that prevalent vertebral deformity was associated with a five-fold increased risk of sustaining a further vertebral deformity; the risk of hip fracture was increased 2.8 fold (95% CI 2.3–3.4) and the risk of any non-vertebral fracture 1.9 fold (95% CI 1.7–2.1), after adjustment for age and calcaneal BMD [43]. Although there was a small increased risk of wrist fracture, this was not significant after adjustment for age and BMD. In the UK, a study has recently shown that 25% of patients with a new low trauma non-vertebral fracture had evidence of a previous vertebral fracture [44].

The number and morphometry of baseline vertebral deformities has also been shown to predict incident vertebral fracture [44]. The greatest risk of subsequent fracture appears to be greatest soon after a fracture, particularly in the first year, with an incidence of a new vertebral fracture at 19.2% [43]. Recent data suggests that the increased risk of virtually all clinical fractures persists for up to 10 years [45].

Economic Cost

The economic cost of fracture is very considerable and has been assessed in the UK and worldwide. The first-year direct cost per hip fracture in the United Kingdom was recently estimated to be between €11,055 and €20,359 [46] while in the United States the combined direct and indirect annual costs for hip fracture have been predicted to rise to US $131.5 billion by 2050 [47]. In a separate analysis it was suggested that patients with osteoporosis-related fractures incurred nearly US $10,000 in excess direct health care costs in the 6 months after fracture, when compared with patients who had not sustained a fracture [48]. The costs associated with other fractures have also recently been calculated, and in the United States, the cost of osteoporotic fractures in 2005 was estimated to be $19 billion in an older estimate of cost [49]. More recently, the cost of osteoporosis, including pharmacologic intervention in the European Union, was estimated to be €37 billion [50]; in the United Kingdom alone, the annual cost to the health care system for osteoporotic fractures was €5.5 billion [46]., highlighting the huge economic burden. Of these costs, hip fractures account for more than one third of the total figure. Since in many countries costs are rising faster than the general rate of inflation, this is a major source of concern and much research is currently focusing on the cost-effectiveness of treatment programs for osteoporosis.

Current Statistics and Future Projections

Currently worldwide, osteoporosis causes more than 8.9 million fractures annually, resulting in an osteoporotic fracture every 3 s [9]; osteoporosis is estimated to affect 200 million women worldwide - approximately one-tenth of women aged 60, one-fifth of women aged 70, two-fifths of women aged 80 and two-thirds of women aged 90 [51], and included in that figure osteoporosis affects an estimated 75 million people in Europe, USA and Japan. In the year 2000, there were an estimated 9 million new osteoporotic fractures, of which 1.6 million were at the hip, 1.7 million were at the forearm and 1.4 million were clinical vertebral fractures. Europe and the Americas accounted for 51% of all these fractures, while most of the remainder occurred in the Western Pacific region and Southeast Asia [9], and the majority of these fractures (61% osteoporotic fractures) occur in women. Overall, 61% of osteoporotic fractures occur in women, with a female-to-male ratio of 1.6 [9]. Importantly nearly 75% of hip, spine and distal forearm fractures occur among patients 65 years old or over [52]. Together these data suggest that as life expectancy is increasing around the globe and the number of elderly individuals is rising within every geographic region. The world population is expected to rise from the current 323 million individuals aged 65 years or over, to 1555 million by the year 2050. These demographic changes alone can be expected to increase the number of hip fractures occurring among people aged 35 years and over worldwide. On the basis of current trends, assuming a constant age-specific rate of fracture, hip fracture rates would be expected to increase in the UK from 46,000 in 1985 to 117,000 in 2016. Likewise, in the US, as the population over 65 increases from 32 million in 1990 to 69 million in 2050, the number of hip fractures in the US is expected to triple [53]. In the US in 2005, the total number of estimated incident fractures was over two million, with 72% of the costs being accounted for by hip fracture alone. By 2005 annual fractures and costs are predicted to rise by almost 50%, with the most rapid growth in 65–74 year age group rising by 87% and Hispanic and other subpopulations increasing by 175% [46].

There is, however, some good news in that there appears to a secular trend toward reducing hip fracture incidence (Figs. 1.3 and 1.4); in a review of studies worldwide, we previously addressed secular trends in the incidence of hip and other fractures [54]. Studies in western populations, whether in North America, Europe or Oceania, have generally reported increases in hip fracture incidence through the second half of the last century, but those researchers continuing to follow trends over the last two decades have found that rates stabilise with age-adjusted decreases being observed in certain centres. By contrast, some studies have suggested that the rate is rising in Asia, highlighting an urgent need to consider strategies to reduce burden in that geographic region. In another study from Framingham [55], researchers examined the decrease in hip fracture incidence over the past 40 years in the US. They studied 4918 men and 5634 women followed up prospectively for the first hip fracture between January 1, 1970, and December 31, 2010; in total the study contained more than 105,000 person-years in 10,552 individuals with a gradual shift toward the offspring participants in the 1980s and 1990s, and women represented more than 55% of the study sample over the years. Adjusted for age, the incidence of hip fracture decreased by 4.4% per year from 1970 to 2010. Interestingly the decrease in hip fracture incidence coincided with a decrease in smoking and heavy drinking while the prevalence of other risk factors for hip fracture, such as being underweight or obese or having had a premature menopause were stable over the study period. The study authors concluded that while better uptake of therapies may contribute, change in lifestyle may also be important and they reinforced the need to treat patients with osteoporosis while continuing to encourage public health interventions for smoking cessation and heavy drinking.

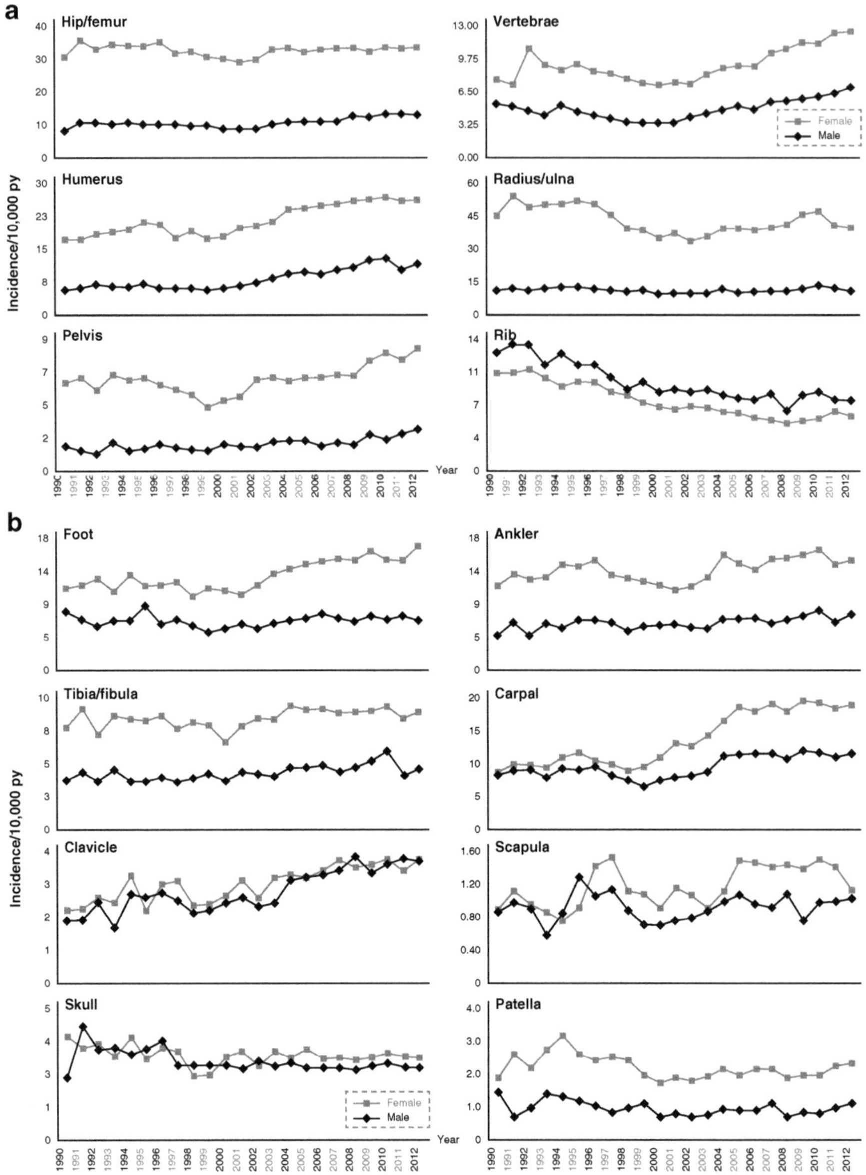

Fig. 1.3 Yearly incidence rates in the years 1990 to 2012 of (**a**) osteoporotic fractures and (**b**) other fracture sites. Secular trends in fracture incidence in the UK between 1990 and 2012. (Reproduced with permission from van der Velde RY, Wyers CE, Curtis EM, Geusens PPMM, van den Bergh JPW, de Vries F, Cooper C, van Staa TP, Harvey NC. Secular trends in fracture incidence in the UK between 1990 and 2012. Osteoporos Int. 2016 Nov;27(11):3197–3206 (Fig. 1.1))

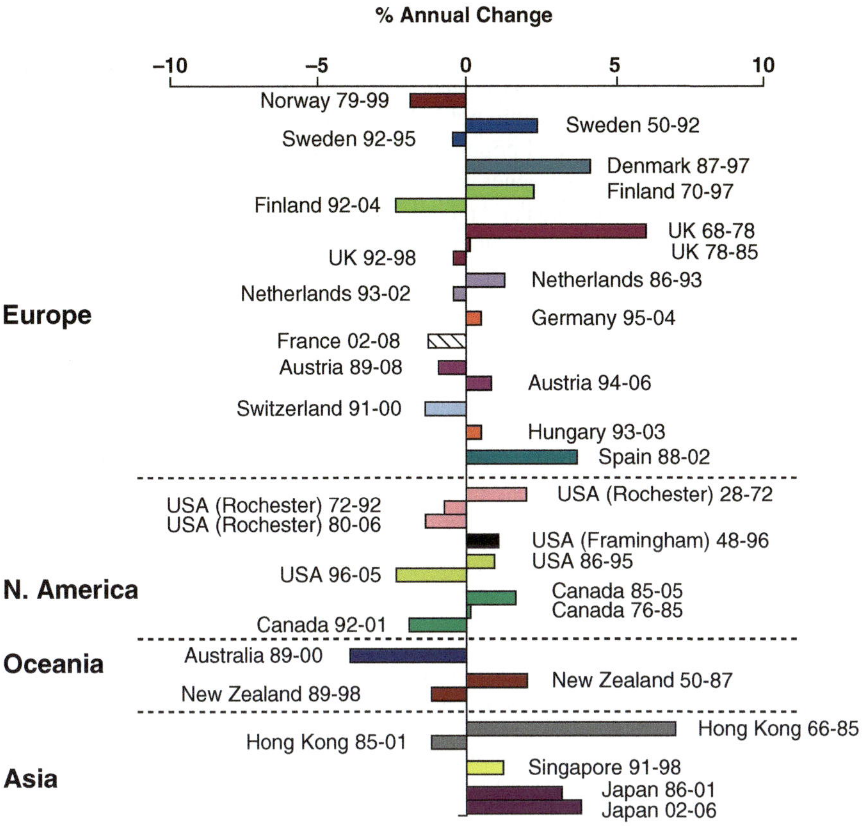

Fig. 1.4 Secular trends in hip fracture worldwide: annual change in age- and sex-adjusted hip fracture incidence. (Reroduced with permission from (Fig. 1.4) Cooper, C., Cole, Z.A., Holroyd, C.R. et al. Secular trends in the incidence of hip and other osteoporotic fractures. *Osteoporos Int* **22,** 1277 (2011))

While half of all hip fractures among elderly people in 1990 took place in Europe and North America, by 2050 the increasingly elderly population in Latin America and Asia could lead to a shift in the geographical distribution of hip fractures, with only a quarter occurring in Europe and North America [53].

Aside from hip fracture, incidence rates for fractures at other skeletal sites are also expected to rise significantly. Studies from Sweden, have suggested that the absolute number of hip fractures among the elderly in Sweden has largely remained constant between 1987 and 2009, while incidence rates have decreased for all age- and sex-specific groups, with the largest changes in the younger age groups and among women. The researchers also reported that the mean age of sustaining a hip fracture has increased for both sexes [56]. Similarly, a Finnish study reported that the number of hip fractures rose sharply till the end of 1990s, but since then, the rise has slowed down and the age-adjusted incidence of hip fracture increased until 1997 but declined thereafter [57].

Conclusion

Osteoporosis is a disease that has a huge effect on public health. The impact of osteoporotic fracture is far-reaching not only for the individual themselves, but for the health service, economy and population as a whole. Osteoporotic fractures are expected to rise in subsequent generations. Recently several of the risk factors for this disease have been elucidated and models are currently being developed to allow a more accurate assessment of fracture risk in patients so as to implement preventative and therapeutic measures appropriately.

References

1. Consensus Development Conference. Prophylaxis and treatment of osteoporosis. Osteoporos Int. 1991;1:114–17.
2. Cooper AP. A treatise on dislocation and fractures of the joints. London: John Churchill; 1842.
3. Department of Health Advisory Group on Osteoporosis. London: Department of Health; 1994.
4. Ruiz-Adame M, Correa M. A systematic review of the indirect and social costs studies in fragility fractures. Osteoporos Int. 2020;31:1205–16.
5. Screening for postmenopausal osteoporosis. WHO technical report series. Geneva: WHO; 1994.
6. Kanis JA, Johnell O, Oden A, et al. Ten year probabilities of osteoporotic fractures according to BMD and diagnostic thresholds. Osteoporos Int. 2001;12:989–95.
7. Van Staa TP, Dennison EM, Leufkens HGM, Cooper C. Epidemiology of fractures in England and Wales. Bone. 2001;29:517–22.
8. Grady D, Rubin SM, Petitti DB, et al. Hormone therapy to prevent disease and prolong life in postmenopausal women. Ann Intern Med. 1992;117:1016–37.
9. Johnell O, Kanis JA. An estimate of the worldwide prevalence and disability associated with osteoporotic fractures. Osteoporos Int. 2006;17(12):1726–33.
10. Johnell O, Kanis JA. An estimate of the worldwide prevalence, mortality and disability associated with hip fracture. Osteoporos Int. 2004;15:897–902.
11. Darbà J, Kaskens L, Pérez-Álvarez N, Palacios S, Neyro JL, Rejas J. Disability-adjusted-life-years losses in postmenopausal women with osteoporosis: a burden of illness study. BMC Public Health. 2015;15:324.
12. Cooper C, Atkinson EJ, Jacobsen SJ, et al. Population-based study of survival after osteoporotic fractures. Am J Epidemiol. 1993;137:1001–5.
13. Hip fracture outcomes in people aged fifty and over: mortality, service use, expenditures, and long-term functional impairment. Washington: Office of Technology Assessment, Congress of the United States; 1993. US Department of Commerce publication NTIS PB94107653.
14. Kado DM, Browner WS, Palermo L, et al. Vertebral fractures and mortality in older women: a prospective study. Arch Intern Med. 1999;159:1215–20.
15. Chrischilles EA, Butler CD, Davis CS, Wallace RB. A model of lifetime osteoporosis impact. Arch Intern Med. 1991;151:2026–32.
16. Kanis JA, Johnell O, Oden A, et al. The risk and burden of vertebral fractures in Sweden. Osteoporos Int. 2004;15:20–6.
17. Baudoin C, Fardellone P, Bean K, et al. Clinical outcomes and mortality after hip fracture: a 2-year follow-up study. Bone. 1996;3(Suppl):149S–57S.
18. Poor G, Atkinson EJ, O'Fallon WM, Melton LJ III. Predictors of hip fractures in elderly men. J Bone Miner Res. 1995;10:1900–7.

19. Johnell O, Gullberg B, Kanis JA, et al. Risk factors for hip fracture in European women: the MEDOS study. J Bone Miner Res. 1995;10:1802–14.
20. Gold DT. The clinical impact of vertebral fractures: quality of life in women with osteoporosis. Bone. 1996;18(suppl 3):S185–9.
21. O'Neill TW, Cockerill W, Matthis C, et al. Back pain, disability, and radiographic vertebral fracture in European women: a prospective study. Osteoporos Int. 2004;15:760–5.
22. Cooper C, Campion G, Melton LJ III. Hip fractures in the elderly: a world-wide projection. Osteoporos Int. 1992;2(6):285–9.
23. Chang K, Center J, Nguyen T, Eisman J. Incidence of hip and other osteoporotic fractures in elderly men and women: Dubbo osteoporosis epidemiology study. J Bone Miner Res. 2004;19:532–6.
24. Falch J, Aho H, Berglund K, et al. Hip fractures in Nordic cities: difference in incidence. Ann Chir Gynaecol. 1995;84:286–90.
25. Hagino H, Yamamoto K, Teshima R, et al. The incidence of fractures of the proximal femur and distal radius in Tottori prefecture Japan. Arch Orthop Trauma Surg. 1990;109:43–4.
26. Yan L, Zhou B, Prentice A, et al. Epidemiological study of hip fracture in Shenyang Peoples Republic China. Bone. 1999;24:151–5.
27. Memon A, Pospula W, Tantawy A, et al. Incidence of hip fracture in Kuwait. Int J Epidemiol. 1998;27:860–5.
28. Solomon L. Osteoporosis and fracture of femoral neck in the South African Bantu. J Bone Joint Surg. 1968;50:2–13.
29. Cooper C, Atkinson EJ, O'Fallon MW, Melton JL. Incidence of clinically diagnosed vertebral fractures: a population-based study in Rochester, Minnesota, 1985–1989. J Bone Miner Res. 1992;7:221–7.
30. Cooper C, Melton LJ III. Vertebral fracture: how large is the silent epidemic? BMJ. 1992;304:793–4.
31. Melton LJ, Lane AW, Cooper C, et al. Prevalence and incidence of vertebral deformities. Osteoporos Int. 1993;3:113–9.
32. O'Neill TW, Felsenberg D, Varlow J, et al. The prevalence of vertebral deformity in European men and women: the European vertebral osteoporosis study. J Bone Miner Res. 1996;11:1010–7.
33. Ross PD, Fujiwara S, Huang C, et al. Vertebral fracture prevalence in women in Hiroshima compared to Caucasians or Japanese in the US. Int J Epidemiol. 1995;24:1171–7.
34. Grados F, Marcelli C, Dargent-Molina P, et al. Prevalence of vertebral fractures in French women older than 75 years from the EPIDOS study. Bone. 2004;34:362–7.
35. Thompson PW, Taylor J, Dawson A. The annual incidence and seasonal variation of fractures of the distal radius in men and women over 25 years in Dorset, UK. Inj Int J Care Inj. 2004;35:462–6.
36. Ensrud KE, Cauley J, Lipschutz R, Cummings SR. Weight change and fractures in older women. Arch Intern Med. 1997;157:857–63.
37. Seeley DG, Browner WS, Nevitt MC, et al. Which fractures are associated with low appendicular bone mass in elderly women? The study of Osteoporotic Fractures Research Group. Ann Intern Med. 1991;115:837–42.
38. Cuddihy MT, Gabriel SE, Crowson CS, et al. Forearm fractures as predictors of subsequent osteoporotic fractures. Osteoporos Int. 1999;9:469–75.
39. Ioannidis G, Flahive J, Pickard L, Papaioannou A, Chapurlat RD, Saag KG, Silverman S, Anderson FA Jr, Gehlbach SH, Hooven FH, Boonen S, Compston JE, Cooper C, Díez-Perez A, Greenspan SL, Lacroix AZ, Lindsay R, Netelenbos JC, Pfeilschifter J, Rossini M, Roux C, Sambrook PN, Siris ES, Watts NB, Adachi JD, GLOW Investigators. Non-hip, non-spine fractures drive healthcare utilization following a fracture: the Global Longitudinal Study of Osteoporosis in Women (GLOW). Osteoporos Int. 2013;24(1):59–67.

40. Ismail AA, Cockerill W, Cooper C, et al. Prevalent vertebral deformity predicts incident hip fracture though not distal forearm fracture: results from the European prospective osteoporosis study. Osteoporos Int. 2001;12:85–90.
41. Black DM, Arden NK, Palermo L, et al. Prevalent vertebral deformities predict hip fractures and new vertebral deformities but not wrist fractures. J Bone Miner Res. 1999;14:821–8.
42. Lunt M, O'Neill T, Armbrecht G, et al. Charcteristics of prevalent vertebral deformity and the risk of incident vertebral fractures. Rheumatology. 2002;41(suppl 1):101–2.
43. Lindsay R, Silverman SL, Cooper C, et al. Risk of new vertebral fracture in the year following a fracture. JAMA. 2001;285:320–3.
44. Gallacher SJ, Gallagher AP, McQuillian C, et al. The prevalence of vertebral fracture amongst patients presenting with non-vertebral fractures. Osteoporos Int. 2007;18(2):185–92.
45. Center JR, Bliuc D, Nguyen TV, et al. Risk of subsequent fracture after low-trauma fracture in men and women. JAMA. 2007;297(4):387–94.
46. Ström O, Borgström F, Kanis JA, et al. Osteoporosis: burden, health care provision and opportunities in the EU: a report prepared in collaboration with the International Osteoporosis Foundation (IOF) and the European Federation of Pharmaceutical Industry Associations (EFPIA). Arch Osteoporos. 2011;6:59–155.
47. Johnell O. The socioeconomic burden of fractures: today and in the 21st century. Am J Med. 1997;103:25S–6S.
48. Viswanathan HN, Curtis JR, Yu J, et al. Direct healthcare costs of osteoporosis-related fractures in managed care patients receiving pharmacological osteoporosis therapy. Appl Health Econ Health Policy. 2012;10:163–73.
49. Burge R, Dawson-Hughes B, Solomon DH, et al. Incidence and economic burden of osteoporosis-related fractures in the United States, 2005-2025. J Bone Miner Res. 2007;22:465–75.
50. Hernlund E, Svedbom A, Ivergård M, et al. Osteoporosis in the European Union: medical management, epidemiology and economic burden. Arch Osteoporos. 2013;8:136.
51. Kanis JA, on behalf of the World Health Organisation Scientific Group. Assessment of osteoporosis at the primary health care level. WHO Collaborating Centre for Metabolic Bone Diseases, University of Sheffield; 2007.
52. Melton LJ 3rd, Crowson CS, O'Fallon WM. Fracture incidence in Olmsted County, Minnesota: comparison of urban with rural rates and changes in urban rates over time. Osteoporos Int. 1999;9:29.
53. Shuit SC, Van Der Klift M, Weel AE, et al. Fracture incidence and association with bone mineral density in elderly men and women: the Rotterdam study. Bone. 2004;34:195–202.
54. Cooper C, Cole ZA, Holroyd CR, et al. Secular trends in the incidence of hip and other osteoporotic fractures. Osteoporos Int. 2011;22(5):1277–88.
55. Swayambunathan J, Dasgupta A, Rosenberg PS, Hannan MT, Kiel DP, Bhattacharyya T. Incidence of hip fracture over 4 decades in the Framingham Heart Study. JAMA Intern Med. 2020;180(9):1225–31.
56. Nilson F, Moniruzzaman S, Gustavsson J, Andersson R. Trends in hip fracture incidence rates among the elderly in Sweden 1987-2009. J Public Health (Oxf). 2013;35(1):125–31.
57. Kannus P, Niemi S, Parkkari J, Sievänen H. Continuously declining incidence of hip fracture in Finland: analysis of nationwide database in 1970-2016. Arch Gerontol Geriatr. 2018;77:64–7.

Chapter 2
How to Identify Individuals Requiring Anti-osteoporosis Therapy: Imaging in Bone Health

Nicholas R. Fuggle and Kate A. Ward

Introduction

Demographic shifts towards older populations are occurring in countries worldwide and are predicted to lead to rapid acceleration in rates of fragility fractures [1]. The individual morbidity, economic cost and societal burden of fragility fractures is therefore set to rise over the coming years and, in order to tackle this forthcoming epidemic, we require the best methods of identifying those who will benefit most from therapy. This involves targeting high risk groups, encouraging a risk assessment approach which allows stratification of therapeutic approaches and effective preventative strategies in those at lower risk, and using imaging modalities to greatest effect. In this chapter we will summarize the rationale behind risk assessment, introduce the key risk assessment tools and a strategy for population-level screening. We will also synthesize the relevant imaging modalities for the assessment of bone mineral density, microarchitecture analysis and fracture risk and consider the most recent developments in the area of computer vision and artificial intelligence.

As mentioned in Chap. 1, the first description of osteoporosis came in 1822 from the British surgeon, Sir Astley Cooper who made comment on the association between abnormal bone and the occurrence of fractures. However, the first use of the term 'osteoporosis' was by Jean Lobstein, a French surgeon in 1835, though it is more likely he was describing osteogenesis imperfecta (OI), as he mentioned the association of blue sclera, a common sequelae of common forms of OI. Moving into the twentieth century, Fuller Albright described a case series of women who had lost ovarian function and subsequently suffered vertebral fractures [2]. However, a comprehensive definition of the condition which could be applied to descriptive epidemiology did not develop until the late twentieth century with the advent of bone imaging.

N. R. Fuggle · K. A. Ward (✉)
MRC Lifecourse Epidemiology Centre, University of Southampton, Southampton, UK
e-mail: nrf@mrc.soton.ac.uk; kw@mrc.soton.ac.uk

E. Dennison (ed.), *Osteoporosis Treatment*, https://doi.org/10.1007/978-3-030-78128-6_2

If one was to aim to identify the members of a population who were at greatest risk of fracture the easiest method would be to ask those who have previously fractured to put their hand up. The old adage "Fractures beget fractures" certainly holds true with those who have suffered a fracture, five times more likely to re-fracture than those who have never fractured [3]. It is therefore highly unfortunate that, in reality, less than 20% of those individuals who sustain a fragility fracture receive treatment to prevent a further fracture from occurring [4, 5]. The figures are even worse for females and those in long-term care institutions and there is also a worrying downward trend in the treatment of osteoporosis in the United Kingdom (UK) and the United States (US) [6, 7]. However, there are ongoing substantial efforts to countermand the treatment gap and identify 'at risk' individuals. These initiatives have included the development of a robust definition of osteoporosis, the development of fracture risk prediction tools, an enhanced comprehension of the role of bone and diagnostic imaging modalities in assessment of risk and Fracture Liaison Services (FLS). The treatment gap and FLS are the subject of later chapters in this book.

The History of Imaging

The assessment of bone loss harks back to the late nineteenth Century with observations published on the osteopenic appearances of dental radiographs. Even in the modern day, it is estimated that a degree of bone loss is crudely quantifiable by a radiologist looking at a radiograph [8] though it should be noted that ~30% bone loss needs to occur before this can be observed on an x-ray. Attempts to better quantify bone loss from radiographs were developed in the 1960's though these lacked precision and repeatability, and led to the development of absorptiometry.

Absorptiometry, generally speaking, describes the generation of an energy source (photon or X-ray) which passes through a test material, and uses a detector to measure the degree of attenuation, known as the linear attenuation coefficient (loss of energy). This can be compared to a standard, control material to calculate the test material density. Depending on the properties of a tissue, it will attenuate radiation differently which allows creation of the image and through image processing, quantification and separation of the tissues (e.g. fat, muscle, bone) from one another.

The origin of absorptiometry lies in the in vivo, single photon absorptiometry (SPA) work of Cameron and Sorenson in 1963 [9]. This early technique used a single energy source of Iridium-125 or Americium 241 to provide a measurement of peripheral bone mineral density at the radius and calcaneum, and involved submerging the wrist or heel in water in order to simulate surrounding of soft-tissue and to improve delineation of soft tissue and bone. This method was precise and affordable but, due to the necessity to submerge the anatomical region to be analysed, could only be performed on peripheral sites, had poor resolution and energy source degradation.

In 1965, gadolinium-153 was employed as a dual-energy source due to its property of emitting photons at two distinct energies, enabling dual photon absorptiometry (DPA). Although this was an improvement upon the single-photon technique and was used to measure BMD at the lumbar spine [10], DPA struggled with issues, similar to those of SPA, including poor resolution, energy source degradation and long (up to 40 min) scan times.

The advent of Dual X-ray Absorptiometry (DXA) by Mazess in 1981 [11] opened up new horizons with increased resolution, precision (1–2% in vivo [12]) and a vastly-reduced scan time. DXA replaced the unstable radioisotope sources with an X-ray radiation source. It uses two different energy sources (at approximately 40 KeV and >70 KeV) to allow discrimination between soft-tissues and bone. The quantitative measures which can be derived from 2D densitometry include bone area (cm^2), bone mineral content (BMC) (grams) and areal bone mineral density (g/cm^2). Areal bone mineral density is calculated using pixel by pixel attenuation values of a test material (in this case bone or calcium hydroxyapatite) against a control phantom. Bone area is calculated by summing the pixels which lie within the bone edges and bone mineral content (in grams) is calculated by multiplying areal BMD (g/cm^2) and bone area (cm^2). In terms of the anatomical location at which to measure BMD, the lumbar spine or proximal femur were the sites the techniques were optimised to measure, being the most common sites of fracture. Ultimately the femoral neck was recognised as the most suitable reference site for use in epidemiological studies [13] and now in clinical practice [14].

DXA remains the gold-standard measure for BMD due to the scientific demonstration of strong correlation with biomechanical bone strength via finite element analysis [15], correlation with the clinical outcome of fracture risk [16] and the relatively low radiation burden [17] which for a proximal femur scan is lower than one day background radiation in the UK. The associations between DXA- measured BMD and fracture risk in post-menopausal women, led, in 1984, to it being included in the working definition of osteoporosis from the World Health Organization.

A limitation of DXA is the aforementioned 2D projection image which limits the ability to measure density (mass/ volume), as the depth of the bone cannot be accounted for. This creates a size-dependence to measurements which is problematic in children and small adults. Several methods exist to account for these inaccuracies in the use of DXA in children and adolescents. These include calculation of a size-corrected lumbar spine BMD from the DXA image, Bone Mineral Apparent Density (BMAD) [18] or regression methods to take into account the size of the child [19, 20].

Over the past decade developments in DXA scanning include vertebral fracture assessment using lateral views of the thoracolumbar spine [21], and trabecular bone scoring (TBS) which provides a measure of bone 'quality' acting as a surrogate for bone miscroarchitecture, rather than the 'quantity' supplied by bone mineral density. Vertebral fracture assessment is now commonly performed in clinical practice, and assessment of iDXA (GE-Waltham-MA) images has been shown to categorise fractures as well as from radiographs in adults and in children [22]. TBS is also now available in some DXA-software and has been incorporated into FRAX™ [23]. An earlier extension to DXA measurements was the incorporation of hip structural analysis, versions of which are available in current software; measurements and use were limited to research use only due to the assumptions made in the translation of two dimensional projection of hip structure.

Using BMD Measurements to Identify Those at Risk

Early work using BMD as a measure of fracture risk, found that the measure predicted hip fracture (age-adjusted risk increase of 2.6 per standard deviation decrease in BMD) [24, 25], that it had a normal distribution within the population and that there was a continuous relationship between fracture risk and BMD with no obvious threshold for designating a step towards higher risk. This made establishing a defined BMD cut-off value for diagnosing osteoporosis difficult. However, in 1994, a committee of the World Health Organisation (WHO) agreed upon a definition of osteoporosis, with a BMD T-score of −2.5 or lower being classified as osteoporosis [26] (a T-score is a standard deviation score derived by comparing an individual's BMD measurement to that of a young-healthy, sex-matched population).

It should be noted that this definition of osteoporosis was for a diagnosis of post-menopausal women, and whilst T-scores are more generically used across the adult population, it is important to consult guidelines as to the correct reference population to use for most accurate diagnosis of osteoporosis in men, pre-menopausal women and in different racial and ethnic groups where population—specific data may not exist [27]. T-scores must never be used in children [28]. The T-score definition is also only applicable to diagnosis by DXA measurements.

In addition, whilst a BMD measure is more effective at predicting future fractures than measures of serum cholesterol are at predicting cardiovascular disease, there are three main reasons why using a T-score as an intervention threshold may be problematic. The first is the low sensitivity of BMD alone to predict fractures, estimated at less than 50%. This was demonstrated in The Rotterdam study [29] in which only 44% of women with non-vertebral fractures (over a follow-up of nearly 7 years) had a BMD T-score less than −2.5 and 12% had a BMD within normal range. This was echoed in a US study which demonstrated that a mere 46% of women who sustained a hip fracture (during the 5 years of follow-up) had a BMD T-score of less than or equal to −2.5 [30]. The second is that a given T-score threshold provides a different significance as age changes. This can be seen in Fig. 2.1.

The third is that fracture rates vary markedly with geography, and to a greater extent than BMD [32]. An example is that a 10 year probability of fracture set a 20% the T score would be −4.6 in Venezuela and −2.0 in Iceland [33]. This highlights the observation that BMD does not take account of the non-skeletal determinants of fracture risk [34], and suggests that other, clinical risk factors should be incorporated into fracture prediction and risk assessment.

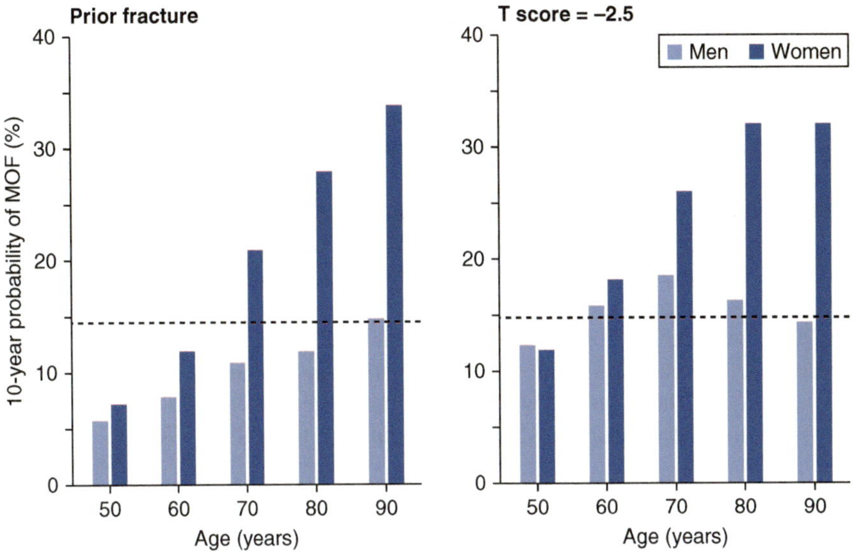

Fig. 2.1 The graph plots 10 year probability of major osteoporotic fracture (MOF; calculated using FRAX) against age The dotted line depicts the treatment threshold based on history of prior fracture (left panel) and a BMD T-score of −2.5 (right panel). A substantially undertreated population is evident, as only individuals whose 10-year probability of MOF falls above the line receive treatment [31]. Also note the different performance fof the thresholds in men versus women

Clinical Prediction Tools for Identification of Risk in Individuals

The balance of risk and benefit is key to many of the decisions made in clinical medicine. The majority of iatrogenic interventions, though benefits are intended, are associated with a possibility of adverse events. Risk assessment is therefore vital to accurately identify those who will benefit from treatment. Substantial scientific resources have been poured into the area of fracture risk assessment over the last 20 years with resultant, highly usable clinical tools to assess a patient's risk of fracture based on clinical parameters. The key tools that currently exist include the Fracture Risk Assessment Tool (FRAX®) [35], Garvan [36] and Q-Fracture [37].

FRAX®

FRAX was devised in 2008, from an original group of 9 cohorts, as a tool to assess the 10 year probability of hip and major osteoporotic fractures (defined as hip, clinical spine, distal forearm and proximal humerus fractures). It utilizes ten clinical risk factors (prior fragility fracture, parental hip fracture, smoking, systemic steroid therapy, excess alcohol consumption, rheumatoid arthritis, secondary causes of osteoporosis, age, sex and body mass index) which were chosen as they were found to predict fractures independent of BMD [35]. BMD at the femoral neck can be included as an input variable, though this is not necessary. The output, fracture probability, is provided taking account of the competing effect of mortality (as many of the risk factors are associated with both risk of fracture and risk of death). This is a unique aspect of the FRAX® algorithm [36, 37].

The robustness of FRAX™ in efficacy for fracture prediction has been demonstrated in 11 independent cohorts [33]. It is the most commonly used of the predictive tools with 80% global coverage and availability in 66 countries [38], in 35 languages and with the FRAX® website receiving three million hits per year [33]. The country-specific models are informed by hip fracture data from the country itself and UN data on mortality, and have been shown to be well-calibrated (effective at predicting fracture risk) in countries including Norway, Canada and the UK [37, 39, 40].

Garvan

The Garvan fracture prediction tool was developed based on ~2500 participants of the Australian Dubbo Osteoporosis Epidemiology Study (DOES) [36]. This tool does not include rheumatoid arthritis, secondary osteoporosis, steroid use, smoking, alcohol, parental hip fracture or secondary osteoporosis in the parameters that are entered into the risk calculation. However, the Garvan tool does include the number of fractures since the age of 50 and the number of falls in the previous year. The tool previously provided a risk of fracture at a large number of sites (including distal femur, pelvis, patella, proximal and distal tibia and fibula, patella, ribs and sternum, hands and feet) but has now focused down to a 5 and 10 year percentage risk of hip fracture and any osteoporotic and/or fragility fracture [36]. The potential disadvantages of the Garvan risk score are that it is based on a single Australian cohort (which could limit its wider applicability), has not been validated more widely, and it does not take the competing hazard of death into account.

Q-Fracture

The QFracture tool was published in 2009 [37]. This tool was derived using Cox proportional hazards models on the data of two million individuals aged between 30 and 85 on the General Practitioner Research Database in the UK. The same dataset was then used to validate the tool. Consequently, QFracture is primarily applicable to the UK population and, although it is only calibrated on hip fracture, the tool does provide estimated incidences of hip, forearm, spinal and shoulder fracture. BMD is not included and QFracture. The number of risk factors was extended in 2012, on the basis of National Institute for Health and Clinical Excellence guidance on the risk assessment for osteoporosis, to include history of previous fracture, presence of epilepsy (or anticonvulsant use), ethnicity and the presence of type 1 diabetes mellitus. The current list of clinical parameters included in the QFracture tool and shown in Table 2.1 (QFracture.org).

Table 2.1 The parameters included in FRAX®, Garvan and QFracture tools [41]. Table reproduced with permission, thanks to the original authors and Elsevier® publishing

Risk factor	FRAX	Garvan	QFracturr	Comments
Age	+	+	+	
Sex	+	+	+	
Height	+	–	+	
Weight	+	+*	+	* Only when BMD is not entered
Ethnicity	+*	–	+	* US and Singapore
Previous fragility fracture	+	+*	+**	* From the age of 50 years * Also number of prior fractures ** Prior hip, spine or shoulder
BMD	+	+*	–	* Site of BMD not specified on website but elsewhere stated to be femoral neck
Parental history of hip fracture	+	–	+*	* Also, parental history of OP
Smoking	+*	–	+**	* Current ** Categories of exposure
Alcohol intake	+*	–	+***	* ≥3 units per day ** Categories of exposure
Taking steroid tablets regularly	+*	–	+	* Currently exposed to oral glucocorticoids or has been exposed to oral glucocorticoids for more than 3 months at a dose of prednisolone of 5 mg daily or more
Osteogenesis imperfecta	+*	–	–	* Grouped as secondary OP
Diabetes	+*	–	+**	* Type 1 grouped as secondary OP ** Type 1. type 2
In nursing home	–	–	+	
Falls history	–	+*	+	* Categories of exposure
Dementia	–	–	+	
Cancer	–	–	+	
Asthma or COPD	–	–	+	
Heart attack, angina, stroke or TIA	–	–	+	
Chronic liver disease	+*	–	+	* Grouped as secondary OP
Chronic kidney disease	–	–	+*	* Stage 4 or 5
Parkinson's disease	–	–	+	

(continued)

Table 2.1 (continued)

Risk factor	FRAX	Garvan	QFracturr	Comments
Rheumatoid arthritis or SLE	+*	–	+	* RA alone
Malabsorption	+*	–	+**	* Grouped as secondary OP ** Crohn's disease, ulcerause colitis, cocliac disease, steatorrhea or blind loop syndrome
Endocrine disorders	+*	–	+**	* Untreated long-standing hyperthyroidism, hypogonadism ** Thyrotoxicosis, hyperparathyroidism, Cushing's syndrome
Premature menopause	+*	–	–	* (<45 years) grouped as secondary OP
Epilepsy or taking anticonvulsants	–	–	+	
Taking antidepressants	–	–	+	
Chronic malnutrition	+*	–	–	* Grouped as secondary OP
HRT	–	–	+*	* Oestrogen only

HRT hormone replacement therapy, *OP* osteoporosis, *SLE* systemic lupus erythematosus

Identifying Who to Assess and when to Treat

It is clear that an individual who has sustained a fragility fracture should be considered for treatment, but in those who have not, the 10-year probability of fracture (acquired via FRAX®) is used as a metric to decide on the necessity for BMD assessment and/or the commencement of treatment in many national guidelines [31]. However, approaches and exact thresholds at which to start treatment vary across the globe. One of the main considerations when comparing these approaches is whether the 10-year probability of fracture is assessed before imaging or simply used to adjudicate on 'borderline' cases which have been identified by imaging.

In the US, the decision to commence anti-osteoporosis medication is indicated by a BMD T-score ≤−2.5 or a previous hip or vertebral fracture [42]. FRAX® is only used as a 'tie-breaker' if the BMD falls in the osteopenic range of T-score −2.5 to −1.0, with treatment commenced if the calculated 10-year probability of major osteoporotic fracture is ≥20% or probability of hip fracture is ≥3%. A similar approach is taken in Japan with BMD assessment and fracture history used initially to commence therapy, and FRAX® used to adjudicate the start of treatment if the BMD is between −1.8 and −2.77 [43]. The National Osteoporosis Guideline Group (NOGG) recommendations in the UK state that treatment should be commenced on the basis of a prior fragility fracture in women or an age-dependent fracture threshold based on 10-year probability of fracture [14]. In contrast to the US and Japanese models, BMD measurement is only indicated if the age-dependent fracture risk falls between the 'treat' and 'lifestyle and reassure' thresholds (Fig. 2.2). This approach

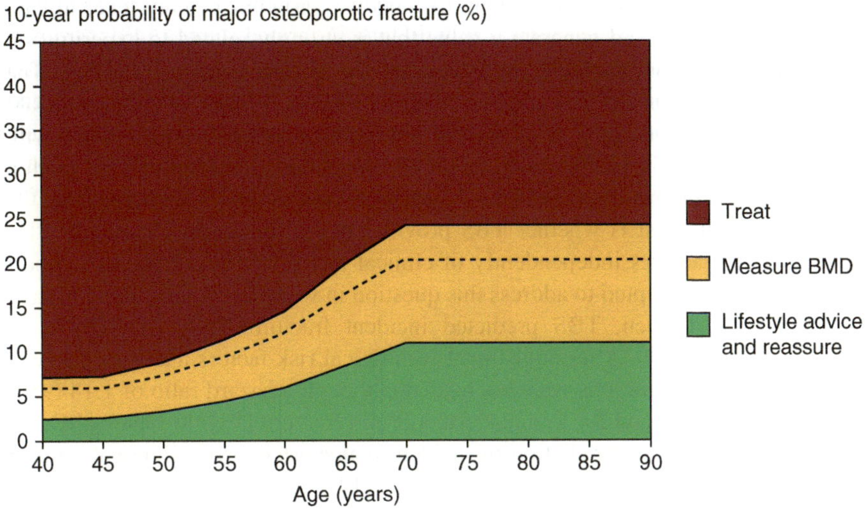

Fig. 2.2 Normogram demonstrating the age-dependent, 10-year probability of major osteoporotic fracture as used in the NOGG recommendations. Those individuals falling in the red area at to be treated, those in the green to be offered lifestyle advice and reassurance and those in the yellow require further assessment of BMD via DXA in order to inform treatment decisions [14]. Note this figure is taken from an article distributed under the terms of the Creative Commons Attribution 4.0 International License (http://creativecommons.org/licenses/by/4.0/)

has the advantage of lowering the demand on imaging resources, with, for example for a woman aged 55, 7 scans would be saved per future hip fracture identified [44]. In this NOGG model, those beneath the lower assessment threshold should receive lifestyle advice, those above the upper assessment threshold should receive anti-osteoporosis medication and those between the thresholds should have BMD assessed via DXA scanning [14]. This approach has been shown to be cost-effective and valid in the treatment of those at risk of fragility fracture in the UK [44, 45].

The International Osteoporosis Foundation (IOF) and European Society for the Clinical and Economic Evaluation of Osteoporosis and Osteoarthritis (ESCEO) have recently advocated the identification of 'very high risk' individuals as those who exceed the intervention threshold by 20% [46]. These patients may benefit from first-line treatment with anabolic therapies, in contrast to the usual first-line treatment of anti-resorprtive therapies.

Trabecular Bone Score

As mentioned previously, TBS is an analytical tool that is applied to data acquired using DXA to provide a surrogate measure of bone microarchitecture, providing information on bone structure above and beyond areal BMD [47]. The tool uses a sequence of experimental variograms to quantify variation in grey-level texture between pixels [48] and generate a value that is strongly related to experimental trabecular separation, trabecular number and connective density [49, 50]. The region of interest is usually an anterior-posterior view of the lumbar spine on DXA; a higher TBS is consistent with fracture-resistant bone and a lower score with weaker bone [51]. Seemingly, there is an age-dependent variation in TBS, with a relative plateau in mid-life (aged 30–45) and a gradual reduction with age [52].

A point of interest is whether TBS provides any information for the effective prediction of fractures independently of clinical risk factors. A study in a cohort from Manitoba attempted to address this question in women [53] and men [54] and found that, in women, TBS predicted incident fractures (HR: 1.36, 95% CI 1.30–1.42, $p < 0.001$). After adjustment for clinical risk factors and femoral neck areal BMD the associations were attenuated, although a hazard ratio of 1.18 (95% CI 1.12–1.23) remained for a major osteoporotic fracture [53]. In males, the area under the curve for the prediction of incident major osteoporotic, hip and clinical vertebral fractures was better than that expected by chance alone [54]. Although TBS has been used to monitor fracture prevention therapy, including bisphosphonates and raloxifene, the percentage change is generally less than that observed in areal BMD [55, 56]. An advantage of TBS is that the tool can be applied to DXA, radiographs, computed tomography and at any skeletal site, although DXA of the lumbar spine is the most common modality. Unlike areal BMD which has artefact in measurement caused by degenerative disease (particularly in the spine), vertebral collapse through fracture, which leads to falsely raised BMD levels, TBS is not affected by degeneration or osteophytes [57].

In 2016, a meta-analysis of 14 cohorts was performed to assess the triangular relationship between clinical risk factors, TBS and areal BMD with regard to fracture prediction. This meta-analysis found that TBS was independently predictive of future major osteoporotic and hip fractures and concluded that the score may have some utility in clinical practice [23]. And in light of this TBS is available as a modifier to the FRAX risk assessment tool online. Hence TBS provides additional information regarding bone quality beyond the quantitative measures provided by 2D densitometry Although DXA is the clinical leader in the image assessment of bone, other scanning modalities have been developed and are used in the research context.

Taking a Population Approach to Screening for those at Risk

The WHO recommendations for screening for fragility fractures include the assessment of fracture risk into high, medium or low risk groups; high-risk individuals are considered for treatment, low-risk individuals are not recommended for treatment and medium-risk individuals are further assessed with a measurement of BMD [58].

The SCreening Of Older women for the Prevention of fractures (SCOOP) trial was designed as a pragmatic, unblinded, randomised controlled UK based trial of women aged 70–85 years, recruiting 12,483 participants. The aim of the study was

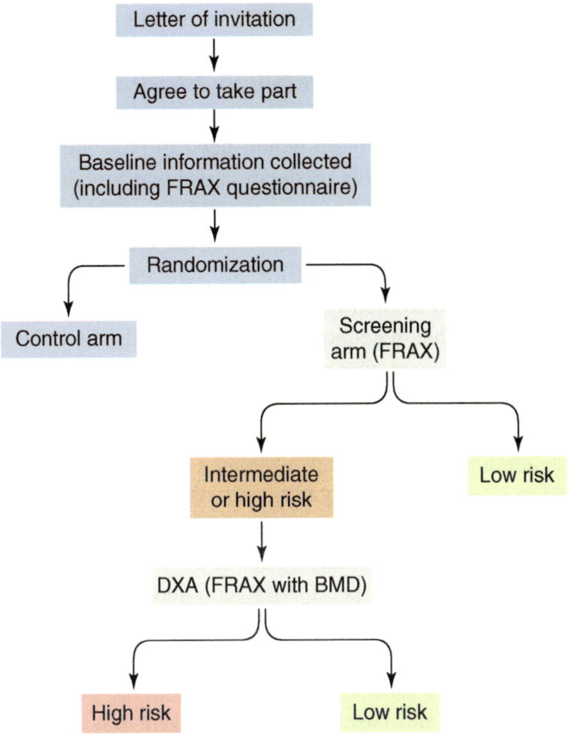

Fig. 2.3 The participant flow for the SCreening of Older wOmen for Prevention of fracture (SCOOP) study [59]

to examine the effectiveness and cost effectiveness of a community-based screening programme to decrease fragility fractures in older women and thereby address the aforementioned 'Treatment Gap' in this population. The structure of the study is depicted in Fig. 2.3.

The control arm comprised individuals receiving 'usual care' (provided in primary care); individuals in the screening arm had their 10 year probability of fracture calculated using FRAX. Those at moderate to high-risk underwent DXA to calculate BMD and treatment decisions were made in primary care based on the above findings.

Previous trials of population screening for osteoporosis had been undertaken, including one based in a population of post-menopausal women, which began in the 1990s and reported in 2010 [60], and reported that screening marginally increased the usage of osteoporosis treatments and reduced fracture incidence. In addition, a more recent RCT of primary-care based screening was reported in 2012 [61], which found that screening for osteoporosis increased prescription of osteoporosis medication at 6 months (OR 2.24, 95% CI 1.16–4.33). The primary difference between these studies and SCOOP is that, with SCOOP the primary outcome was fracture incidence and not treatment uptake.

Although there were no significant differences in the primary outcome measure of all osteoporosis-related fractures between the screening arm and control arm (HR

0.94; CI, 0.85–1.03) or the rate of all clinical fractures (HR 0.94; CI 0.86–1.03) [62], in a pre-specified analysis, the rate of hip fracture was statistically significantly lower in the screening arm (HR 0.72; CI, 0.59–0.89). In terms of numbers needed to treat, the absolute size in hip fracture rate reduction was 0.9%, which means that 111 women aged 70–85 would need to be screened in order to avert a single hip fracture. Osteoporosis medication use was higher in the screening group compared to controls at the end of year one (15% vs 4%), with medication use being particularly high in the high risk group at the 6 month time point (78%). The qualitative work performed as part of the SCOOP study demonstrated that the screening was acceptable to women [63].

The key heath economic finding from the SCOOP study was that the screening model trialed was cost-effective. There was an increase of 0.0237 Quality-Adjusted Life Years (QALYs) for participants in the active arm of the trial with an £2772 incremental cost per QALY in the screening arm versus the control arm [64]. The screening intervention also reduced fractures with a cost per osteoporosis-related fracture prevented was £4478 and a cost per hip fracture prevented via the screening programme was £7694. The cost-effectiveness acceptability curves suggested that there was a 93% probability of the screening intervention being cost-effective, at a value of >£20,000 per QALY, concluding that the screening programme was a highly cost-effective strategy [64].

A post-hoc analysis focusing on those who are at high risk of fracture was published in 2018 [65], which aimed to examine possible interactions between screening efficacy and baseline FRAX 10 year risk of fracture and fracture outcomes. Interactions were observed between the history of prior fracture, parental fracture history, smoking and the efficacy of screening [65]. Importantly, in individuals at highest risk of fracture the estimated reduction in hip fracture risk was greater than 50% [65]. Despite the limitation that not all participants included in the SCOOP trial had BMD measurements at baseline or during follow-up the conclusion of the post-hoc analysis was that those women who are at high risk of hip fracture based on FRAX probability are responsive to appropriate osteoporosis management [65]. The greater reduction in hip fracture risk in those who had higher baseline risk strongly suggests that treatment rather than other factors explained the observed effect.

The effect of screening was greatest in those with the risk factors of prior history of fracture and parental history of fracture [65]. These two groups represent the most relevant clinical risk factors. These factors might have had some bearing on persistence and uptake of medications by study participants. The presence of these two factors might also have driven increased treatment rates in the screening arm.

Since the initial study, further analyses have demonstrated that this approach to population screening led to increased use of and adherence to anti-osteoporosis medications [66], gains in quality of life and life years, and reductions in fracture costs which exceed the costs of taking this new approach to population screening [67].

In summary, if the SCOOP screening strategy were to be adopted in the UK in 70–85 year old women (assuming the size of this population is similar to that estimated in 2016 of 3.7 million), it could prevent 8000 hip fractures each year, would be cost-effective in doing so and result in considerably better treatment adherence at 5 years of follow-up. This gives a window into a potentially effective and cost-efficient approach to population screening for osteoporosis, and identifying those in need of treatment. Determining effectiveness of such a method in older men or in other groups and populations is an important next step.

Extended Roles for Imaging in Assessments of Risk

DXA imaging, which forms the mainstay of bone imaging in clinical practice, has been described above. Beyond DXA, other imaging modalities which can provide a more granular depiction of bone microarchitecture and strength. One of the aforementioned limitations of DXA is its lack of sensitivity to predict individual fracture risk and that in part is likely due to the 2D nature of measurements and lack of assessment of separate bone compartments which may differentially respond to treatments and disease, and measures of physiological cross sections which provide assessment of bone size, shape, distribution and strength.

In 2001, Rauch and Schonau proposed a model to enhance the comprehension and interpretation of bone densitometry measures in children and adolescents [68] though they can also be employed in the understanding of adult bone physiology. The model focuses on three key areas material BMD, compartmental BMD and total BMD. Material BMD refers to the mineralization of a small volume of organic bone matrix. The small volume is due to the necessity to exclude marrow, lacunae, canaliculi and osteonal canals from the sample. This can be performed invasively via bone biopsy, or, more recently, via the virtual bone biopsy afforded by High Resolution Peripheral Quantitative Computed Tomography (HRpQCT) which will be described further below. Compartmental BMD refers to the amount of mineral in the cortical or trabecular compartments and can be assessed by QCT methods (central, peripheral and HRpQCT). Because DXA is two-dimensional it does not provide measures of compartment BMD. DXA therefore provides an integrated measure of total bone mineral density which refers to the entire density of the material within the periosteal envelope.

Alternative Scanning Modalities

As previously attested, DXA is the current gold standard for predicting those at high risk of fragility fractures though this method does have some issues and limitations. These issues include the lack of estimates of compartmental and material BMD, the fact that BMD measurements are size dependent (as they are calculated using a 2D projection of a 3D structure with no adjustments for object depth) and that the measures of BMD are susceptible to changes in body composition [69]. In order to counter these issues and to provide additional measures of bone structure, morphometry and biomechanics, other, non-DXA scanning techniques have developed and are employed, largely in the research setting. Indeed, elements of bone microarchitecture have been shown to be predictive of incident fracture independent of BMD [70]. These scanning modalities include central quantitative QCT, peripheral QCT (pQCT) and High Resolution pQCT (HRpQCT).

Central QCT

Central QCT was first developed in the 1970s [71] but came to wider usage in the 1980s [72]. Central QCT is a modality which uses multiple 2D slices or a 3D volume scan and the 'central' description of the modality refers to the fact the regions of interest are the lumbar spine (particularly the L1–L3 vertebrae), the proximal femur and peripheral sites, and central QCT also provides a measure of muscle mass or composition [73]. The advantages of central QCT over DXA include the ascertainment of mean volumetric BMD measured in mg per cm^3. This measurement is less sensitive to changes in bone size than areal BMD and measures compartmental BMD, bone geometry and biomechanical measures of bone strength [73]. Compared to DXA, the main disadvantages of central QCT are the increased burden of ionizing radiation [74] and potential issues exist with confounding by changes in bone marrow fat owing to the majority of scanners being single-energy devices [75].

Peripheral QCT

The next scanning modality in the QCT family is peripheral QCT, which became commercially available in the 1990s [76], with the most common model being the XCT 2000 (Stratec, Pforzheim, Germany). This method takes 2D slices (1–2 mm thick) of the radius and tibia, which (owing to the very low radiation burden) can be performed at multiple sites along the bone. Not only does this modality provide valuable data on volumetric BMD, compartmental BMD, bone geometry and bone strength but peripheral QCT also provides muscle measures including cross-sectional area and muscle density [77]. Measurements of muscle provide the opportunity to calculate a bone to muscle ratio, which is relevant when considering some hypotheses for bone strength and loading (for example, the 'mechanostat theory' [78]).

High-Resolution Peripheral QCT

The most recently developed QCT scanning modality is HRpQCT (XtremeCT I and II, Scanco Medical, Bruttisellen, Switzerland) which allows multiple 2D slices (most commonly of the radius or tibia) to be recreated into a 3D 'virtual bone biopsy'. The enhanced spatial resolution afforded by this modality is in excess of that provided by standard peripheral QCT, QCT or MRI [79]. HRpQCT imparts a low dose of radiation (<3 microSv) and owing to semi-automated contouring and segmentation of tissue this method provides data on densitometry, morphometry and biomechanic parameters. A recent prospective study by the Bone Microarchitecture Consortium found that HRpQCT measurements (particularly peripheral skeleton failure load, which is the prediction of the external force required to cause failure of the bone) were statistically significantly associated with future risk of fracture over ~4.5 year follow-up after adjustment for femoral neck BMD [70]. al measures (including stiffness and elastic modulus) through finite element analysis) [80, 81].

Non-DXA Scanning in Clinical Practice

It should be emphasized that although 'non-DXA' scanning modalities provide valuable data to drive forward densitometric research, they are not currently used in clinical practice due to a lack of routine accessibility and robust data to show improvement, independently of DXA assessed BMD, in fracture risk prediction prediction. The diagnostic criteria for osteoporosis, osteopenia from the WHO are also not applicable to other techniques [82].

Ultrasound is probably the technology most widely used beside DXA in centres where QCT is not available. Whilst quantitative ultrasound was used extensively in research and epidemiological studies, particularly in the 1990s, and had the advantages of being portable and using non-ionising radiation, the practical limitations of this technology and inferior ability to predict individual fracture status (compared to DXA) led to diminishing use. Quantitative ultrasonography (similar to other imaging modalities) also lacks coherent standardization across different models [83]. This method does, however, have a potential utility in low-resource settings where DXA is unavailable, and new developments include ultrasound of the hip and lumbar spine, currently being evaluated in clinical trials. Interestingly, MRI has also been used to assess bone density and microstructure but was limited due to technical and proprietary software in the clinical or research settings [84].

Artificial Intelligence Approaches

There is great interest, both from research and industry, in the ability of automated fracture detection from forms of imaging performed for other reasons. For example, a possible source of vertebral fracture case detection are CT scans of the thorax, pelvis and abdomen. These images include spinal sections but vertebral fractures are often not picked up. Indeed, studies have shown that only 13–16% of CT vertebral fractures are reported in routine reporting [85–87]. This is probably due to the incidental nature of these findings, as they were not primarily performed to identify fractures. A high correlation between CT-acquired trabecular vertebral attenuation values and DXA scores has been demonstrated [88–90], however the high dose of radiation (typical effective dose for an adult abdominal CT is 8 mSv) [91] and greater financial cost, make this approach most appropriate for opportunistic screening for vertebral fracture, clinically the most prevalent yet often clinically silent until multiple fractures occur causing pain, morbidity and disability. The importance of identification is an individual with a vertebral fracture is 5 times more likely to suffer a subsequent MOF. Similar approaches have been used with magnetic resonance imaging (MRI) [92].

Substantial advances in processing power and computer vision have resulted in a rise in interest in algorithms and deep learning (e.g. convolutional and recurrent neural networks) to identify fractures. First, sagittal plane images of the spine are constructed from the original coronal CT scan and secondly, the images are classified by neural networks according to the probability of the presence of a vertebral fracture. The accuracy afforded by this approach is 89–97% [93, 94]. An alternative method uses active appearance modelling for assessing the contours of the vertebra and reports an accuracy of 93%, though in a limited data set of 50 CT scans [95]. A recent study in China, incorporating about 1500 CT scans, developed an algorithm to opportunistically abdominal or spinal CTs for the presence of osteoporosis and osteopenia [96].

Of course, similar deep learning methods can be used for VFA, and a recent study including over 12,000 VFAs has reported an area under the receiver operating characteristic curve of 0.94 (95% confidence interval [CI]: 0.93, 0.95) for vertebral fracture detection (corresponding to a sensitivity of 87.4% (534 of 611) and specificity of 88.4% (2838 of 3211)) and performed comparably to the study radiologists (all who had in excess of 10 years of experience) [97].

These innovative approaches have the potential to heighten accuracy or diagnosis whilst providing reporting clinicians with more time to interpret the more complex radiological images. It is important to acknowledge that these innovations are relatively nascent and rigorous validation is required. It should also be noted that curated, experimental test sets may differ from those in a real-world clinical environment, and this possible bias is the subject of substantial work which is on-going.

Conclusions

In conclusion, there is a growing burden of osteoporosis and fragility fractures across the globe. Making identification of those in need of treatment imperative. This requires an approach based on history of fragility fracture, assessment of clinical risk and the use of opportunistic screening. Imaging modalities other than DXA may offer an advantage to predicting those at risk of fracture but they are not accessible for widespread clinical use at present, and artificial intelligence approaches to computer vision may hold benefits in the future.

Acknowledgments Professor Ward and Dr Fuggle would like to thank Elsevier publishing for their permission to use Table 1 and acknowledge that a substantial proportion of this chapter was taken from a review article entitled 'Fracture Prediction, Imaging and Screening' co-authored by Nicholas Fuggle, Elizabeth Curtis, Kate Ward, Nicholas Harvey, Elaine Dennison, Cyrus Cooper published in Nature Reviews in Endocrinology. Figures 2.1 and 2.3 are re-drawn from this publication.

References

1. Cooper C, Campion G, Melton LJ 3rd. Hip fractures in the elderly: a world-wide projection. Osteoporos Int. 1992;2:285–9.
2. Albright F, Burnett CH, Cope O, et al. Acute atrophy of bone (osteoporosis) simulating hyperparathyroidism12. J Clin Endocrinol Metabol. 1941;1:711–6. https://doi.org/10.1210/jcem-1-9-711.
3. van Geel TA, van Helden S, Geusens PP, et al. Clinical subsequent fractures cluster in time after first fractures. Ann Rheum Dis. 2009;68:99–102. https://doi.org/10.1136/ard.2008.092775.
4. Kanis JA, Svedbom A, Harvey N, et al. The osteoporosis treatment gap. J Bone Miner Res. 2014;29:1926–8. https://doi.org/10.1002/jbmr.2301.
5. Giangregorio L, Papaioannou A, Cranney A, et al. Fragility fractures and the osteoporosis care gap: an international phenomenon. Semin Arthritis Rheum. 2006;35:293–305. https://doi.org/10.1016/j.semarthrit.2005.11.001.
6. Solomon DH, Johnston SS, Boytsov NN, et al. Osteoporosis medication use after hip fracture in U.S. patients between 2002 and 2011. J Bone Miner Res. 2014;29:1929–37. https://doi.org/10.1002/jbmr.2202.
7. van der Velde RY, Wyers CE, Teesselink E, et al. Trends in oral anti-osteoporosis drug prescription in the United Kingdom between 1990 and 2012: variation by age, sex, geographic location and ethnicity. Bone. 2017;94:50–5. https://doi.org/10.1016/j.bone.2016.10.013.
8. Lenchik L, Leib ES, Hamdy RC, et al. Executive summary International Society for Clinical Densitometry position development conference Denver, Colorado July 20-22, 2001. J Clin Densitom. 2002;5 Suppl:S1–3.
9. Cameron JR, Sorenson J. Measurement of bone mineral in vivo: an improved method. Science. 1963;142:230–2.
10. Roos BO, Sköldborn H. Dual photon absorptiometry in lumbar vertebrae. I. Theory and method. Acta Radiol Ther Phys Biol. 1974;13:266–80. https://doi.org/10.3109/02841867409129883.
11. Mazess RB, Peppler WW, Harrison JE, et al. Total body bone mineral and lean body mass by dual-photon absorptiometry. III. Comparison with trunk calcium by neutron activation analysis. Calcif Tissue Int. 1981;33:365–8.
12. Crabtree NJ, Arabi A, Bachrach LK, et al. Dual-energy X-ray absorptiometry interpretation and reporting in children and adolescents: the revised 2013 ISCD pediatric official positions. J Clin Densitom. 2014;17:225–42. https://doi.org/10.1016/j.jocd.2014.01.003.
13. Kanis JA, Adachi JD, Cooper C, et al. Standardising the descriptive epidemiology of osteoporosis: recommendations from the Epidemiology and Quality of Life Working Group of IOF. Osteoporos Int. 2013;24:2763–4. https://doi.org/10.1007/s00198-013-2413-7.
14. Compston J, Cooper A, Cooper C, et al. UK clinical guideline for the prevention and treatment of osteoporosis. Arch Osteoporos. 2017;12:43. https://doi.org/10.1007/s11657-017-0324-5.
15. Lotz JC, Cheal EJ, Hayes WC. Fracture prediction for the proximal femur using finite element models: part I—Linear analysis. J Biomech Eng. 1991;113:353–60.
16. Nielson CM, Marshall LM, Adams AL, et al. BMI and fracture risk in older men: the osteoporotic fractures in men study (MrOS). J Bone Miner Res. 2011;26:496–502. https://doi.org/10.1002/jbmr.235.
17. Shepherd JA, Schousboe JT, Broy SB, et al. Executive summary of the 2015 ISCD position development conference on advanced measures from DXA and QCT: fracture prediction beyond BMD. J Clin Densitom. 2015;18:274–86. https://doi.org/10.1016/j.jocd.2015.06.013.
18. Fewtrell MS, Gordon I, Biassoni L, et al. Dual X-ray absorptiometry (DXA) of the lumbar spine in a clinical paediatric setting: does the method of size-adjustment matter? Bone. 2005;37:413–9. https://doi.org/10.1016/j.bone.2005.04.028.
19. Kroger H, Kotaniemi A, Vainio P, et al. Bone densitometry of the spine and femur in children by dual-energy x-ray absorptiometry. Bone Miner. 1992;17:75–85.
20. Crabtree NJ, Shaw NJ, Bishop NJ, et al. Amalgamated reference data for size-adjusted bone densitometry measurements in 3598 children and young adults—the ALPHABET study. J Bone Miner Res. 2017;32:172–80. https://doi.org/10.1002/jbmr.2935.

21. Adams JE. Advances in bone imaging for osteoporosis. Nat Rev Endocrinol. 2013;9:28–42. https://doi.org/10.1038/nrendo.2012.217.
22. Crabtree NJ, Chapman S, Högler W, et al. Vertebral fractures assessment in children: evaluation of DXA imaging versus conventional spine radiography. Bone. 2017;97:168–74. https://doi.org/10.1016/j.bone.2017.01.006.
23. McCloskey EV, Oden A, Harvey NC, et al. A meta-analysis of trabecular bone score in fracture risk prediction and its relationship to FRAX. J Bone Miner Res. 2016;31:940–8. https://doi.org/10.1002/jbmr.2734.
24. Cummings SR, Black DM, Nevitt MC, et al. Bone density at various sites for prediction of hip fractures. The Study of Osteoporotic Fractures Research Group. Lancet. 1993;341:72–5. https://doi.org/10.1016/0140-6736(93)92555-8.
25. Marshall D, Johnell O, Wedel H. Meta-analysis of how well measures of bone mineral density predict occurrence of osteoporotic fractures. BMJ. 1996;312:1254–9. https://doi.org/10.1136/bmj.312.7041.1254.
26. Assessment of fracture risk and its application to screening for postmenopausal osteoporosis. Report of a WHO Study Group. World Health Organ Tech Rep Ser. 1994;843:1–129.
27. Shuhart CR, Yeap SS, Anderson PA, et al. Executive summary of the 2019 ISCD position development conference on monitoring treatment, dxa cross-calibration and least significant change, spinal cord injury, peri-prosthetic and orthopedic bone health, transgender medicine, and pediatrics. J Clin Densitom. 2019;22:453–71.
28. Weber DR, Boyce A, Gordon C, et al. The utility of DXA assessment at the forearm, proximal femur, and lateral distal femur, and vertebral fracture assessment in the pediatric population: 2019 ISCD official position. J Clin Densitom. 2019;22:567–89. https://doi.org/10.1016/j.jocd.2019.07.002.
29. Schuit SC, van der Klift M, Weel AE, et al. Fracture incidence and association with bone mineral density in elderly men and women: the Rotterdam Study. Bone. 2004;34:195–202.
30. Wainwright SA, Marshall LM, Ensrud KE, et al. Hip fracture in women without osteoporosis. J Clin Endocrinol Metab. 2005;90:2787–93. https://doi.org/10.1210/jc.2004-1568.
31. Kanis JA, Harvey NC, Cooper C, et al. A systematic review of intervention thresholds based on FRAX: a report prepared for the National Osteoporosis Guideline Group and the International Osteoporosis Foundation. Arch Osteoporos. 2016;11:25. https://doi.org/10.1007/s11657-016-0278-z.
32. Kanis JA, McCloskey EV, Harvey NC, et al. Intervention thresholds and the diagnosis of osteoporosis. J Bone Miner Res. 2015;30:1747–53. https://doi.org/10.1002/jbmr.2531.
33. Kanis JA, Harvey NC, Johansson H, et al. A decade of FRAX: how has it changed the management of osteoporosis? Aging Clin Exp Res. 2020;32:187–96. https://doi.org/10.1007/s40520-019-01432-y.
34. Kanis JA. Diagnosis of osteoporosis and assessment of fracture risk. Lancet. 2002;359:1929–36. https://doi.org/10.1016/s0140-6736(02)08761-5.
35. Kanis JA, Johnell O, Oden A, et al. FRAX and the assessment of fracture probability in men and women from the UK. Osteoporos Int. 2008;19:385–97. https://doi.org/10.1007/s00198-007-0543-5.
36. Nguyen ND, Frost SA, Center JR, et al. Development of prognostic nomograms for individualizing 5-year and 10-year fracture risks. Osteoporos Int. 2008;19:1431–44. https://doi.org/10.1007/s00198-008-0588-0.
37. Hippisley-Cox J, Coupland C. Predicting risk of osteoporotic fracture in men and women in England and Wales: prospective derivation and validation of QFractureScores. BMJ. 2009;339:b4229. https://doi.org/10.1136/bmj.b4229.
38. Kanis JA, Johansson H, Oden A, et al. Worldwide uptake of FRAX. Arch Osteoporos. 2014;9:166. https://doi.org/10.1007/s11657-013-0166-8.
39. Hoff M, Meyer HE, Skurtveit S, et al. Validation of FRAX and the impact of self-reported falls among elderly in a general population: the HUNT study, Norway. Osteoporos Int. 2017;28:2935–44. https://doi.org/10.1007/s00198-017-4134-9.

40. Fraser LA, Langsetmo L, Berger C, et al. Fracture prediction and calibration of a Canadian FRAX® tool: a population-based report from CaMos. Osteoporos Int. 2011;22:829–37. https://doi.org/10.1007/s00198-010-1465-1.
41. Kanis JA, Harvey NC, Johansson H, et al. Overview of fracture prediction tools. J Clin Densitom. 2017;20:444–50. https://doi.org/10.1016/j.jocd.2017.06.013.
42. Cosman F, de Beur SJ, LeBoff MS, et al. Clinician's guide to prevention and treatment of osteoporosis. Osteoporos Int. 2014;25:2359–81. https://doi.org/10.1007/s00198-014-2794-2.
43. Hajime O, Toshitaka N, Takayuki H, et al. Japanese 2011 guidelines for prevention and treatment of osteoporosis--executive summary. Arch Osteoporos. 2012;7(1):3–20. PMID: 23203733, PMCID: PMC3517709. https://doi.org/10.1007/s11657-012-0109-9.
44. Johansson H, Kanis JA, Oden A, et al. A comparison of case-finding strategies in the UK for the management of hip fractures. Osteoporos Int. 2012;23:907–15. https://doi.org/10.1007/s00198-011-1864-y.
45. Kanis JA, Adams J, Borgström F, et al. The cost-effectiveness of alendronate in the management of osteoporosis. Bone. 2008;42:4–15. https://doi.org/10.1016/j.bone.2007.10.019.
46. Kanis JA, Harvey NC, McCloskey E, et al. Algorithm for the management of patients at low, high and very high risk of osteoporotic fractures. Osteoporos Int. 2020;31:1–12. https://doi.org/10.1007/s00198-019-05176-3.
47. Silva BC, Leslie WD, Resch H, et al. Trabecular bone score: a noninvasive analytical method based upon the DXA image. J Bone Miner Res. 2014;29:518–30. https://doi.org/10.1002/jbmr.2176.
48. Dalle Carbonare L, Giannini S. Bone microarchitecture as an important determinant of bone strength. J Endocrinol Invest. 2004;27:99–105.
49. Hans D, Goertzen AL, Krieg MA, et al. Bone microarchitecture assessed by TBS predicts osteoporotic fractures independent of bone density: the Manitoba study. J Bone Miner Res. 2011;26:2762–9. https://doi.org/10.1002/jbmr.499.
50. Winzenrieth R, Michelet F, Hans D. Three-dimensional (3D) microarchitecture correlations with 2D projection image gray-level variations assessed by trabecular bone score using high-resolution computed tomographic acquisitions: effects of resolution and noise. J Clin Densitom. 2013;16:287–96. https://doi.org/10.1016/j.jocd.2012.05.001.
51. Harvey NC, Gluer CC, Binkley N, et al. Trabecular bone score (TBS) as a new complementary approach for osteoporosis evaluation in clinical practice. Bone. 2015;78:216–24. https://doi.org/10.1016/j.bone.2015.05.016.
52. Simonelli C, Leib E, Mossman N, et al. Creation of an age-adjusted, dual-energy x-ray absorptiometry-derived trabecular bone score curve for the lumbar spine in non-Hispanic US White women. J Clin Densitom. 2014;17:314–9. https://doi.org/10.1016/j.jocd.2013.09.002.
53. Leslie WD, Johansson H, Kanis JA, et al. Lumbar spine texture enhances 10-year fracture probability assessment. Osteoporos Int. 2014;25:2271–7. https://doi.org/10.1007/s00198-014-2761-y.
54. Leslie WD, Aubry-Rozier B, Lix LM, et al. Spine bone texture assessed by trabecular bone score (TBS) predicts osteoporotic fractures in men: the Manitoba Bone Density Program. Bone. 2014;67:10–4. https://doi.org/10.1016/j.bone.2014.06.034.
55. Popp AW, Guler S, Lamy O, et al. Effects of zoledronate versus placebo on spine bone mineral density and microarchitecture assessed by the trabecular bone score in postmenopausal women with osteoporosis: a three-year study. J Bone Miner Res. 2013;28:449–54. https://doi.org/10.1002/jbmr.1775.
56. Krieg MA, Aubry-Rozier B, Hans D, et al. Effects of anti-resorptive agents on trabecular bone score (TBS) in older women. Osteoporos Int. 2013;24:1073–8. https://doi.org/10.1007/s00198-012-2155-y.
57. Padlina I, Gonzalez-Rodriguez E, Hans D, et al. The lumbar spine age-related degenerative disease influences the BMD not the TBS: the Osteolaus cohort. Osteoporos Int. 2017;28:909–15. https://doi.org/10.1007/s00198-016-3829-7.
58. Kanis JA. The World Health Organization Scientific Group Assessment of osteoporosis at the primary health-care level, technical report. World Health Organization Collaborating Centre for Metabolic Bone Diseases, University of Sheffield; 2007.

59. Shepstone L, Fordham R, Lenaghan E, et al. A pragmatic randomised controlled trial of the effectiveness and cost-effectiveness of screening older women for the prevention of fractures: rationale, design and methods for the SCOOP study. Osteoporos Int. 2012;23:2507–15. https://doi.org/10.1007/s00198-011-1876-7.
60. Barr RJ, Stewart A, Torgerson DJ, et al. Population screening for osteoporosis risk: a randomised control trial of medication use and fracture risk. Osteoporos Int. 2010;21:561–8. https://doi.org/10.1007/s00198-009-1007-x.
61. Clark EM, Gould V, Morrison L, et al. Randomized controlled trial of a primary care-based screening program to identify older women with prevalent osteoporotic vertebral fractures: Cohort for Skeletal Health in Bristol and Avon (COSHIBA). J Bone Miner Res. 2012;27:664–71. https://doi.org/10.1002/jbmr.1478.
62. Shepstone L, Lenaghan E, Cooper C, et al. Screening in the community to reduce fractures in older women (SCOOP): a randomised controlled trial. Lancet. 2018;391:741–7. https://doi.org/10.1016/s0140-6736(17)32640-5.
63. Emmett CL, Redmond NM, Peters TJ, et al. Acceptability of screening to prevent osteoporotic fractures: a qualitative study with older women. Fam Pract. 2012;29:235–42. https://doi.org/10.1093/fampra/cmr069.
64. Turner DA, Khioe RFS, Shepstone L, et al. The cost-effectiveness of screening in the community to reduce osteoporotic fractures in older women in the UK: economic evaluation of the SCOOP study. J Bone Miner Res. 2018;33:845–51. https://doi.org/10.1002/jbmr.3381.
65. McCloskey E, Johansson H, Harvey NC, et al. Management of patients with high baseline hip fracture risk by FRAX reduces hip fractures—a post hoc analysis of the SCOOP study. J Bone Miner Res. 2018;33:1020–6. https://doi.org/10.1002/jbmr.3411.
66. Parsons CM, Harvey N, Shepstone L, et al. Systematic screening using FRAX(®) leads to increased use of, and adherence to, anti-osteoporosis medications: an analysis of the UK SCOOP trial. Osteoporos Int. 2020;31:67–75. https://doi.org/10.1007/s00198-019-05142-z.
67. Söreskog E, Borgström F, Shepstone L, Clarke S, Cooper C, Harvey I, Harvey NC, Heawood A, Howe A, Johansson H, Marshall T, O'Neill TW, Peters T, Redmond N, Torgerson D, Turner D, McCloskey E, Kanis JA, the SCOOP Study. Long-term cost-effectiveness of screening for fracture risk in a UK primary care setting. Osteoporos Int. 2020;31(8):1499–506.
68. Rauch F, Schoenau E. Changes in bone density during childhood and adolescence: an approach based on bone's biological organization. J Bone Miner Res. 2001;16:597–604. https://doi.org/10.1359/jbmr.2001.16.4.597.
69. Ward KA, Mughal Z, Adams JE. Tools for measuring bone in children and adolescents. In: Sawyer AJ, Bachrach LK, Fung EB, editors. Bone densitometry in growing patients current clinical practice. Totowa: Humana Press; 2007.
70. Samelson EJ, Broe KE, Xu H, et al. Cortical and trabecular bone microarchitecture as an independent predictor of incident fracture risk in older women and men in the Bone Microarchitecture International Consortium (BoMIC): a prospective study. Lancet Diabetes Endocrinol. 2019;7:34–43. https://doi.org/10.1016/s2213-8587(18)30308-5.
71. Isherwood I, Rutherford RA, Pullan BR, et al. Bone-mineral estimation by computer-assisted transverse axial tomography. Lancet. 1976;2:712–5.
72. Guglielmi G, Schneider P, Lang TF, et al. Quantitative computed tomography at the axial and peripheral skeleton. Eur Radiol. 1997;7:32–42.
73. Engelke K. Quantitative computed tomography-current status and new developments. J Clin Densitom. 2017;20:309–21. https://doi.org/10.1016/j.jocd.2017.06.017.
74. Link TM, Lang TF. Axial QCT: clinical applications and new developments. J Clin Densitom. 2014;17:438–48. https://doi.org/10.1016/j.jocd.2014.04.119.
75. Sfeir JG, Drake MT, Atkinson EJ, et al. Evaluation of cross-sectional and longitudinal changes in volumetric bone mineral density in postmenopausal women using single- versus dual-energy quantitative computed tomography. Bone. 2018;112:145–52. https://doi.org/10.1016/j.bone.2018.04.023.

76. Ruegsegger P, Durand EP, Dambacher MA. Differential effects of aging and disease on trabecular and compact bone density of the radius. Bone. 1991;12:99–105.
77. Griffith JF, Genant HK. Bone mass and architecture determination: state of the art. Best Pract Res Clin Endocrinol Metab. 2008;22:737–64. https://doi.org/10.1016/j.beem.2008.07.003.
78. Frost HM. The mechanostat: a proposed pathogenic mechanism of osteoporoses and the bone mass effects of mechanical and nonmechanical agents. Bone Miner. 1987;2:73–85.
79. Krug R, Burghardt AJ, Majumdar S, et al. High-resolution imaging techniques for the assessment of osteoporosis. Radiol Clin North Am. 2010;48:601–21. https://doi.org/10.1016/j.rcl.2010.02.015.
80. Burghardt AJ, Kazakia GJ, Ramachandran S, et al. Age- and gender-related differences in the geometric properties and biomechanical significance of intracortical porosity in the distal radius and tibia. J Bone Miner Res. 2010;25:983–93. https://doi.org/10.1359/jbmr.091104.
81. Liu XS, Zhang XH, Sekhon KK, et al. High-resolution peripheral quantitative computed tomography can assess microstructural and mechanical properties of human distal tibial bone. J Bone Miner Res. 2010;25:746–56. https://doi.org/10.1359/jbmr.090822.
82. Miller PD. Controversies in bone mineral density diagnostic classifications. Calcif Tissue Int. 2000;66:317–9. https://doi.org/10.1007/s002230010066.
83. Gong B, Mandair GS, Wehrli FW, et al. Novel assessment tools for osteoporosis diagnosis and treatment. Curr Osteoporos Rep. 2014;12:357–65. https://doi.org/10.1007/s11914-014-0215-2.
84. Chang G, Boone S, Martel D, et al. MRI assessment of bone structure and microarchitecture. J Magn Reson Imaging. 2017;46:323–37. https://doi.org/10.1002/jmri.25647.
85. Bartalena T, Giannelli G, Rinaldi MF, et al. Prevalence of thoracolumbar vertebral fractures on multidetector CT: underreporting by radiologists. Eur J Radiol. 2009;69:555–9. https://doi.org/10.1016/j.ejrad.2007.11.036.
86. Carberry GA, Pooler BD, Binkley N, et al. Unreported vertebral body compression fractures at abdominal multidetector CT. Radiology. 2013;268:120–6. https://doi.org/10.1148/radiol.13121632.
87. Williams AL, Al-Busaidi A, Sparrow PJ, et al. Under-reporting of osteoporotic vertebral fractures on computed tomography. Eur J Radiol. 2009;69:179–83. https://doi.org/10.1016/j.ejrad.2007.08.028.
88. Buckens CF, Dijkhuis G, de Keizer B, et al. Opportunistic screening for osteoporosis on routine computed tomography? An external validation study. Eur Radiol. 2015;25:2074–9. https://doi.org/10.1007/s00330-014-3584-0.
89. Loffler MT, Jacob A, Valentinitsch A, et al. Improved prediction of incident vertebral fractures using opportunistic QCT compared to DXA. Eur Radiol. 2019;29:4980–9. https://doi.org/10.1007/s00330-019-06018-w.
90. Pickhardt PJ, Pooler BD, Lauder T, et al. Opportunistic screening for osteoporosis using abdominal computed tomography scans obtained for other indications. Ann Intern Med. 2013;158:588–95. https://doi.org/10.7326/0003-4819-158-8-201304160-00003.
91. Damilakis J, Adams JE, Guglielmi G, et al. Radiation exposure in X-ray-based imaging techniques used in osteoporosis. Eur Radiol. 2010;20:2707–14. https://doi.org/10.1007/s00330-010-1845-0.
92. Adams JE, Lenchik L, Roux C, et al. Vertebral fracture initiative, Part II, Radiological assessment of vertebral fracture; 2010.
93. Lessmann N, van Ginneken B, de Jong PA, et al. Iterative fully convolutional neural networks for automatic vertebra segmentation and identification. Med Image Anal. 2019;53:142–55. https://doi.org/10.1016/j.media.2019.02.005.
94. Tomita N, Cheung YY, Hassanpour S. Deep neural networks for automatic detection of osteoporotic vertebral fractures on CT scans. Comput Biol Med. 2018;98:8–15. https://doi.org/10.1016/j.compbiomed.2018.05.011.
95. Al-Helo S, Alomari RS, Ghosh S, et al. Compression fracture diagnosis in lumbar: a clinical CAD system. Int J Comput Assist Radiol Surg. 2013;8:461–9. https://doi.org/10.1007/s11548-012-0796-0.

96. Fang Y, Li W, Chen X, et al. Opportunistic osteoporosis screening in multi-detector CT images using deep convolutional neural networks. Eur Radiol. 2021;31(4):1831–42. https://doi.org/10.1007/s00330-020-07312-8.
97. Derkatch S, Kirby C, Kimelman D, et al. Identification of vertebral fractures by convolutional neural networks to predict nonvertebral and hip fractures: a registry-based cohort study of dual X-ray absorptiometry. Radiology. 2019;293:405–11. https://doi.org/10.1148/radiol.2019190201.

Chapter 3
The Role of Nutrition in Bone Health

D. Sanchez-Rodriguez, L. Lengelé, Charlotte Beaudart, J. -Y. Reginster, and O. Bruyère

Introduction

As demographic changes occur globally and conditions such as osteoporosis that typically occur in later life become more prevalent, The World Health Organization (WHO) has developed a plan of action that will facilitate optimal ageing [1], that includes a focus on functional status, and has led to the Decade of Healthy Ageing from 2020 to 2030 [2]. To this end, several European organisms and scientific societies' aim to improve health status by providing nutritional advice; the European Food Safety Agency periodically revisits the Dietary Reference Intakes, which is the list of nutrients and their quantity required to cover the needs of the different organs and systems in the human body, established by the National Institute of Medicine of the United States [3]. The European Society of Clinical Nutrition and Metabolism

D. Sanchez-Rodriguez (✉)
WHO Collaborating Center for Public Health Aspects of Musculo-Skeletal health and Ageing, Division of Public Health, Epidemiology and Health Economics, University of Liège, Liège, Belgium

Geriatrics Department, Rehabilitation Research Group, Hospital del Mar Medical Research Institute (IMIM). Universitat Pompeu Fabra, Barcelona, Spain
e-mail: dolores.sanchez@uliege.be

L. Lengelé · C. Beaudart · O. Bruyère
WHO Collaborating Center for Public Health Aspects of Musculo-Skeletal health and Ageing, Division of Public Health, Epidemiology and Health Economics, University of Liège, Liège, Belgium
e-mail: llengele@uliege.be; C.Beaudart@uliege.be; Olivier.Bruyere@uliege.be

J.-Y. Reginster
WHO Collaborating Center for Public Health Aspects of Musculo-Skeletal health and Ageing, Division of Public Health, Epidemiology and Health Economics, University of Liège, Liège, Belgium

Biochemistry Department, College of Science, King Saud University, Riyadh, KSA

E. Dennison (ed.), *Osteoporosis Treatment*, https://doi.org/10.1007/978-3-030-78128-6_3

(ESPEN) revisits these recommendations and adapts them to the needs of different populations, such as older people to produce clinical guidelines [4], and accompanies other published recommendations regarding nutritional intakes and bone and muscle health [5–15]. This chapter highlights intakes of dietary elements that are associated with better bone health according to available level of evidence [16].

Nutrients with Important Impact on Bone Health

Nutrients are defined as substances needed by an organism to survive, grow, and reproduce. Human requirements vary according to age, gender, and different conditions (weight, acute and chronic diseases, etc.). Despite all nutrients being necessary, not all of them have the same impact on the different organs and systems of the human body. In this chapter, we will review the nutrients that have been shown to have a more direct impact on bone mineral density (BMD) and risk of fracture, namely, proteins, calcium, and vitamin D [17, 18]. Other nutrients, such as vitamin A, vitamin K, magnesium, phosphates, phosphorus, and zinc may also have some influence on BMD and risk of fracture, but the evidence is less compelling [19, 20] and therefore will not be discussed here.

Proteins

Dietary proteins play a key role in muscle and bone health. Bone is composed of a protein matrix that contributes up to 50% of its volume and a third of its mass, therefore, an adequate protein intake is crucial to maintain this matrix [21, 22]. The biological pathways that explain the role of dietary proteins in bone anabolism and mineralization are mediated by calcium-phosphate metabolism, vitamin D regulation (intestinal absorption and renal excretion), and insulin-like growth factor 1 (IGF-1) [6, 23]. Diets rich in proteins are associated with higher calcium absorption in the intestine, and this process involves vitamin D. Despite a higher intestinal absorption of calcium being linked to an increase in renal excretion of calcium, the overall balance of calcium level associated with the absorption of proteins is positive and therefore, both, calcium and proteins levels increase and contribute to bone formation [23]. Moreover, diets rich in proteins have shown an anabolic effect on bone, mediated by the activation of osteoblasts by the insulin-like growth factor 1 (IGF-1) [23].

General adult population at any age and general older populations (Primary prevention): The European Food and Safety Agency recommended daily allowance (RDA) of protein intake, in general adult populations, at any age, for men and women, is 0.8–0.83 g/kg/body weight/day [24]. Moreover, the recommended minimum intake of proteins should provide 10% of the total calories intake per day, calculated for energy requirements of 2.000–2.200 Kcal/day and based on the nitrogen balance resulting from the amino acids provided by those proteins [22]. There are insufficient data about the tolerable and recommended maximum intake of proteins and the percentage of calories it would provide varies between 20% and 35%, both for general and older populations [6, 22, 25–27] (Table 3.1).

Table 3.1 Summary table with protein, calcium, and vitamin D doses, and some examples of a dietary intake

Nutrient	Doses	Examples of dietary intake
Proteins	**General:** 0.8 g/kg/body weight/day **Older people (≥65-year-old), subject with osteoporosis or fractures:** 1.0–1.2 g/kg/body weight/day	*Example*: A healthy postmenopausal woman 65-year-old, 160 cm, and 60 kg should achieve 60 g of protein/day, distributed in 3 servings per day Red meat: 26 g of proteins/100 g of red meat Poultry: 27 g of proteins/100 g of poultry Fish: 23 g of proteins/100 g of fish Seafood: 19 g of proteins/100 g of seafood Eggs: 7 g of proteins/50 g (1 egg) *Dairy products* Skimmed or whole milk: 6 g of proteins/one glass of 200 mL Hard cheese (e.g. Gouda, Emmental, Gruyère, etc.): 28 g/100 g: 9 g of proteins/33 g (one slice) Soft-paste cheese (e.g. Brie, Camembert, etc.): 21 g of proteins/100 g: 7 g of proteins/30 g (one portion) Yoghurt: 4 g of proteins/125 g *Vegetable sources* Legumes (beans, chickpeas): 8 g of proteins/100 g cooked Soy-derived products (soymilk): 6 g of proteins/one glass of 200 mL Nuts: 13 g of proteins/100 g: 3 g/ 25 g (a handful) Seeds: 20 g of proteins/100 g
Calcium	≥1200 mg/day	Preferable from dietary sources and dairy products: Up to 3 intakes of dairy products per day *Fishes with eatable bones (a can of fish usually contains from 85 to 120 g)* Sardines: 130 mg of calcium/100 g Anchovies: 87 mg of calcium/100 g Pilchards: 250 mg of calcium/100 g *Dairy products* Whole milk: 240 mg of calcium/one glass of 200 mL Semi-skimmed milk: 230 mg of calcium/one glass of 200 mL Skimmed milk: 210 mg of calcium/one glass of 200 mL Hard cheese (e.g. Gouda, Emmental, Gruyère, etc.): 946 mg of calcium/100 g: 315 mg of calcium/33 g (one slice) Soft-paste cheese (e.g. Brie, Camembert, etc.): 534 mg of calcium/100 g: 160 mg of calcium/30 g (one portion) Yoghurt: 128 mg of calcium/125 g *Vegetables sources* Broccoli: 43 mg of calcium/100 g cooked Cabbage: 50 mg of calcium/100 g cooked Kale: 72 mg of calcium/100 g *Legumes* Okra: 77 mg of calcium/100 g Soybeans: 220 mg of calcium/100 g Nuts: 75 mg of calcium/100 g: 19 mg/ 25 g (a handful)

(continued)

Table 3.1 (continued)

Nutrient	Doses	Examples of dietary intake
Vitamin D	800–1000 IU/day	*Oily Fishes* Smoked or cooked salmon: 220 UI of vitamin D/100 g Sardines: 480 UI of vitamin D/100 g Herrings: 440 UI of vitamin D/100 g Cod: 160 UI of vitamin D/100 g Tuna: 80 UI of vitamin D/100 g Canned tuna in oil: 160 UI of vitamin D/100 g Egg yolk: 80 UI of vitamin D/100 g: One egg yolk: 14.4 UI of vitamin D/18 g *Dairy products* Whole milk: 40 UI of vitamin D/one glass of 200 mL Semi-skimmed milk: 40 UI of vitamin D/one glass of 200 mL Skimmed milk: 0 UI of vitamin D/one glass of 200 mL Hard cheese (e.g. Gouda, Emmental, Gruyère, etc.): 12 UI of vitamin D/100 g: 4 UI/ 33 g (one slice) Soft-paste cheese (e.g. Brie, Camembert, etc.): 40 UI of vitamin D/100 g: 12 UI/ 30 g (one portion) Yoghurt: 40 UI of vitamin D/125 g

In general, for older people without any specific deficiency, the ESPEN guideline on clinical nutrition and hydration in geriatrics [4] recommends the same intake as the one recommended for the general adult population at any age. This dose was higher in the position paper from the PROT-age group, which reviewed the literature and concluded that a protein intake of 1.0–1.2 g/kg/body weight/day obtained the greatest benefits in musculoskeletal health [6]. The recommendations regarding optimal protein intake may underestimate the needs of older people [28], who might have additional requirements to optimize the effects of exercise programs [29], therefore, maybe a higher intake might be more appropriate. Moreover, the absorption of macro and micronutrients in the digestive system and the anabolic stimuli in muscles are affected by age, and may be less effective in older people, leading to higher requirements than the general population [30].

Patients with osteoporosis and fractures (Secondary and Tertiary prevention): Associations have been found between higher protein intake and better bone health, with positive trends in BMD at all sites [21, 31] and reduced risk of hip fracture [31]. Based on these results, protein intake should not be limited to the RDA [25, 31]. Indeed, a protein intake accounting for 24% of the total calories intake per day has been recommended for patients with osteoporosis [6] and an intake above 1.0–1.2 g/kg/body weight/day was found to produce greater benefits in BMD in patients ≥65-year-old with osteoporosis and in patients with hip fracture [6].

A systematic review of the literature has found that intake might need to be adapted in some populations. For example, an intake of proteins of 0.6–0.8 g/kg/day was found to have the greatest benefits in patients with severe chronic kidney disease [if glomerular filter rate (GFR <30 mL/min/1.73 m^2)]. Higher intakes (1.2–1.5 g/kg/day) were found to be more effective in patients with acute and chronic illnesses (diseases which involve inflammation and increased catabolism) [6, 32], and patients with severe illnesses, injuries or malnutrition (e.g. pressure ulcers) derive benefits from intake of proteins up to 2 g/kg/day [6, 33]. These recommendations for special populations are consistent in all studies and have been adopted by most updated guidelines: ESPEN guideline on nutrition and hydration in geriatrics [4], the ESPEN recommendations for protein intake [32], and the consensus statement from the ESCEO [14], among others [33].

Dietary sources of proteins: Animal-based foods are the most important dietary source of proteins, i.e., red meat, poultry, viscera, fish, seafood, eggs, dairy products (milk, cheese, yoghurt and similar), and animal proteins contain all the essential amino acids required by human beings (high quality proteins). The available evidence suggests that the greatest benefits for bone health are obtained from proteins provided by dairy products [34]. There are also vegetable sources of proteins, i.e., legumes (chickpeas, beans), soy-derived products, cereals, nuts, and seeds. However, despite the fact that certain plants (e.g. soy beans) may contain higher amount of proteins than animal sources, rare (or very rare) (e.g. quinoa) [35] are the vegetable sources that provide all the essential amino acids required by human beings (low quality proteins). Moreover, the bioavailability of vegetable proteins is lower due to lower intestinal absorption. Therefore, vegetarian, and more particularly vegan, diets do not compare with the amount of proteins and more specifically, of amino acids provided by high quality proteins, which are necessary for bone health. Those diets have been associated with lower BMD and higher risk of fracture [36] although other authors have reported slightly different results. For example, a meta-analysis found no differences in the relationship between BMD and either animal vs. isoflavone-rich soy protein intake [37]. However this meta-analysis did not consider relationships between protein intake and the risk of fracture and thus the topic still remains controversial. Hence while we await further research careful review of individuals who follow a vegetarian or vegan diet may be appropriate.

Distribution of the protein intake: Distribution of protein intake as 3 meals per day, including high quality proteins in each meal, has been recommended by ESCEO as well as ingesting these proteins after physical exercise for greater benefits [14, 38].

Vitamin D

Vitamin D is essential for the correct regulation and functioning of several systems of the human body. Maintaining correct levels of vitamin D during the life course has an impact on bone health [13]. The association between serum levels of vitamin D and bone health has been described as follows: vitamin D deficiency (<25 nmol/L) produces a mineralization defect; vitamin D insufficiency (<50 nmol/L) produces increased parathyroid hormone levels and an increase in bone turnover; levels from 50 to 75 nmol/L (or at least 75 nmol/L in older people) are defined as vitamin D sufficiency and have neutral or desirable effects, with benefits for BMD and risk of fracture [13]. The target level is considered by many to be around 125 nmol/L; higher levels than this are not recommended, as they can produce undesirable effects [39]. The oral daily intake of vitamin D generally required to achieve these serum levels in a substantial proportion of subjects [13] is 800–1000 IU or its equivalent on a weekly or monthly basis. This intake of vitamin D is adequate for primary prevention in the general population, but also for secondary, and tertiary prevention in individuals receiving pharmacological treatment for osteoporosis. Moreover, vitamin D is considered to have a wide range of extra-skeletal effects, including on muscular function and on the immune system [40].

Doses of vitamin D ≥ 3000 IU daily should be avoided [39], as well as administration by large periodic bolus e.g., 250,000–1000,000 IU every 3–12 months as these have been shown to lead to a higher risk of falls and fractures in older patients. Other secondary effects of large doses of vitamin D, such as renal stones and hypercalciuria have also been described [41]. Supplementation with vitamin D does not increase cardiovascular risk and no association between ischemic cardiac events and supplementation with vitamin D has been found. Work using the UK Biobank Cohort, a cohort of 502,637 participants, did not find any association between the use of vitamin D and increased risk of hospital admission or death following ischemic cardiovascular events [42].

Sources of vitamin D: Vitamin D is the only nutrient naturally produced by the human body through exposure to sunlight. Dietary sources of vitamin D are fish, such as salmon, with higher content in wild than in farmed salmon [43], sardines, herrings, cod, tuna (all fresh or canned) [44], and in fish oil (in particular, in cod liver oil) [44]. Other dietary sources with high content of vitamin D are egg yolk and dairy products, but only if they are not "low-fat", because vitamin D is a fat-soluble vitamin. Vegetables do not naturally contain vitamin D, but soy milk artificially enriched with vitamin D is available. Dietary sources of vitamin D may be insufficient to reach the recommended intake.

Calcium

Calcium is the main constituent of bone. It provides strength and structure to the bone tissue. Moreover, the skeleton acts as a dynamic reservoir of calcium. Apart from its role in bone health, calcium is necessary to maintain the correct function of several systems and organs of the human body, i.e., to regulate the flow of molecules through cell membranes, to produce electric impulse of the muscular cells and myocytes of the heart, and to regulate contraction of arterial vessels [45].

Intestinal absorption and renal excretion of calcium are based on feedback mechanisms, mediated by phosphate and vitamin D [6, 23]. If the intake of calcium is insufficient, the level of calcium decreases in the blood and the release of parathyroid hormone (PTH) is activated. This triggers catabolism, osteoclastic bone resorption and, thus, releases calcium from the bone matrix into the blood to maintain an adequate circulating level of calcium. Therefore, a sufficient dietary intake that ensures physiological levels of calcium is required for bone health [46].

The European Food and Safety Agency RDA of calcium intake is at least 1200 mg/day, preferably from dairy products (Table 3.1). This recommendation is suitable for the general adult population, older populations, and patients at any risk of fracture (primary, secondary, and tertiary prevention) [10, 17, 47]. If this daily intake is not achieved by food intake, oral supplements should be considered; calcium supplementation is recommended to be given in combination with vitamin D, as calcium supplementation alone has not shown a decrease in the loss of BMD or the risk of fracture [48]. The benefits of calcium are not only skeletal, but also extra-skeletal. A decrease in hypertension, with reduction in systolic and diastolic blood pressure, and reduction of total and LDL cholesterol have been observed in patients following diets fortified with calcium [49], among other protective effects on cardiovascular diseases [40]. Despite previous controversies about divalent cations, recent studies show no association between risk of cardiovascular diseases and calcium supplementation in physiological doses, which can be considered safe [42]. An intake of calcium above 2000 mg/day is above physiological doses and is thus not recommended, especially considering that higher intake does not involve higher benefit for bone health and are associated with secondary effects, such as kidney stones [40].

Dietary sources of calcium: Sources of calcium are milk and other dairy products, fish with eatable bones such as sardines, mackerel, anchovies, and pilchards, vegetables such as broccoli, cabbage, kale, legumes, okra, and soybeans [50] (Table 3.1).

Calcium and Vitamin D: Better Together

Individuals who do not achieve the recommended dietary intake of calcium or vitamin D, especially those who are taking anti-osteoporosis medication are recommended to take supplements [51, 52].

In those individuals taking therapy for osteoporosis, two network meta-analyses (NMA) [51, 52] of randomised controlled trials of calcium and vitamin D supplementation are of interest. In the first NMA, calcium in combination with vitamin D reduced the risk of hip fracture if they were administered together (odds ratio, 0.81; 95% confidence interval, 0.68–0.96), but not separately [52]. In the second NMA [51], Barrionuevo et al. compared the effective estimates for various interventions aimed at reducing the risk of fracture. This NMA showed that calcium in combination with vitamin D produced a reduction in hip fractures but with a considerably lower efficacy than the reduction obtained by the anabolic therapy and antiresorptive treatments included in the analysis [51]. These results are consistent with those reported in another NMA by Yao et al., 2019, where daily supplementation with combined calcium and vitamin D showed a reduction in the risk of hip fracture, but neither daily nor intermittent supplements of vitamin D alone were effective for the reduction of the risk of fracture [53].

Safety of supplementation with calcium and vitamin D: Calcium and vitamin D supplementation can be considered relatively safe. In a recent systematic review from the US Preventive Services Task Force, an association between calcium and vitamin D supplementation and the risk of kidney stones compared with placebo (absolute risk difference 0.33% [95% CI, 0.06–0.60%]) was found, without any other risks associated [54]. Despite some controversial effects on vascular calcification, the risk is not clinically relevant, and calcium and vitamin D are safe and do not increase coronary heart disease or all-cause mortality risk [55–58].

Diets and Dietary Patterns with Significant Impact on Bone Health

Mediterranean Diet

This is an ancient pattern of dietary intake related to the local products traditionally available on the Mediterranean coast. The Mediterranean diet is based on a reduced intake of saturated fatty acids and red meat, and an increased intake of fish, legumes, vegetables, fruits, whole grains, nuts, and olive oil. Several studies have reported benefits of a Mediterranean diet on all health outcomes [59, 60], including bone health [61]. The mechanisms that produce the beneficial effects of Mediterranean diet on bone health are not well established. Some authors suggest these effects might be mediated by decrease in inflammation and oxidative stress, decrease in the incidence of cardiovascular risk factors, and overall improvement in cardiovascular health [26, 62]. A higher adherence to Mediterranean diet has been shown to be related to a higher BMD and lower risk of hip fracture (RR 0.95, 95% CI 0.92–0.98, $p = 0.01$) [26].

Western Patterns and Other Dietary Patterns

A meta-analysis of cohort, case-control, and cross-sectional studies assessed the effect of dietary patterns and diets on BMD and risk of fracture. Diets defined as "unhealthy", "Western", or "processed", composed of "hamburgers and fried foods, pickles, snacks, cola beverages, coffee, and sugar", were compared with diets defined as "Healthy", "Health conscious", "Prudent", "Dairy and fish", "Milk and root vegetables" or "Fruit, milk, and whole grains", composed of "fish, low-fat milk, dairy products, legumes, vegetables, fruits, whole grains, nuts, and olive oil". The second pattern appeared to have a protective effect on bone health in all ages (children and adolescents, adults, and older ages) and both sexes. For example, in cohort studies, in older ages, a decrease of the risk of low BMD with a RR of 0.58 (95% CI: 0.43, 0.78; $p < 0.001$) and of risk of fracture with a RR of 0.81 (95% CI: 0.69, 0.95; $p = 0.01$) were observed [63].

Diets Rich in Dairy Products

Diets rich in dairy products have a high protein, calcium and vitamin D content. They decrease urine calcium and increase calcium retention, with benefits in bone health as shown in all MA that assessed these diets [64]. An intake of dairy products that include three servings per day has been considered safe and beneficial for bone health [65]. Milk consumption has been shown to increase BMD and decrease the risk of fracture at any age [66]. Moreover, systematic reviews have shown the cost-effectiveness and positive economic impact on public health of dairy products, in terms of prevention of osteoporosis and decrease in the risk of fracture [67–69]. A recent study considering the beneficial effects of dairy products intake on musculoskeletal health has been published; the authors found that the intake of whole dairy products has higher effects than the sum of each single individual nutrient of dairy products [34]. The consumption of dairy products has been recommended by guidelines that address this topic [17, 70].

Other Dietary Patterns

In the last decade, new diets such as very-low-carbohydrate ketogenic diets, intermittent fasting or calorie restriction have emerged, aimed at weight control. Very-low-carbohydrate ketogenic diets were initially developed as a way to control intractable epilepsy and have been used for losing weight more latterly. They are composed of high contents of proteins and fat and a very low carbohydrate content. The physiological effect of a ketogenic diet is based on (1) the body's consumption of ketonic bodies produced from the fat mass as a source of energy, instead of using glucose; (2) the satiety signals from fat intake; (3) the decrease in appetite due to protein intake, and (4) the absence of hunger-promoting carbohydrates such as fructose and/or sucrose in the diet [71]. The progressive loss of BMD produced by a ketogenic diet has been observed in children with intractable epilepsy, but the effects of ketogenic diets on bone metabolism in adults remain unexplored [71]. Similarly, the effects of intermittent fasting on BMD or fracture risk still require further research.

Dietary patterns, such as vegetarianism and veganism have also gained in popularity. The level of restriction of these diets vary widely. For example, a recent cohort study, among Greek adults found that "'vegetables-fruit" dietary patterns were very heterogeneous in their content and levels of vitamin D intake [44]. Systematic reviews and meta-analyses have highlighted the potential dangers of intermittent fasting, calorie restrictions, vegetarianism and veganism for bone health [36, 71, 72]. Vegetarian and in particular vegan diets have been shown to be associated with lower values of BMD and higher risk of fracture [36]. Guidelines therefore recommend that individuals who follow special diets should be assessed, and supplementation of the nutrients that do not reach the dietary recommendations, such as proteins, calcium or vitamin D considered [36, 70, 71] in order to avoid possible damages in musculoskeletal health.

Conclusions

This chapter provides an overview of the role of different nutrients in bone health. Strong evidence exists for the importance of adequate intake of protein, calcium and vitamin D. A protein intake of 0.8 g/kg/body weight/day in a general adult population and from 1.0 to 1.2 g/kg/body weight/day in older populations is recommended, which should be distributed as 3 servings per day and if possible, after physical exercise. Moreover, a vitamin D intake of 800–1000 IU/24 h (suitable to maintain serum 25-hydroxyvitamin D levels >50 nmol/L), and a calcium intake of 1200 mg/24 h, preferably obtained from dietary sources [14] is required to maintain bone health. The Mediterranean diet has shown the highest benefits in musculoskeletal health [61].

References

1. Beard JR, Officer A, de Carvalho IA, Sadana R, Pot AM, Michel J-P, et al. The world report on ageing and health: a policy framework for healthy ageing. Lancet. 2016;387(10033):2145–54.
2. World Health Organisation. Global strategy and action plan on ageing and health (2016–2020). Geneva: World Health Organisation; 2016.
3. Dietary reference values for nutrients summary report. EFSA Support Publ. 2017;14(12).
4. Volkert D, Beck AM, Cederholm T, Cruz-Jentoft A, Goisser S, Hooper L, et al. ESPEN guideline on clinical nutrition and hydration in geriatrics. Clin Nutr. 2019;38(1):10–47.
5. Blain H, Masud T, Dargent-Molina P, Martin FC, Rosendahl E, van der Velde N, et al. A comprehensive fracture prevention strategy in older adults: the European Union Geriatric Medicine Society (EUGMS) statement. Aging Clin Exp Res. 2016;28(4):797–803.
6. Bauer J, Biolo G, Cederholm T, Cesari M, Cruz-Jentoft AJ, Morley JE, et al. Evidence-based recommendations for optimal dietary protein intake in older people: a position paper from the prot-age study group. J Am Med Dir Assoc. 2013;14(8):542–59.
7. Perkisas S, Baudry S, Bauer J, Beckwée D, De Cock A-M, Hobbelen H, et al. The SARCUS project: evidence-based muscle assessment through ultrasound. Eur Geriatr Med. 2019;10(1):157–8.
8. Sanchez-Rodriguez D, Bruyère O. The international registry of patients with sarcopenia: applying research in sarcopenia to clinical practice. Eur Geriatr Med. 2018;9(6):735–8.
9. Cruz-Jentoft AJAAJ, Bahat GGG, Bauer JJJJ, Boirie Y, Bruyère O, Cederholm T, et al. Sarcopenia: revised European consensus on definition and diagnosis. Age Ageing. 2019;48(4):601.
10. Harvey NC, Biver E, Kaufman J-M, Bauer J, Branco J, Brandi ML, et al. The role of calcium supplementation in healthy musculoskeletal ageing. Osteoporos Int. 2017;28(2):447–62.

11. Al-Daghri NM, Al-Saleh Y, Aljohani N, Sulimani R, Al-Othman AM, Alfawaz H, et al. Vitamin D status correction in Saudi Arabia: an experts' consensus under the auspices of the European Society for Clinical and Economic Aspects of Osteoporosis, Osteoarthritis, and Musculoskeletal Diseases (ESCEO). Arch Osteoporos. 2017;12(1):1.
12. Cianferotti L, Cutolo M, Kaufman J-M, Bischoff-Ferrari HA, Rizzoli R, Reginster J-Y, et al. Vitamin D supplementation in the prevention and management of major chronic diseases not related to mineral homeostasis in adults: research for evidence and a scientific statement from the European Society for Clinical and Economic Aspects of Osteoporosis. Endocrine. 2017;56(2):245–61.
13. Rizzoli R, Boonen S, Brandi M-L, Bruyère O, Cooper C, Kanis JA, et al. Vitamin D supplementation in elderly or postmenopausal women: a 2013 update of the 2008 recommendations from the European Society for Clinical and Economic Aspects of Osteoporosis and Osteoarthritis (ESCEO). Curr Med Res Opin. 2013;29(4):305–13.
14. Rizzoli R, Stevenson JC, Bauer JM, Van Loon LJC, Walrand S, Kanis JA, et al. The role of dietary protein and vitamin D in maintaining musculoskeletal health in postmenopausal women: a consensus statement from the European Society for Clinical and Economic Aspects of Osteoporosis and Osteoarthritis (ESCEO). Maturitas. 2014;79(1):122–32.
15. Bauer JM, Mikušová L, Verlaan S, Bautmans I, Brandt K, Donini LM, et al. Safety and tolerability of 6-month supplementation with a vitamin D, calcium and leucine-enriched whey protein medical nutrition drink in sarcopenic older adults. Aging Clin Exp Res. 2020;12:1–14.
16. Explanation of the 2011 Oxford Centre for Evidence-Based Medicine (OCEBM) Levels of Evidence (Background Document). Oxford Cent Evidence-Based Med; 2011. https://www.cebm.net/index.aspx.
17. Body J-J, Bergmann P, Boonen S, Boutsen Y, Bruyere O, Devogelaer J-P, et al. Non-pharmacological management of osteoporosis: a consensus of the Belgian Bone Club. Osteoporos Int. 2011;22(11):2769–88.
18. Kanis JA, Cooper C, Rizzoli R, Reginster J-Y. Executive summary of European guidance for the diagnosis and management of osteoporosis in postmenopausal women. Aging Clin Exp Res. 2019;31(1):15–7.
19. Farsinejad-Marj M, Saneei P, Esmaillzadeh A. Dietary magnesium intake, bone mineral density and risk of fracture: a systematic review and meta-analysis. Osteoporos Int. 2016;27(4):1389–99.
20. Vorland CJ, Stremke ER, Moorthi RN, Hill Gallant KM. Effects of excessive dietary phosphorus intake on bone health. Curr Osteoporos Rep. 2017;15(5):473–82.
21. Shams-White MM, Chung M, Du M, Fu Z, Insogna KL, Karlsen MC, et al. Dietary protein and bone health: a systematic review and meta-analysis from the National Osteoporosis Foundation. Am J Clin Nutr. 2017;105(6):ajcn145110.
22. Gaffney-Stomberg E, Insogna KL, Rodriguez NR, Kerstetter JE. Increasing dietary protein requirements in elderly people for optimal muscle and bone health. J Am Geriatr Soc. 2009;57(6):1073–9.
23. Rizzoli R, Biver E, Bonjour J-P, Coxam V, Goltzman D, Kanis JA, et al. Benefits and safety of dietary protein for bone health—an expert consensus paper endorsed by the European Society for Clinical and Economical Aspects of Osteopororosis, Osteoarthritis, and Musculoskeletal Diseases and by the International Osteoporosis Foundation. Osteoporos Int. 2018;29(9):1933–48.
24. Scientific opinion on dietary reference values for protein. EFSA J. 2012;10(2):2557.
25. Wolfe RR, Cifelli AM, Kostas G, Kim I-Y. Optimizing protein intake in adults: interpretation and application of the recommended dietary allowance compared with the acceptable macronutrient distribution range. Adv Nutr. 2017;8(2):266–75.
26. Malmir H, Saneei P, Larijani B, Esmaillzadeh A. Adherence to Mediterranean diet in relation to bone mineral density and risk of fracture: a systematic review and meta-analysis of observational studies. Eur J Nutr. 2018;57(6):2147–60.
27. Van Elswyk ME, Weatherford CA, McNeill SH. A systematic review of renal health in healthy individuals associated with protein intake above the US recommended daily allowance in randomized controlled trials and observational studies. Adv Nutr. 2018;9(4):404–18.

28. Volpi E, Campbell WW, Dwyer JT, Johnson MA, Jensen GL, Morley JE, et al. Is the optimal level of protein intake for older adults greater than the recommended dietary allowance? J Gerontol A Biol Sci Med Sci. 2013;68(6):677–81.
29. Daly RM. Exercise and nutritional approaches to prevent frail bones, falls and fractures: an update. Climacteric. 2017;20(2):119–24.
30. Pennings B, Koopman R, Beelen M, Senden JMG, Saris WHM, Van Loon LJCC. Exercising before protein intake allows for greater use of dietary protein-derived amino acids for de novo muscle protein synthesis in both young and elderly men. Am J Clin Nutr. 2011;93(2):322–31.
31. Groenendijk I, den Boeft L, van Loon LJC, de Groot LCPGM. High versus low dietary protein intake and bone health in older adults: a systematic review and meta-analysis. Comput Struct Biotechnol J. 2019;17:1101–12.
32. Deutz NEPP, Bauer JMJM, Barazzoni R, Biolo G, Boirie Y, Bosy-Westphal A, et al. Protein intake and exercise for optimal muscle function with aging: recommendations from the ESPEN Expert Group. Clin Nutr. 2014;33(6):929–36.
33. Cruz-Jentoft AJ, Dawson Hughes B, Scott D, Sanders KM, Rizzoli R. Nutritional strategies for maintaining muscle mass and strength from middle age to later life: a narrative review. Maturitas. 2020;132:57–64.
34. Geiker NRW, Mølgaard C, Iuliano S, Rizzoli R, Manios Y, van Loon LJC, et al. Impact of whole dairy matrix on musculoskeletal health and aging-current knowledge and research gaps. Osteoporos Int. 2020;31(4):601–15.
35. Mota C, Santos M, Mauro R, Samman N, Matos AS, Torres D, et al. Protein content and amino acids profile of pseudocereals. Food Chem. 2016;193:55–61.
36. Veronese N, Reginster J-YY. The effects of calorie restriction, intermittent fasting and vegetarian diets on bone health. Aging Clin Exp Res. 2019;31(6):753–8.
37. Shams-White MM, Chung M, Fu Z, Insogna KL, Karlsen MC, LeBoff MS, et al. Animal versus plant protein and adult bone health: a systematic review and meta-analysis from the National Osteoporosis Foundation. PLoS One. 2018;13(2):e0192459.
38. Xia W, Cooper C, Li M, Xu L, Rizzoli R, Zhu M, et al. East meets west: current practices and policies in the management of musculoskeletal aging. Aging Clin Exp Res. 2019;31(10):1351–73.
39. Bouillon R. Safety of high-dose vitamin D supplementation. J Clin Endocrinol Metab. 2020;105(4):1290–1.
40. Body J-JJ, Bergmann P, Boonen S, Devogelaer J-PP, Gielen E, Goemaere S, et al. Extraskeletal benefits and risks of calcium, vitamin D and anti-osteoporosis medications. Osteoporos Int. 2012;23(S1):1–23.
41. Schousboe JT, Lix LM, Morin SN, Derkatch S, Bryanton M, Alhrbi M, et al. Vertebral fracture assessment increases use of pharmacologic therapy for fracture prevention in clinical practice. J Bone Miner Res. 2019;34(12):2205–12.
42. Harvey NC, D'Angelo S, Paccou J, Curtis EM, Edwards M, Raisi-Estabragh Z, et al. Calcium and vitamin D supplementation are not associated with risk of incident ischemic cardiac events or death: findings from the UK biobank cohort. J Bone Miner Res. 2018;33(5):803–11.
43. Jakobsen J, Smith C, Bysted A, Cashman KD. Vitamin D in wild and farmed atlantic salmon (salmo salar)—what do we know? Nutrients. 2019;11(5):982.
44. Grigoriou E, Trovas G, Papaioannou N, Dontas I, Makris K, Apostolou-Karampelis K, et al. Dietary patterns of Greek adults and their associations with serum vitamin D levels and heel quantitative ultrasound parameters for bone health. Nutrients. 2020;12(1):123.
45. Weaver CM, Gordon CM, Janz KF, Kalkwarf HJ, Lappe JM, Lewis R, et al. The National Osteoporosis Foundation's position statement on peak bone mass development and lifestyle factors: a systematic review and implementation recommendations. Osteoporos Int. 2016;27(4):1281–386.
46. Goltzman D, Mannstadt M, Marcocci C. Physiology of the calcium-parathyroid hormone-vitamin D Axis. Front Horm Res. 2018;50:1–13.
47. Aspray TJ, Bowring C, Fraser W, Gittoes N, Javaid MK, Macdonald H, et al. National Osteoporosis Society vitamin D guideline summary. Age Ageing. 2014;43(5):592–5.

48. Bailey RL, Zou P, Wallace TC, McCabe GP, Craig BA, Jun S, et al. Calcium supplement use is associated with less bone mineral density loss, but does not lessen the risk of bone fracture across the menopause transition: data from the study of women's health across the nation. JBMR Plus. 2020;4(1):e10246.
49. Bostick RM. Effect of calcium supplementation on serum cholesterol and blood pressure: a randomized, double-blind, placebo-controlled, clinical trial. Arch Fam Med. 2000;9(1):31–9.
50. Public Health England. Government recommendations for energy and nutrients for males and females aged 1–18 years and 19+ years. Gov Diet Recomm. 2016;1–12.
51. Barrionuevo P, Kapoor E, Asi N, Alahdab F, Mohammed K, Benkhadra K, et al. Efficacy of pharmacological therapies for the prevention of fractures in postmenopausal women: a network meta-analysis. J Clin Endocrinol Metab. 2019;104(5):1623–30.
52. Murad MH, Drake MT, Mullan RJ, Mauck KF, Stuart LM, Lane MA, et al. Comparative effectiveness of drug treatments to prevent fragility fractures: a systematic review and network meta-analysis. J Clin Endocrinol Metab. 2012;97(6):1871–80.
53. Yao P, Bennett D, Mafham M, Lin X, Chen Z, Armitage J, et al. Vitamin D and calcium for the prevention of fracture: a systematic review and meta-analysis. JAMA Netw Open. 2019;2(12):e1917789.
54. Kahwati LC, Weber RP, Pan H, Gourlay M, LeBlanc E, Coker-Schwimmer M, et al. Vitamin D, calcium, or combined supplementation for the primary prevention of fractures in community-dwelling adults: evidence report and systematic review for the US preventive services task force. JAMA. 2018;319(15):1600–12.
55. Lewis JR, Radavelli-Bagatini S, Rejnmark L, Chen JS, Simpson JM, Lappe JM, et al. The effects of calcium supplementation on verified coronary heart disease hospitalization and death in postmenopausal women: a collaborative meta-analysis of randomized controlled trials. J Bone Miner Res. 2015;30(1):165–75.
56. Grossman DC, Curry SJ, Owens DK, Barry MJ, Caughey AB, Davidson KW, et al. Vitamin D, calcium, or combined supplementation for the primary prevention of fractures in community-dwelling adults. JAMA. 2018;319(15):1592.
57. Avenell A, Mak JCS, O'Connell D. Vitamin D and vitamin D analogues for preventing fractures in post-menopausal women and older men. Cochrane Database Syst Rev. 2014;2014(4):CD000227.
58. Kopecky SL, Bauer DC, Gulati M, Nieves JW, Singer AJ, Toth PP, et al. Lack of evidence linking calcium with or without vitamin D supplementation to cardiovascular disease in generally healthy adults: a clinical guideline from the National Osteoporosis Foundation and the American Society for Preventive Cardiology. Ann Intern Med. 2016;165(12):867.
59. Eleftheriou D, Benetou V, Trichopoulou A, La Vecchia C, Bamia C. Mediterranean diet and its components in relation to all-cause mortality: meta-analysis. Br J Nutr. 2018;120(10):1081–97.
60. Tsartsou E, Proutsos N, Castanas E, Kampa M. Network meta-analysis of metabolic effects of olive-oil in humans shows the importance of olive oil consumption with moderate polyphenol levels as part of the mediterranean diet. Front Nutr. 2019;12:6.
61. Mohseni R, Aliakbar S, Abdollahi A, Yekaninejad MS, Maghbooli Z, Mirzaei K. Relationship between major dietary patterns and sarcopenia among menopausal women. Aging Clin Exp Res. 2017;29(6):1241–8.
62. Franquesa M, Pujol-Busquets G, García-Fernández E, Rico L, Shamirian-Pulido L, Aguilar-Martínez A, et al. Mediterranean diet and cardiodiabesity: a systematic review through evidence-based answers to key clinical questions. Nutrients. 2019;11(3):655.
63. Denova-Gutiérrez E, Méndez-Sánchez L, Muñoz-Aguirre P, Tucker K, Clark P. Dietary patterns, bone mineral density, and risk of fractures: a systematic review and meta-analysis. Nutrients. 2018;10(12):1922.
64. Fenton TR, Lyon AW, Eliasziw M, Tough SC, Hanley DA. Phosphate decreases urine calcium and increases calcium balance: a meta-analysis of the osteoporosis acid-ash diet hypothesis. Nutr J. 2009;8(1):41.

65. Rozenberg S, Body J-JJ, Bruyère O, Bergmann P, Brandi ML, Cooper C, et al. Effects of dairy products consumption on health: benefits and beliefs—a commentary from the Belgian Bone Club and the European Society for Clinical and Economic Aspects of Osteoporosis, Osteoarthritis and Musculoskeletal Diseases. Calcif Tissue Int. 2016;98(1):1–17.
66. Fardellone P. The effect of milk consumption on bone and fracture incidence, an update. Aging Clin Exp Res. 2019;31(6):759–64.
67. Ethgen O, Hiligsmann M, Burlet N, Reginster JY. Public health impact and cost-effectiveness of dairy products supplemented with vitamin D in prevention of osteoporotic fractures. Arch Public Health. 2015;73(1):48.
68. Ethgen O, Hiligsmann M, Burlet N, Reginster JY. Cost-effectiveness of personalized supplementation with vitamin D-rich dairy products in the prevention of osteoporotic fractures. Osteoporos Int. 2016;27(1):301–8.
69. Shi Y, Zhan Y, Chen Y, Jiang Y. Effects of dairy products on bone mineral density in healthy postmenopausal women: a systematic review and meta-analysis of randomized controlled trials. Arch Osteoporos. 2020;15(1):48.
70. Sanchez-Rodriguez D, Bergmann P, Body JJ, Cavalier E, Gielen E, Goemaere S, et al. The Belgian Bone Club 2020 guidelines for the management of osteoporosis in postmenopausal women. Maturitas. 2020;139(0):69–89.
71. Caprio M, Infante M, Moriconi E, Armani A, Fabbri A, Mantovani G, et al. Very-low-calorie ketogenic diet (VLCKD) in the management of metabolic diseases: systematic review and consensus statement from the Italian Society of Endocrinology (SIE). J Endocrinol Invest. 2019;42(11):1365–86.
72. Iguacel I, Miguel-Berges ML, Gómez-Bruton A, Moreno LA, Julián C. Veganism, vegetarianism, bone mineral density, and fracture risk: a systematic review and meta-analysis. Nutr Rev. 2019;77(1):1–18.

Chapter 4
The Bone Turnover Cycle

Sarah Carter and Elaine Dennison

The Human Skeleton

The skeleton serves several critical roles in the human body: it provides structure and support, protects vital organs like the brain and the heart, and allows muscle attachment necessary for movement. In addition, the skeleton holds the body's calcium and mineral reserves and produces bone marrow and white blood cells [1].

Nearly all bones in the skeleton contain both cortical bone and trabecular bone in proportions that allow them to provide structural support while being light enough to maintain a range of movement [2]. The mixture of mineral reserves and flexible collagen matrix consisting of type I collagen fibres, proteins, and water allows for the strength, flexibility, and durability of bone. In adults, the skeleton is 20% spongy inner trabecular bone and 80% outer cortical bone. As about 60% of cortical bone is dense mineral reserve, it is mostly responsible for providing support and protection [2]. In contrast, trabecular bone is less dense, covers a larger surface area, and is the site of marrow production [1].

Bone is always being turned over, in an effort to maintain the structural integrity of the skeleton and ensure that mineral reserves are in equilibrium throughout the lifecourse. The cycle of bone turnover should be in balance, but disequilibrium can occur during illness or osteoporosis. Bone turnover rates can be assessed through the measurement of bone turnover markers, which will be discussed later in this chapter.

S. Carter
MRC Lifecourse Epidemiology Centre, Southampton, UK
e-mail: sc3@mrc.soton.ac.uk

E. Dennison (✉)
MRC Lifecourse Epidemiology Centre,
University of Southampton, Southampton, UK
e-mail: emd@mrc.soton.ac.uk

E. Dennison (ed.), *Osteoporosis Treatment*, https://doi.org/10.1007/978-3-030-78128-6_4

Remodelling: Bone Cells

Bone formation begins in utero, around 6–7 foetal weeks, and continues until young adulthood. This process, called osteogenesis, occurs in two different ways: in the clavicles and bones of the face, it is the creation of new bone from mesenchymal tissue; in long bones and ribs, it is the replacement of cartilage bone models with mineral osteoid and bone. Osteogenesis is only completed when growth plates in long bones, the skull, and the clavicle fuse in late adolescence.

The only time in adulthood when bone formation usually occurs is when bones must be repaired after fracture [2]. Unlike in childhood, when bones are both formed and remodeled as an individual grows, adult bones are remodeled almost entirely in order to maintain the health of the skeleton. This continuous remodelling renews bone, repairs compromised areas, and maintains the strength and function of the skeleton. Remodelling also contributes to calcium and phosphate homeostasis by providing access to the mineral reservoir in the skeleton [3]. The bone turnover cycle is a constant, rapid process during childhood, adolescence, and young adulthood, only slowing down when an individual is 40 years of age.

While a site-specific bone turnover cycle takes around 200 days, bone remodeling is a lifelong process, with about 5–10% of the adult skeleton remodelled every year. Studies have estimated that, at any given time, the adult skeleton is undergoing remodeling by up to one million bone remodeling units (BRUs), with three to four million units initiated every year [4]. These bone remodeling units are defined by the interplay of two different types of cells: osteoclasts and osteoblasts. Osteoclasts are exocrine cells responsible for breaking down bone mineral structure and dissolving extracellular matrix (ECM) proteins. Osteoblasts produce bone matrix and support mineralization by secreting type I collagen, which accounts for nearly all of the protein in the bone matrix. These two cell types are responsible for removing compromised bone and laying down new bone at damage sites, which they are able to do with the help of osteocytes.

Nearly 95% of all bone cells are osteocytes. Osteocytes are former osteoblasts that have survived bone formation cycles without undergoing apoptosis. After becoming surrounded by calcified bone tissue, these cells can remain in lacunae in the bone matrix for many years, functioning as a signal network between their origin site and bone areas in which repair is necessary. Bone microdamage caused by mechanical forces like compression causes osteocyte apoptosis at the damage site, which signal both bone resorption by osteoclasts and bone remodelling by osteoblasts, allowing for bone repair.

As seen in Fig. 4.1, the bone turnover cycle can be organized into four waves of osteoclast and osteoblast involvement: *activation*, the recruitment of osteoclasts to damage sites; *resorption*, the dissolving of bone by osteoclasts; *reversal,* the apoptosis of osteoclasts and the recruitment of osteoblasts; and *formation*, the production of new bone by osteoblasts, which is then mineralized [5]. This process is continuous and ongoing in adulthood, and is kept in equilibrium by the endocrine system.

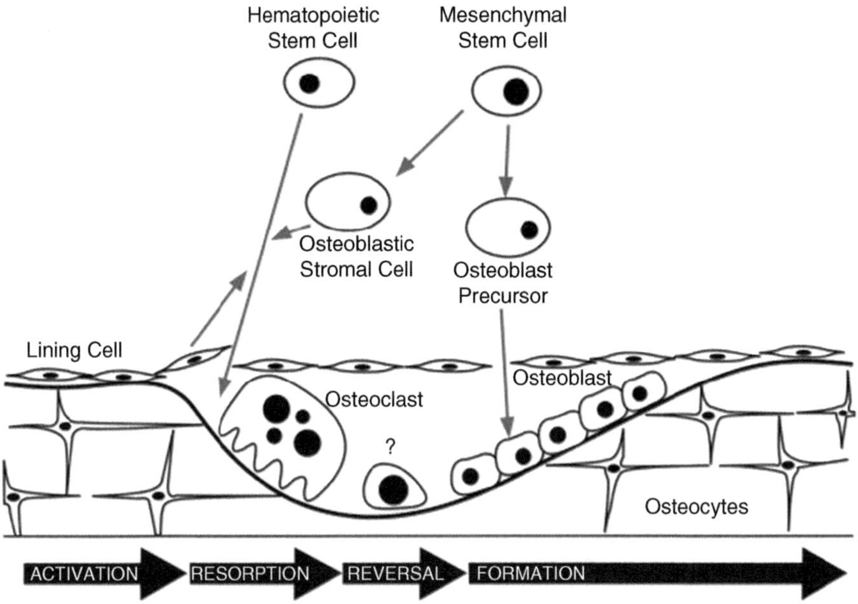

Fig. 4.1 The four stages of osteoclast and osteoblast involvement in the bone turnover cycle. (Reproduced with permission from Bone Health and Osteoporosis: A Report of the Surgeon General. Office of the Surgeon General (US). Rockville (MD): Office of the Surgeon General (US); 2004)

Regulation of the Bone Turnover Cycle

Osteoclast and osteoblast activity—and therefore bone remodeling in general—is controlled by the endocrine system. Osteoclast differentiation and activation is driven primarily by macrophage colony-stimulating factor (M-CSF) and nuclear factor-KB (RANK) ligand. Endocrine involvement in osteoblast formation and function is multifaceted. Osteoblastogenesis and the formation of bone matrix is controlled by bone morphogenic proteins (BMPs) and Wnt signalling. Additionally, the action of osteocytes, the post-mitotic cells formed from osteoblasts, relies almost fully on endocrine involvement.

Bone remodeling is therefore highly regulated, such that in normal circumstances, bone resorption and formation will occur in equal amounts. A critical regulator of the bone turnover cycle is the RANK/RANK ligand (RANKL) process: osteoclast cell membranes contain RANK receptors, which begin osteoclast activity when stimulated, and osteoblasts secrete RANKL, which activates bone remodeling. This process is illustrated by Fig. 4.2.

When RANKL excreted from the bone matrix activates RANK receptors in osteoclast precursors, these join together, becoming multinucleated cells which form specific resorption sites on the surface of bone: the sealing zone, the ruffled border, and the functional secretory domain [6]. Osteoclasts use actin-rich

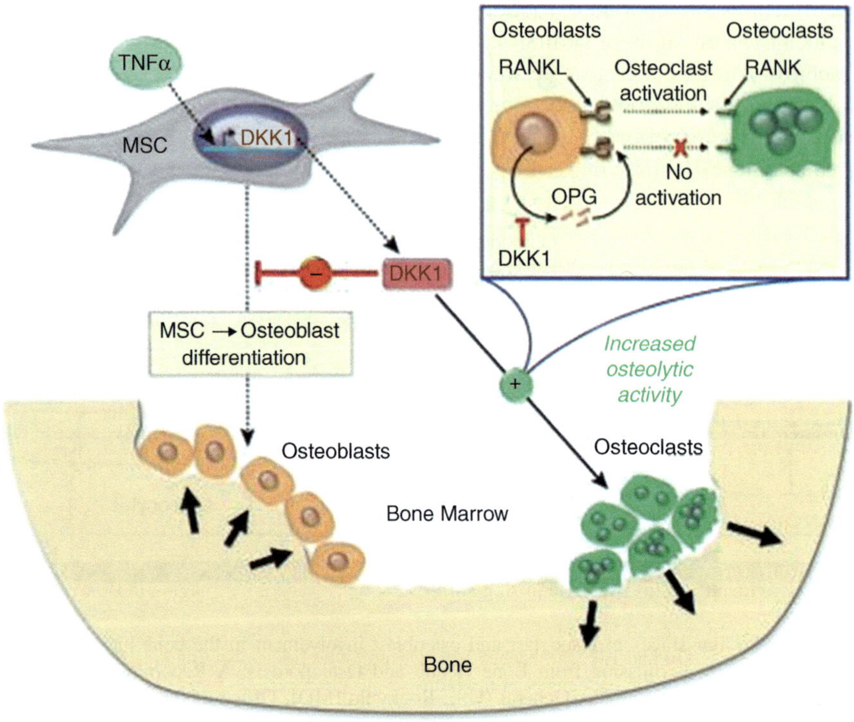

Fig. 4.2 The Role of RANK/RANKL in the bone turnover cycle. (Reproduced with permission from Pinzone, J.J., et al. The role of Dickkopf-1 in bone development, homeostasis, and disease. Blood. 2009. 113(3): 517–525)

podosomes to attach themselves to the surface of bone, allowing them to form seals with the bone matrix. These tight sealing zones permit the development of the ruffled border, which is built from osteoclastic cytoplasm. Utilizing their cytoplasm in this way, osteoclasts increase their surface area, allow for more efficient degrading of the underlying bone matrix, and protect surrounding bone cells from dissolution. The ruffled border allows for the transport of endosomes and lysosomes vital to osteoclast survival, and provides a key avenue through which cathepsin K, proteolytic enzyme, and hydrochloric acid can be secreted by osteoclasts onto the surface of bone, enabling the destruction of old or compromised bone matrix. Bone resorption forms a small depression called a Howship lacuna.

After osteoclasts remove damaged osteocytes, osteoblasts are activated to begin bone formation. Wnt signalling is crucial to this stage of the bone turnover cycle, as Wnt is a glycoprotein that inhibits the death of osteoblast precursor cells, thus allowing for the proliferation and differentiation of osteoblasts [6]. Without Wnt signalling, there would be few osteoblasts with which to begin bone formation since Wnts act on osteoblast precursor cells and promote their differentiation into mature osteoblasts through the β-catenin-dependent canonical pathway. In addition, Wnts suppress bone resorption by regulating the receptor activator of NF-κB ligand

(RANKL)/osteoprotegerin (OPG) ratio through the same pathway in mature osteoblasts. (There are actually two pathways of Wnt signaling: the β-catenin-dependent canonical pathway described above, and the β-catenin-independent non-canonical pathway, activation of which enhances the RANKL-induced osteoclast formation in mouse macrophage cultures).

Once osteoblasts are activated, organic unmineralized bone matrix containing collagen, called osteoid, is produced by osteoblasts and laid down in straight lines. Osteoblasts are also responsible for controlling the mineralization of bone, by releasing calcium and phosphate into the osteoid and destroying pyrophosphate and proteoglycans, which inhibit mineralization [7]. Two weeks after osteoblasts lay down osteoid, the first phase of hydroxyapatite crystal mineralization begins. This initial mineralization can last for up to 6 months after the osteoid is produced. Mineralization of the new bone then continues for up to 3 years, as mineral and hydroxyapatite crystal deposits slowly build up the bone structure [1].

The Bone Turnover Cycle and Disequilibrium

The bone remodeling cycle is in equilibrium for about 20 years after peak bone mass attainment, after which bone remodeling slows and age-related bone loss may begin [5]. Changing endocrine levels can be a major contributor to the development of skeletal pathology. Disequilibrium in the RANK and RANKL system is associated with bone loss, and may show marked perturbations in some conditions associated with accelerated bone loss such as rheumatoid arthritis, and hyperparathyroidism. In these conditions, changes in hormone levels or amount of inflammatory cytokines present increase the number of BRUs actively resorbing bone.

Lower levels of estrogen are associated with greater osteocyte apoptosis, which, in turn, stimulates more bone remodeling, resulting in lower bone mass (as seen in osteoporosis). Deficiencies in estrogen are also associated with IL-7 upregulation, which can lead to increases in tumor necrosis factor (TNF) and RANKL production. TNF promotes osteoclast differentiation, possibly by altering RANK expression in osteoclastic precursors, and impedes osteoblast formation by suppressing IGF-1. Anti-osteoporosis medications, such as bisphosphonates, Denosumab, and hormone replacement therapies, work to counteract osteoclast proliferation and decrease the rate of bone resorption [1], and are detailed in later chapters.

As mentioned above, comorbidities traditionally associated with poorer bone health such as rheumatoid arthritis may impact RANKL expression in synovial cells, where it contributes to the destruction of joints [8]. There is also evidence that joint destruction is associated with TNF; the upregulation of TNF has been shown to contribute to the development of rheumatoid arthritis by inhibiting Wnt signalling, which leads to the erosion of bone and prevention of new bone formation [9]. Finally TNF also allows the movement of osteoclast precursors to areas of joint inflammation, where it can stimulate them to differentiate into osteoclasts [9]. Secondary osteoporosis is described in greater detail in a later chapter.

Bone Turnover in Osteoporosis

Osteoporosis is a disease that disproportionately impacts women, with up to 52% of women over 80 years old experiencing osteoporotic fracture [10]. As osteoporosis is a bone disease caused by disequilibrium of the bone turnover cycle, the link between estrogen and bone turnover is one explanation for why postmenopausal women are at such greater risk of osteoporosis.

Estrogen stimulates osteoprotegerin (OPG) secretion and decreases macrophage colony-stimulating factor (M-CSF) and RANK production, promoting osteoblastic activity. Estrogen deficiency associated with menopause disrupts the bone turnover cycle by lowering OPG secretion and increasing M-CSF, TNF, and RANK levels, thereby allowing unbalanced bone resorption by osteoclasts. This causes a swift increase in bone loss, beginning a year before a final menstrual period, continuing at the same rate for up to 3 years post-menopause, and lasting to some degree for up to 8 years after [11]. Menopausal bone loss can be so fast that, on average, women lose around 10% of their BMD during this period [10]. Loss of estrogen can also contribute to decreases in calcium absorption for women aged 60 and above, which in turn can lead to secondary hyperparathyroidism, another avenue through which bone can be lost post-menopause.

Bone Loss in Other Endocrine Conditions

Hyperparathyroidism occurs when the parathyroid glands, which regulate blood calcium and phosphorus with parathyroid hormone (PTH), produce too much PTH. Increased PTH stimulates bones to release greater amounts of calcium into the bloodstream, leading to an excess of calcium in the blood and increased bone remodelling. In this way, hyperparathyroidism can contribute to osteoporosis and osteoporotic fracture. Cortisol is also associated with poorer bone health, as it reduces osteoblast differentiation. The role of high cortisol levels in accelerated bone loss is discussed in more detail in the chapter on secondary osteoporosis.

An imbalance in Vitamin D also has implications for bone health, but in the opposite way to that of PTH. Vitamin D is protective for bone mass, as it supports osteoblast differentiation and therefore increases bone formation [12]. In addition to allowing for osteoblast differentiation, there is evidence that vitamin D inhibits osteoclast activity, further underscoring its role in protecting bone mass. Further, estradiol, testosterone, and insulin-like growth factor 1 (IGF1) also all contribute to osteoblast proliferation and differentiation and have been associated with the maintenance of bone health [12]. While IGF1 has been linked to osteoclast activity in ex-vivo studies, decreased levels of IGF1 are linked to low bone mass, indicating that it is generally protective for bone.

Bone Turnover Markers

Bone turnover markers are molecules that allow for monitoring of the bone turnover cycle. As these markers are present in blood or urine, testing is relatively easy and can be repeated more often than more invasive measures of bone density, such as DXA scans. In addition, biomarkers of bone turnover can be used to assess bone turnover in response to anti-osteoporosis medication, assessing response much faster than through other measures [13]. It is possible to measure levels of both the endocrine stimulators of bone formation or resorption and the mineral material released during these processes, making bone turnover markers more dynamic measures of bone health than DXA. Bone turnover markers allow for the measurement of baseline bone health, the prediction of fracture risk, and the monitoring of anti-osteoporosis treatment. The role of bone turnover markers in the management of osteoporosis has been discussed in several position statements which suggest that these biomarkers are effective measures of the efficacy of (and the compliance with) anti-osteoporosis medications [14]. The most commonly used bone turnover markers are presented both in the following text and in Table 4.1 below.

Markers of Bone Resorption

Urinary bone turnover markers can be used to estimate postmenopausal bone loss. One sign of type I collagen breakdown, urinary N-terminal telopeptide of type I collagen (U-NTX), has been used to predict bone loss in the lumbar spine and femoral neck in menopausal women. U-NTX increases in the 2 years before menopause and peaks and plateaus about 18 months after a woman's final period, meaning it mirrors post-menopausal bone loss [11]. Research has shown that U-NTX levels in late perimenopause and early postmenopause can predict rate of bone loss after this period. However, this turnover marker is less reliable in the perimenopausal period [11].

Table 4.1 Bone turnover markers for clinical practice

Recommended assay type	Bone resorption	Bone formation
Urine	N-terminal telopeptide of type I collagen (U-NTX)	N- and C-terminal propeptides (PINP and PICP)
	Deoxy-pyridinoline (DPD)	
Serum	Serum carboxy-terminal collagen crosslinks (CTX)	Osteocalcin
	Tartrate-resistant acid phosphatase 5b (TRACP-5b)	Bone-specific alkaline phosphatase (BAP)

Adapted from [15]

Another type I collagen structural material associated with bone resorption is deoxy-pyridinoline (DPD), a collagen cross-link released from bone when it is resorbed and passed in the urine, providing evidence of the rate of bone turnover [13]. Much like NTX and DPD, serum carboxy-terminal collagen crosslinks (CTX) is evidence of osteoclastic activity. CTX is another by-product of the breakdown of type I collagen, and is removed from the body through the kidneys, allowing assessment via urinalysis. CTX and NTX perform similarly in clinical efficacy tests, and are both regularly used in practice. While both can be measured in serum and urine, NTX is generally analysed in urine samples and CTX is tested via serum [13]. Like most biomarkers of bone resorption, NTX and CTX are linked to circadian variation and therefore, any serum measurements should be taken in the morning after fasting [13].

While NTX, DPD, and CTX are measures of the breakdown of collagen in bone, thereby identifying the activity of osteoclasts, tartrate-resistant acid phosphatase 5b (TRACP-5b) is an enzyme secreted by osteoclasts that is associated with the number of osteoclasts present at testing. Bone turnover markers of bone resorption can therefore measure both osteoclast activity and quantity. Although TRACP-5b is a less consistent measure than NTX or CTX, it is one of very few biomarkers of bone resorption that is not found in urine, making it a bone turnover marker useful in patients experiencing renal failure [13].

Markers of Bone Formation

In addition to identifying potential bone loss, bone turnover markers can be used to measure bone formation by osteoblasts, by using both type I collagen and non-collagen byproducts. N- and C-terminal propeptides (PINP and PICP) form part of the collagen molecule produced by osteoblasts. As PINP and PICP eventually enter circulation during the bone turnover cycle, their levels can be assessed by urinalysis [13]. Studies have shown that PINP may be a more sensitive measure than PICP, as it is cleared more directly through the liver, allowing it to more effectively report bone turnover [15].

Osteocalcin is another analyte that can be used to measure the rate of bone turnover. As it is a non-collagen peptide that binds to calcium, nearly all osteocalcin produced during bone formation remains in the matrix and is ossified into bone. Enough osteocalcin is released during osteoblastic activity that it is possible to use it as a bone formation marker. However, osteoclastic bone resorption can release osteocalcin from the bone matrix, meaning that the full efficacy of osteocalcin as a bone turnover marker is an avenue for future research. Additionally, serum osteocalcin can degrade quickly, making it difficult to produce comparable samples [15].

A second non-collagen bone turnover marker associated with bone formation is serum bone-specific alkaline phosphatase (BAP), which is a glycoprotein associated with osteoblastic activity during mineralization. The amount of BAP released into circulation is proportional to the amount of osteoblasts active at a given time, making it a key indicator of bone formation. However, BAP measurements may be influenced by the presence of liver alkaline phosphatase, meaning that, if possible, other bone turnover markers should be tested in people with liver disease [13].

Bone Turnover Markers and the Prediction of Fracture

Additionally, there have been several reported associations between bone turnover markers and fracture risk, with the relationship between decreasing bone turnover markers and lower risk of fracture considered more correlated than that between biomarkers and BMD [16]. In studies investigating the relationship between bone turnover markers and fracture in patients treated with antiresorptive medications, stronger associations have been reported for biomarkers of bone formation than for those signalling bone resorption [17], indicating that bone formation biomarkers could be used to predict fracture risk in those undergoing antiresorptive treatment. Indeed, research has determined that larger decreases in bone turnover markers are associated with equivalently lower risk of fracture [13].

A review of studies of bone turnover markers determined that in addition to allowing for the monitoring of osteoporosis treatment, these biomarkers may predict fracture risk in postmenopausal women, independent of BMD [18]. High bone turnover is associated with increased fracture risk when the disequilibrium in the cycle leads to more bone resorption, and thus lower bone mineral density. However, bone turnover may also be associated with risk of fracture due to the very nature of the cycle itself; it may be that increased bone remodelling, and therefore more resorption lacunae, degrades skeletal integrity by weakening bone architecture, removing key mineralized bone, and increasing the amount of trabecular bone that is unmineralized and less robust [18].

However, a lack of standardization in measurement, small sample sizes, and variability in the test results between individuals means that there is as of yet no clinical standard. Differences between studies in how and when specific biomarkers were measured, which fracture locations they were linked to, and what statistical analyses were used to make determinations means that prediction of fracture risk using bone turnover markers remains unclear. Developing international measurement references to allow more widespread use of bone turnover markers for fracture prediction in clinical practice is an avenue for future studies.

Therefore, while research has shown that there are associations between bone turnover markers and fracture, measurements of bone turnover are not currently considered as risk factors for osteoporotic fracture in fracture prediction tools like FRAX® [19]. This represents a broader conflict in the use of bone turnover markers in research versus clinical practice. Biomarkers of the bone turnover cycle provide ample information about bone health in individuals, but due to potential irregularities in measurements across individuals, it is difficult to use bone turnover markers in more general clinical assessment.

Use of Bone Turnover Markers in Clinical Practice

While monitoring of bone turnover markers should not take the place of regular BMD measurements, response to treatment reported in serum or urine tests might be used to predict BMD change. In a study using Fracture Intervention Trial data, changes in CTX and NTX levels after 6 months of treatment with alendronate predicted lumbar spine BMD changes up to 4 years later [20]. Another study of the association between bone turnover markers and BMD found that early changes in PICP and PINP during treatment with teriparatide predicted changes in lumbar spine BMD after 18 months [21].

Bone turnover markers, then, are crucial tools in the diagnosis and monitoring of bone disorders. However, markers of both bone resorption and formation are present when bone turnover occurs, regardless of whether the cycle ends with bone loss or bone gain [11], and there are issues with reproducibility and standardization of measures, meaning that the clinical utility of bone turnover markers may vary by individual patient. Reproducibility and standardization of results can be facilitated by repeating measurements at the same time of day, which is especially important for urine samples, as bone turnover markers can vary with circadian rhythms [15]. Difficulty in standardization of biomarker measurements has inspired current research on the development of a bone balance index. This bone balance index combines markers of bone formation and bone resorption into one measure reporting net bone loss, and research has reported that it may be possible to predict bone loss using the proportion of U-NTX to serum osteocalcin [22].

However, until such a bone balance index is validated, individual bone turnover markers are most useful in clinical practice. Recent recommendations cite PINP and serum CTX as the key markers of bone formation and resorption, as research suggests they are the most consistent measures [16]. Current best practice is to use bone turnover biomarkers in conjunction with BMD measurements to monitor bone health in patients with suspected or diagnosed osteoporosis.

The bone turnover markers recommended for use by the International Osteoporosis Foundation are CTX and PINP, both due to their consistency in measurement and their ability to monitor adherence to medication [17]. As discussed above, serum samples need to be taken after a period of fasting, and repeated urine samples should be measured at the same time of day, to ensure reliability of the results.

Anti-osteoporosis Medication and Bone Turnover Response

A detailed exposition of the change in BTM associated with therapy for osteoporosis is shown in the therapeutics chapters of this book. For the past several decades, bisphosphonates have been prescribed as the first line to combat osteoporosis. These medications bind to hydroxyapatite crystals in the organic bone matrix, most readily in locations of bone turnover, making them key treatments for bone turnover disorders [18]. Bisphosphonates prevent hydroxyapatite destruction and inhibit osteoclast function, thus slowing bone resorption. In addition, bisphosphonates support bone formation by osteoblasts and extend bone mineral deposition, increasing bone density and improving trabecular structure. Research has reported that bone turnover is so sensitive to bisphosphonates that telopeptides decrease by 50–70% and PINP decreases by more than 60% during the first 3 months of bisphosphonate treatment [19].

Another commonly used osteoporosis treatment is denosumab a monoclonal antibody against RANKL, which blocks osteoclast activity and reduces bone resorption, with proven anti-fracture efficacy. Therapy is associated with rapid change in bone turnover markers associated with denosumab treatment led to subsequent BMD change [10]. Importantly, the cessation of denosumab is associated with an increase in bone remodelling and possible rebound fractures. Research has reported that osteocytes can inhibit WNT signalling by secreting sclerostin, which has led to the development of a monoclonal antibody against sclerostin as another therapeutic avenue [10].

Conversely, steroids can contribute to bone loss. While glucocorticoids are effective treatments against autoimmune and chronic inflammatory conditions, they can limit bone formation by inhibiting osteoblastogenesis and increasing the rate of osteoblast and osteocyte apoptosis. Glucocorticoids may also support osteoclast survival, therefore promoting bone resorption while suppressing bone formation. Finally, there is evidence that glucocorticoids can contribute to the development of secondary hyperparathyroidism, by promoting loss of calcium via the kidneys. This, in turn, also negatively impacts bone health, as it stimulates the removal of more calcium from the bones [23]. The detrimental effect of glucocorticoids on bone can be accelerated if treatment lasts for more than 3 months or if a daily dose of 5 mg of prednisone is prescribed three to four times a day [24]. Careful steroid dosing, ongoing monitoring of bone turnover, and prevention of hyperparathyroidism are opportunities for combating steroid-related bone loss. Steroid induced osteoporosis is described in detail in the chapter on secondary osteoporosis.

BTM in Drug Monitoring

There is some evidence to suggest that it is possible to use measurement of bone turnover markers to assess adherence to anti-osteoporosis medication, specifically when that medication is oral bisphosphonates [25]. This is discussed further in the chapter by Beaudart and colleagues later in this book. Given the efficacy of oral bisphosphonates to slow bone turnover, it may be possible to identify those patients who are not complying with their medications by analysing how quickly bone turnover slows, as represented by decreases in PINP and CTX measurements [17]. Studies reporting an association between PINP or CTX and adherence to anti-osteoporosis medications conclude that determining whether or not a patient has adhered to their medication requires repeated testing of bone biomarkers, with particular care given to securing a measurement of bone turnover markers before the start of treatment [26]. While there are no standard measurements against which to compare individual patients, research has determined that decreases of nearly 80% in CTX and nearly 70% in PINP are associated with good adherence to medication [17]. It is worth noting, however, that there must be very low adherence to medication for there to be little decrease in CTX or PINP. Current studies provide evidence that bone turnover markers are promising guides for monitoring adherence to medication, but future research is needed to examine the full clinical utility of the use of biomarkers to measure compliance with anti-osteoporosis medication.

Conclusion

The bone turnover cycle is a process vital to the maintenance of skeletal integrity throughout the lifecourse, with disruptions to the cycle in mid and later life often leading to osteoporosis. Mapping of the bone turnover cycle has allowed for the development of several anti-osteoporosis medications targeting bone resorption, which have been shown to effectively preserve bone mineral density. The identification and testing of bone turnover markers released in urine and blood allow for repeated monitoring of the remodelling cycle and therefore of bone health, as serum and urine measurements can be taken much more easily than those obtained via bone scan. This repeated testing of markers within individuals may provide useful information about both a patient's baseline bone health and their response to treatment.

In addition to enabling the tracking of treatment response, bone turnover markers have also been shown to provide evidence of adherence to anti-osteoporosis medication and may 1 day be able to predict fracture risk. Studies have reported that a sizable percentage decrease in markers of bone turnover after the start of bisphosphonate treatment may point to the consistency of medication compliance, crucial information in the treatment of osteoporosis, as adherence to medication is a common barrier. Research also indicates that bone turnover markers may someday be able to supplement BMD measurements in fracture risk prediction, if international reference categories can be established [25].

References

1. Walsh MC, Choi Y. Biology of the RANKL-RANK-OPG system in immunity, bone, and beyond. Front Immunol. 2014;5:511.
2. Crockett JC, et al. Bone remodelling at a glance. J Cell Sci. 2011;124(Pt 7):991–8.
3. Kenkre JS, Bassett J. The bone remodelling cycle. Ann Clin Biochem. 2018;55(3):308–27.
4. Manolagas SC. Birth and death of bone cells: basic regulatory mechanisms and implications for the pathogenesis and treatment of osteoporosis. Endocr Rev. 2000;21(2):115–37.

5. Langdahl B, Ferrari S, Dempster DW. Bone modeling and remodeling: potential as therapeutic targets for the treatment of osteoporosis. Ther Adv Musculoskelet Dis. 2016;8(6):225–35.
6. Boyce BF, Xing L. Functions of RANKL/RANK/OPG in bone modeling and remodeling. Arch Biochem Biophys. 2008;473(2):139–46.
7. Clarke B. Normal bone anatomy and physiology. Clin J Am Soc Nephrol. 2008;3(Suppl 3):S131–9.
8. Kearns AE, Khosla S, Kostenuik PJ. Receptor activator of nuclear factor kappaB ligand and osteoprotegerin regulation of bone remodeling in health and disease. Endocr Rev. 2008;29(2):155–92.
9. Goldring SR, et al. Bone remodelling in inflammatory arthritis. Ann Rheum Dis. 2013;72(Suppl 2):ii52–5.
10. Tella SH, Gallagher JC. Prevention and treatment of postmenopausal osteoporosis. J Steroid Biochem Mol Biol. 2014;142:155–70.
11. Karlamangla AS, Burnett-Bowie SM, Crandall CJ. Bone health during the menopause transition and beyond. Obstet Gynecol Clin N Am. 2018;45(4):695–708.
12. Cannarella R, et al. Osteoporosis from an endocrine perspective: the role of hormonal changes in the elderly. J Clin Med. 2019;8(10):1564.
13. Greenblatt MB, Tsai JN, Wein MN. Bone turnover markers in the diagnosis and monitoring of metabolic bone disease. Clin Chem. 2017;63(2):464–74.
14. Delmas PD, et al. The use of biochemical markers of bone turnover in osteoporosis. Committee of Scientific Advisors of the International Osteoporosis Foundation. Osteoporos Int. 2000;11(Suppl 6):S2–S17.
15. Blumsohn A, Eastell R. The performance and utility of biochemical markers of bone turnover: do we know enough to use them in clinical practice? Ann Clin Biochem. 1997;34(Pt 5):449–59.
16. Vasikaran S, et al. International Osteoporosis Foundation and International Federation of Clinical Chemistry and Laboratory Medicine position on bone marker standards in osteoporosis. Clin Chem Lab Med. 2011;49(8):1271–4.
17. Diez-Perez A, et al.; International Osteoporosis Foundation and European Calcified Tissue Society Working Group. Recommendations for the screening of adherence to oral bisphosphonates. Osteoporos Int. 2017;28(3):767–774.
18. Drake MT, Clarke BL, Khosla S. Bisphosphonates: mechanism of action and role in clinical practice. Mayo Clin Proc. 2008;83(9):1032–45.
19. Eastell R, Hannon RA. Biomarkers of bone health and osteoporosis risk. Proc Nutr Soc. 2008;67(2):157–62.
20. Bauer DC, et al. Change in bone turnover and hip, non-spine, and vertebral fracture in alendronate-treated women: the fracture intervention trial. J Bone Miner Res. 2004;19(8):1250–8.
21. Chen P, et al. Early changes in biochemical markers of bone formation predict BMD response to teriparatide in postmenopausal women with osteoporosis. J Bone Miner Res. 2005;20(6):962–70.
22. Shieh A, et al. Urinary N-telopeptide and rate of bone loss over the menopause transition and early postmenopause. J Bone Miner Res. 2016;31(11):2057–64.
23. Mushtaq T, Ahmed SF. The impact of corticosteroids on growth and bone health. Arch Dis Child. 2002;87(2):93–6.
24. Klein GL. The effect of glucocorticoids on bone and muscle. Osteoporos Sarcopenia. 2015;1(1):39–45.
25. Fontalis A, Eastell R. The challenge of long-term adherence: the role of bone turnover markers in monitoring bisphosphonate treatment of osteoporosis. Bone. 2020;136:115336.
26. Tan RZ, Loh TP, Vasikaran S. Bone turnover marker monitoring in osteoporosis treatment response. Eur J Endocrinol. 2020;183(1):C5–7. https://doi.org/10.1530/EJE-19-0970. PMID: 32504486.

Chapter 5
Anti-resorptive Therapies

Michael Clynes and Elaine Dennison

Introduction

The bone turnover cycle was described in the previous chapter. Drugs used to treat osteoporosis are typically classified as anabolic (bone forming) or anti-resorptive: until recently, most drugs used in the treatment of osteoporosis were anti-resorptive, which means that they modulate fracture risk by inhibiting bone resorption. Anti-resorptive agents predominantly act to prevent post-menopausal and age-related bone loss and examples include the bisphosphonates, denosumab, raloxifene and selective oestrogen receptor modulators. The widespread adoption of anti-resorptive therapies in westernised countries has contributed to a significant reduction in the incidence of fragility fracture [1]. Upon initiation of anti-resorptive therapy there is classically an initial increase in bone mineral density (BMD) as bone formation 'catches up'. Following this there is increased secondary mineralization of bone which can induce a sustained yet smaller increase in BMD, as seen with more potent anti-resorptive agents such as alendronate, or alternatively BMD plateaus. This chapter discusses some of the most commonly used anti-resorptive agents, in addition to calcium and vitamin D supplementation which are often used as adjunctive therapy.

Calcium and Vitamin D

Supplementary calcium and vitamin D are often prescribed alongside anti-osteoporosis medication, and are also discussed in the previous chapter. In the first

M. Clynes
MRC Lifecourse Epidemiology Centre, Southampton, UK
e-mail: mc@mrc.soton.ac.uk

E. Dennison (✉)
MRC Lifecourse Epidemiology Centre, University of Southampton, Southampton, UK
e-mail: emd@mrc.soton.ac.uk

E. Dennison (ed.), *Osteoporosis Treatment*, https://doi.org/10.1007/978-3-030-78128-6_5

randomised controlled trial to consider the efficacy of these agents, Chapuy and colleagues showed that a daily dose of calcium (1200 mg) and vitamin D3 (800 IU) in community dwelling elderly women normalized serum parathyroid hormone and 25(OH)D levels [2] and apparently led to a reduced bone loss and decreased risk of hip fracture. In a subsequent study [3] which used a 400 IU daily vitamin D dose, a non-significant reduction in hip fractures was observed, possibly as a consequence of the lower doses used.

Studies of calcium supplementation have given conflicting results, with some but not all studies suggesting that there may be an increased risk of cardiovascular disease among women prescribed calcium supplements [3–5]. The most recent systematic review of the effectiveness of calcium and vitamin D combined supplementation by Eleni and colleagues [6] observed a reduction in hip and total fracture which appeared more marked in the elderly, patients with low body weight and increased fracture risk and concluded that the minimum effective dose of calcium is 1200 mg while daily vitamin D intake should not be below 800 IU. In this systematic review, supplementation of institutionalised patients and patients with a low dietary calcium intake demonstrated greater risk reduction. This most recent systematic review supplements two previous reviews; one by Yao and colleagues which also reported a beneficial effect of the combination of calcium and vitamin D on osteoporotic fractures [7] while Zhao et al. [8] concluded the opposite. Methodological factors may be the explanation for these differing results, highlighting the need to look at the details of each study, specifically the nutritional status of the population being supplemented and the route of administration of supplementation (bolus or daily supplementation). In general, the combination of calcium with vitamin D is well tolerated, although increased frequency of urinary and renal tract stones has been reported and many patients report mild gastrointestinal irritation with calcium supplementation.

Bisphosphonates

Bisphosphonates such as alendronate, risedronate and zoledronate are typically used as the first line treatment for osteoporosis. Bisphosphonates have been used clinically to treat disorders of calcium metabolism over the past 50 years but chemically the first bisphosphonates were synthesised in the 1800s, with etidronate, the first bisphosphonate used in humans, synthesised over a century ago [9]. Bisphosphonates reduce bone resorption via the inhibition of farnesyl pyrophosphate synthase in the mevalonate pathway, which results in apoptosis of the osteoclasts and increases in BMD [10]. The key trials to assess efficacy of alendronic acid are the Fracture Intervention Trial (FIT) and Fracture Intervention Trial Long-Term Extension (FLEX) studies. FIT demonstrated significant reductions in the incidence of vertebral fractures in postmenopausal women treated with alendronate 10 mg per day for 3–4 years with existing fractures, or a femoral T-score of less than −2.5 [11]. The FLEX study was a continuation of FIT that compared outcomes among postmenopausal women who received alendronate for either 5 or 10 years. It found that women who discontinued alendronate after 5 years did not suffer significantly more non-vertebral fractures (18.9% for placebo versus 19% for alendronate; 95% confidence interval [CI], 0.76–1.32 or morphometric vertebral fractures (11.3% for placebo versus 9.8% for alendronate; 95% CI, 0.60–1.22) but there was a significantly lower risk in clinically recognized vertebral fractures for those who continued alendronate (5.3% for placebo versus 2.4% for alendronate; 95% CI, 0.24–0.85). These results suggest that while for a proportion of women 5 years of treatment with alendronate may be sufficient initially, women who have very low BMD and/or a very high risk of developing vertebral fractures may benefit from continuing alendronate beyond 5 years [12].

Risedronate is the other commonly used oral bisphosphonate. Its anti-fracture efficacy has been shown in several randomized phase III controlled studies. The first key trial is the VERT study of postmenopausal women, conducted multinationally [13, 14]. A significant reduction was observed in the risk of new vertebral fractures by about 60% after the first year of treatment with risedronate and this effect was maintained throughout the treatment period (3 years), with significant reduction in the incidence of new vertebral fractures of over 40%. Risedronate has also been shown to significantly reduce the risk of non-vertebral fractures. In other work, the Hip Intervention Program of 9.331 patients [15] demonstrated that treatment with risedronate significantly reduces the risk of hip fractures in osteoporotic women; the risk reduction was 41% versus placebo over 3 years in women with low bone mineral density at the femoral neck and 60% versus placebo in women with low bone mineral density at the femoral neck and at least one prevalent vertebral fracture. A particular benefit of risedronate therapy is its fast action; risedronate is the only bisphosphonate that has been shown to significantly reduce the risk of both vertebral and non-vertebral fractures within 6 months of therapy [16].

However, if oral bisphosphonates are contraindicated, or an individual is unable to tolerate them (for example malabsorption or dysphagia), then an alternative intravenous bisphosphonate, for example zoledronate, can be given [17]. Zoledronate is usually administered as a yearly infusion but a recent trial has demonstrated that in patients with osteopenia an infusion every 18 months can be efficacious [18]. The main randomised controlled trial of zoledronate efficacy is the HORIZON study, with data available at different study time points. Hence Black and colleagues compared the effects of 3 versus 6 years zoledronic acid in the HORIZON Pivotal Study [19], and found that, while femoral neck BMD remained constant in women randomised to 6 years of intravenous bisphosphonate, it decreased slightly in those randomised to placebo after 3 years with similar effects at other sites. Biochemical markers tended to rise in those subjects randomised to the placebo group but still remained below pre-treatment levels, and the researchers reported that new morphometric vertebral fractures increased about two-fold after zoledronate was stopped at 3 years as compared to women maintained 6 years on therapy (OR 0.51 for 6 versus 3 years; $p = 0.035$). However, no rise in risk of non-vertebral fractures was observed among those who went on placebo after 3 years compared to those who continued therapy for 6 years. In a further study, a randomised second extension provided data regarding 9 years versus 6 years of treatment [20]. From year 6 to 9, the mean change in total hip BMD was −1.31% versus −0.54% in those randomised to placebo after 6 years of treatment compared to those who continued to receive infusions (difference 0.78%; 95% confidence interval [CI]: −0.37%, 1.93%; $p = 0.183$) while bone turnover markers showed small, non-significant increases in those who discontinued after 6 years compared with those who continued for 9 years. The number of fractures was low and did not significantly differ by treatment. The researchers noted that there was a small increase in cardiac arrhythmias in the continued treatment group but no other safety signals were detected, and concluded that almost all patients who have received six annual zoledronate infusions can stop medication for up to 3 years without apparent adverse consequences.

Gastrointestinal Side Effects

The most commonly prescribed bisphosphonate is alendronate which is usually given orally once weekly. Oral bisphosphonates must be given on an empty stomach as gastrointestinal absorption is inhibited by food and liquid. Suboptimal administration can result in oesophageal irritation, dysphagia and heartburn. These side effects potentially limit the tolerance and adherence of oral bisphosphonates but trial data show they are rare. A meta-analysis of adverse effects comprising several randomised controlled trials (RCTs) demonstrated that alendronate is associated with an increased risk of mild upper gastrointestinal side effects (odds ratio (OR) 1.07, 95% confidence interval (CI) 1.01–1.14) [21]. Furthermore, a meta-analysis exploring the comparative gastrointestinal safety of bisphosphonates showed no significant difference in discontinuation rates due to adverse events between alendronate, risedronate, and zolendronic acid [22].

There is conflicting evidence linking bisphosphonates to an increased risk of oesophageal cancer. A meta-analysis comprising seven studies, with 19,700 oesophageal cancer cases showed a positive relationship between exposure to bisphosphonates and oesophageal cancer, with an OR of 1.74 with a 95% CI of 1.19–2.55 [23]. However, a further meta-analysis of four cohort studies and three case-control studies showed bisphosphonate treatment was not associated with risk of oesophageal cancer in both cohort studies [pooled relative risk (RR) 1.23, 95% CI 0.79–1.92] and case-control studies [pooled odds ratio (OR) 1.24, 95% CI 0.98–1.57] [24]. Based on these findings the FDA believes that the benefits of oral bisphosphonate drugs in reducing the risk of serious fractures in people with osteoporosis continue to outweigh the potential risk of oesophageal cancer [25].

Osteonecrosis of the Jaw

In recent years there has been concern regarding a rare but very serious complication that has been associated with anti-resorptive therapy. Concerns in patients has led to recommendations from the American Society for Bone and Mineral Research

(ASBMR) that patients should be informed that there is a low risk of development of osteonecrosis of the jaw (ONJ) with bisphosphonate therapy and that health providers should encourage patients to practice good oral hygiene and have regular dental visits [10]. Osteonecrosis of the jaw was first recorded in relation to bisphosphonate therapy in 2003 [26]. Cases of ONJ have been predominantly observed in larger doses of bisphosphonates given to oncology patients for metastatic disease [26, 27], and the risk of those being treated for osteoporosis is very low; The ASBMR has estimated ONJ incidence as between 1 in 10,000–100,000 patient-treatment years [28]. Studies have suggested that the strongest risk factors for developing ONJ whilst on bisphosphonates are pre-existing dental disease and prior dental extraction [29, 30].

Atypical Femoral Fracture

Atypical fracture is now a recognized potential complication of bisphosphonates although they have also been observed in patients not treated with anti-osteoporosis medications. Atypical fractures can occur spontaneously with or without prodromal pain. These fractures are located in the subtrochanteric region or femoral shaft, are usually not comminuted, and include a transverse fracture line at the point of origination in the lateral cortex [31]. Atypical femoral fractures are rare with a recent meta-analysis of five case-controlled studies finding an overall pooled risk ratio of 1.70 (1.22–2.37) [32]. The risk of atypical femoral fracture increases with the length of treatment with bisphosphonates; a study of in excess of one million women has shown that the incidence rate of atypical femoral fracture increases from 1.78 per 100,000 in women receiving 2 years or less of bisphosphonate therapy, to over 100 per 100,000 following 8 years or more of treatment [33]. To reduce the risk of atypical femoral fracture after prolonged use of bisphosphonates, patient reassessment is now recommended after 3–5 years of treatment. Unfortunately widespread media reports of this very rare complication, like for ONJ, has led many patients to discontinue therapies that would greatly reduce the risk of fragility fracture.

Other Adverse Effects

Use of bisphosphonates is associated with nephrotoxicity, with alendronate and zoledronate being contraindicated in patients with a creatinine clearance less than 35 mL/min/1.73 m^2 and below 30 mL/min/1.73 m^2 for risedronate and ibandronate [34]. Intravenous bisphosphonates have been associated with transient symptoms related to an acute phase response including fever, myalgia, arthralgia and headache. These symptoms usually resolve within 72 h and occur in an estimated 12–42% of patients [35]. As bisphosphonates inhibit osteoclastic bone resorption they reduce calcium efflux from bone and potentially decrease serum calcium. Data from the HORIZON-PFT (Health Outcomes and Reduced Incidence with Zolendronic Acid Once Yearly Pivotal Fracture Trial) showed that zoledronate is associated with transient and asymptomatic hypocalcaemia in 1.3% of patients [29].

Denosumab

Another commonly used anti-resorptive medication is the human monoclonal antibody denosumab, which targets RANKL (receptor activator of NFκB ligand). RANKL is a major activator of osteoclastic bone resorption which is secreted by osteoblasts and mimics the action of osteoprotegerin (OPG) [17]. Denosumab is administered by a subcutaneous injection every 6 months and has been shown to be efficacious in patients with renal impairment, commonly useful in clinical practice. The main trial assessing efficacy of denosumab therapy was the FREEDOM trial [36]. Through this, denosumab has been shown to be effective in improving BMD and reducing fracture among women who received up to 10 years of treatment [37]; in the long-term treatment group, BMD increased from FREEDOM baseline by 21·7% at the lumbar spine, 9·2% at total hip, 9·0% at femoral neck, and 2·7% at the one-third radius. In the same study, the annual incidence of new vertebral fractures (ranging from 0·90% to 1·86%) and non-vertebral fractures (ranging from 0·84% to 2·55%) remained low during the extension, and were noted to be similar to rates observed in the denosumab group during the first 3 years of the FREEDOM study, and lower than rates projected for a virtual long-term placebo cohort [37]. However, very importantly for clinical practice, several studies have suggested that denosumab withdrawal may be associated with accelerated bone loss and vertebral fractures [38–40]. In one of these studies, an analysis of 797 subjects withdrawing from the study drug (placebo or denosumab) during the original FREEDOM study, researchers reported 42% versus 28% of placebo- and denosumab-treated subjects, respectively, initiated another therapy (mostly bisphosphonates). Following discontinuation, similar percentages of subjects in both groups sustained a new fracture (9% placebo, 7% denosumab) [36]. Of note, in the FREEDOM extension trial, the risk of multiple vertebral fractures upon discontinuation after 3 years of denosumab was more than three-fold higher among those with a prevalent vertebral fracture (incidence 5.9%, compared to 4.1% off placebo in this high risk group). The risk also increased with the duration off therapy, the gain in hip BMD on therapy, and the loss of hip BMD off therapy [37], possibly reflecting association between fracture risk and BMD.

Adverse Effects

Apart from the risk of rebound bone loss and fracture on discontinuation, side effects with denosumab are uncommon and over 3 years in the FREEDOM study, there was no significant difference between denosumab and placebo in the proportion of patients who experienced treatment-emergent adverse events [36]. Denosumab can rarely be associated with skin infections, predominantly cellulitis. This is likely secondary to an immunomodulatory effect of the drug not typically seen at the injection site [17]. Hypocalcaemia can also be a risk, particularly if the patient is vitamin D deficient, or has renal impairment. In the extension of the FREEDOM trial over up to 10 years' therapy, two atypical femoral fractures (AFFs) were recorded and there were 13 cases of ONJ, predominantly occurring after invasive oral surgery [41]. Denosumab can be associated with hypocalcaemia and therefore it is recommended that calcium level monitoring is performed prior to each dose in all patients, in addition to within 2 weeks of a dose in patients predisposed to hypocalcaemia (e.g. patients with severe renal impairment) [42].

Strontium Ranelate

Strontium ranelate is a less commonly used anti-resorptive agent as its use has been recently restricted secondary to concerns regarding cardiovascular risks [43]. Strontium ranelate is a compound made up of ranelic acid bound with two atoms of the element strontium which sits below calcium on the periodic table and is incorporated into bone at the same rate as calcium. The relative risks and benefits of strontium ranelate were reviewed by the European Medicines Agency in March 2014, who advised that strontium ranelate should be used only in individuals with severe osteoporosis for which other treatment options have been exhausted [44]. Following this there has been a large decline in the use of strontium ranelate [10]. Its mechanism of action remains uncertain, and its inclusion in a chapter on anti-resorptive therapy might be challenged, but there is evidence that it increases bone strength by altering bone material properties. Although strontium ranelate therapy leads to a substantial increase in BMD at the spine and hip, it is recognised that part of this increase is artefactual, due to incorporation of strontium (which has a greater atomic weight than calcium) into bone. Reassuringly however, studies have shown a 36% relative risk reduction in hip fracture over 3 years in osteoporotic patients treated with this therapy, suggesting that it does have beneficial effects on bone mass [45].

Selective Oestrogen Receptor Modulators

Raloxifene is used less commonly than bisphosphonates for the treatment and prevention of osteoporosis in postmenopausal women and for glucocorticoid induced osteoporosis. It was approved for clinical use in the United States in 1997. It is a mixed agonist and antagonist at the oestrogen receptor and acts as an agonist in bone, but an antagonist in other areas of the body such as the uterus and breast. Raloxifene therefore has positive oestrogenic effects on bone without the unwanted side effects of oestrogen elsewhere. The main study evaluating the efficacy of this therapy was the Multiple Outcomes of Raloxifene Evaluation (MORE) study, which was based on 7705 women aged 31 to 80 years in 25 countries, who had been postmenopausal for at least 2 years, and who met WHO criteria for osteoporosis. This study demonstrated that raloxifene increases BMD in the spine and femoral neck and reduces the risk of vertebral fracture [46]; the study demonstrated a four-year cumulative relative risk of 0.7 (95% CI, 0.5–0.8) for new vertebral fractures and relative risk of 0.9 (95% CI, 0.8–1.1) that was not significant for nonvertebral fractures. Treatment with raloxifene is, however, associated with an increased risk of venous thrombo-embolic events and so patients need to be assessed prior to commencing treatment with regard to their risk, as its use is contraindicated in patients with active or past history of venous thrombo-embolic events, including deep vein thrombosis, pulmonary embolism and retinal vein thrombosis [10]. It has therefore been suggested that raloxifene can be used as the first line for less severe osteoporosis, predominantly of the spine, or may be considered as a weaker antiresorptive therapy for higher-risk patients during a bisphosphonate holiday [47] [48]. Finally a substudy of the MORE trial by Ettinger et al. reported an increase in BMD of 2.1% and 2.6% at the femoral neck and spine, respectively, in women who received raloxifene 60 mg per day compared with women who received placebo. The results of this study confirmed a relative risk of 0.7 (95% CI, 0.5–0.8) for vertebral fractures among treated women and a relative risk of 0.9 (95% CI, 0.8–1.1) for nonvertebral fractures in women receiving raloxifene 60 mg per day [46].

The Role of HRT

While hormone replacement therapy used to be a commonly used therapy to prevent osteoporosis, the recognition that long term therapy is associated with adverse health consequences has meant that it is now recommended only for the prevention of osteoporosis in high-risk postmenopausal women and should be used only after all nonestrogenic osteoporotic treatments have been considered inappropriate [49].

The main trial that considered its efficacy, after a raft of observational studies, was the Women's Health Initiative (WHI), which was a randomized controlled trial of 16,608 postmenopausal patients that demonstrated a statistically significant reduction in fractures with estrogen-progestin combination therapy. Unfortunately the WHI study data also reported an increase in the risk of cardiovascular events, stroke, VTE, and invasive breast cancer associated with the estrogen-progestin groups [50] and because of this, hormonal replacement therapy is no longer recommended as first line for the treatment and prevention of osteoporosis in postmenopausal and premenopausal women [47].

Drug Holidays

The recognition of rare side events associated with anti-resorptive therapies has led to the common practice of 'drug holidays' for bisphosphonates, whereby patients who have been on treatment for 3–5 years are considered for their suitability for an intermission in treatment, typically for 1–2 years as detailed in Fig. 5.1. Drug holidays are becoming the norm in many countries, which is of concern as some high-risk patients might derive more benefit than harm from ongoing therapy [51]. A systematic review by Dennison and colleagues showed that the risk of new clinical fractures was 20–40% higher in subjects who stopped bisphosphonate treatment, and vertebral fracture risk was approximately doubled [52]. As detailed earlier in this chapter, following denosumab discontinuation a fall in BMD is often observed, with an associated incidence

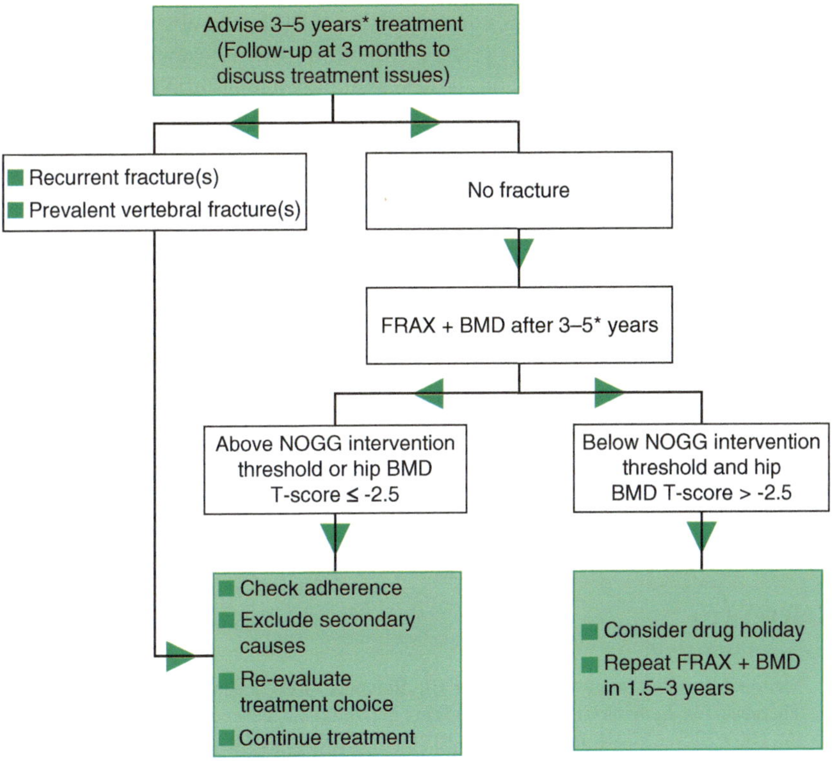

* 3 years for zoledronic acid; 5 years for other bisphosphonates
BMD=bone mineral density.
Reproduced with kind permission from the WHO Collaborating Centre for Metabolic Bone Diseases, www. shef.ac.uk/FRAX

Fig. 5.1 Algorithm for treatment monitoring with the use of bisphosphonates from the National Osteoporosis Guideline Group (NOGG)

of multiple vertebral fractures around 5% [52]. Importantly studies which have considered long-term continuation did not identify increased fracture risk, and reported very low rates of adverse skeletal events such as atypical femoral fracture [29, 37]. The view that all patients on long-term treatment for osteoporosis should be offered a drug holiday is therefore not supported by the existing evidence and individuals on long term bisphosphonates should be assessed on a case by case basis.

This position is becoming increasingly widespread, with the publications of a number of position papers and guidelines [53–56], which generally reinforce the importance of continuing therapy among women who remain at high risk of fracture. Despite these recommendations, however, more than 1 in every two patients stops therapy after 2 years and most physicians would stop therapy regardless of risk evaluation after 3–5 years. A particular concern of patients and physicians alike is the apparent association of osteoporosis treatment with atypical femoral fractures and ONJ. However, this risk remains less than 1 in 1000 subjects treated even for 10 years according to most long-term extensions of RCTs and observational studies. Although the long-term benefits remain difficult to exactly evaluate in absence of large placebo-controlled extension studies, assuming a long-term reduction of fracture risk in the order of 30% with anti-resorptive therapy, as suggested by the available evidence, particularly among high risk subjects, would result in a benefit: risk ratio (fractures prevented: adverse skeletal event) of at least 100:1.

Conclusion

Anti-resorptive agents have been widely shown to reduce the incidence of fragility fractures in patients with osteoporosis, with bisphosphonates being the most commonly prescribed. Some rare but serious side effects (osteonecrosis of the jaw and atypical fracture) have been reported, but in patients with a high risk of fragility fracture their benefits far outweigh their risks.

References

1. Melton LJ 3rd, Kearns AE, Atkinson EJ, Bolander ME, Achenbach SJ, Huddleston JM, Therneau TM, Leibson CL. Secular trends in hip fracture incidence and recurrence. Osteoporos Int. 2009;20(5):687–94. https://doi.org/10.1007/s00198-008-0742-8.
2. Chapuy MC, Pamphile R, Paris E, Kempf C, Schlichting M, Arnaud S, Garnero P, Meunier PJ. Combined calcium and vitamin D3 supplementation in elderly women: confirmation of reversal of secondary hyperparathyroidism and hip fracture risk: the Decalyos II study. Osteoporos Int. 2002;13(3):257–64. https://doi.org/10.1007/s001980200023.
3. Prentice RL, Pettinger MB, Jackson RD, Wactawski-Wende J, Lacroix AZ, Anderson GL, Chlebowski RT, Manson JE, Van Horn L, Vitolins MZ, Datta M, LeBlanc ES, Cauley JA, Rossouw JE. Health risks and benefits from calcium and vitamin D supplementation: Women's Health Initiative clinical trial and cohort study. Osteoporos Int. 2013;24(2):567–80. https://doi.org/10.1007/s00198-012-2224-2.

4. Bolland MJ, Avenell A, Baron JA, Grey A, MacLennan GS, Gamble GD, Reid IR. Effect of calcium supplements on risk of myocardial infarction and cardiovascular events: meta-analysis. BMJ. 2010;341:c3691. https://doi.org/10.1136/bmj.c3691.
5. Jenkins DJA, Spence JD, Giovannucci EL, Kim YI, Josse R, Vieth R, Blanco Mejia S, Viguiliouk E, Nishi S, Sahye-Pudaruth S, Paquette M, Patel D, Mitchell S, Kavanagh M, Tsirakis T, Bachiri L, Maran A, Umatheva N, McKay T, Trinidad G, Bernstein D, Chowdhury A, Correa-Betanzo J, Del Principe G, Hajizadeh A, Jayaraman R, Jenkins A, Jenkins W, Kalaichandran R, Kirupaharan G, Manisekaran P, Qutta T, Shahid R, Silver A, Villegas C, White J, Kendall CWC, Pichika SC, Sievenpiper JL. Supplemental vitamins and minerals for CVD prevention and treatment. J Am Coll Cardiol. 2018;71(22):2570–84. https://doi.org/10.1016/j.jacc.2018.04.020.
6. Eleni A, Panagiotis P. A systematic review and meta-analysis of vitamin D and calcium in preventing osteoporotic fractures. Clin Rheumatol. 2020;39(12):3571–9. https://doi.org/10.1007/s10067-020-05122-3.
7. Yao P, Bennett D, Mafham M, Lin X, Chen Z, Armitage J, Clarke R. Vitamin D and calcium for the prevention of fracture: a systematic review and meta-analysis. JAMA Netw Open. 2019;2(12):e1917789. https://doi.org/10.1001/jamanetworkopen.2019.17789.
8. Zhao JG, Zeng XT, Wang J, Liu L. Association between calcium or vitamin D supplementation and fracture incidence in community-dwelling older adults: a systematic review and meta-analysis. JAMA. 2017;318(24):2466–82. https://doi.org/10.1001/jama.2017.19344.
9. Russell RG. Bisphosphonates: the first 40 years. Bone. 2011;49(1):2–19. https://doi.org/10.1016/j.bone.2011.04.022.
10. Chan CK, Mason A, Cooper C, Dennison E. Novel advances in the treatment of osteoporosis. Br Med Bull. 2016;119(1):129–42. https://doi.org/10.1093/bmb/ldw033.
11. Black DM, Thompson DE, Bauer DC, Ensrud K, Musliner T, Hochberg MC, Nevitt MC, Suryawanshi S, Cummings SR. Fracture risk reduction with alendronate in women with osteoporosis: the fracture intervention trial. FIT Research Group. J Clin Endocrinol Metab. 2000;85(11):4118–24. https://doi.org/10.1210/jcem.85.11.6953.
12. Black DM, Schwartz AV, Ensrud KE, Cauley JA, Levis S, Quandt SA, Satterfield S, Wallace RB, Bauer DC, Palermo L, Wehren LE, Lombardi A, Santora AC, Cummings SR. Effects of continuing or stopping alendronate after 5 years of treatment: the fracture intervention trial long-term extension (FLEX): a randomized trial. JAMA. 2006;296(24):2927–38. https://doi.org/10.1001/jama.296.24.2927.
13. Harris ST, Watts NB, Genant HK, McKeever CD, Hangartner T, Keller M, Chesnut CH 3rd, Brown J, Eriksen EF, Hoseyni MS, Axelrod DW, Miller PD. Effects of risedronate treatment on vertebral and nonvertebral fractures in women with postmenopausal osteoporosis: a randomized controlled trial. Vertebral Efficacy with Risedronate Therapy (VERT) Study Group. JAMA. 1999;282(14):1344–52. https://doi.org/10.1001/jama.282.14.1344.
14. Reginster J, Minne HW, Sorensen OH, Hooper M, Roux C, Brandi ML, Lund B, Ethgen D, Pack S, Roumagnac I, Eastell R. Randomized trial of the effects of risedronate on vertebral fractures in women with established postmenopausal osteoporosis. Vertebral Efficacy with Risedronate Therapy (VERT) Study Group. Osteoporos Int. 2000;11(1):83–91. https://doi.org/10.1007/s001980050010.
15. McClung MR, Geusens P, Miller PD, Zippel H, Bensen WG, Roux C, Adami S, Fogelman I, Diamond T, Eastell R, Meunier PJ, Reginster JY. Effect of risedronate on the risk of hip fracture in elderly women. Hip Intervention Program Study Group. N Engl J Med. 2001;344(5):333–40. https://doi.org/10.1056/nejm200102013440503.
16. Roux C, Seeman E, Eastell R, Adachi J, Jackson RD, Felsenberg D, Songcharoen S, Rizzoli R, Di Munno O, Horlait S, Valent D, Watts NB. Efficacy of risedronate on clinical vertebral fractures within six months. Curr Med Res Opin. 2004;20(4):433–9. https://doi.org/10.1185/030079903125003125.

17. Liu J, Curtis EM, Cooper C, Harvey NC. State of the art in osteoporosis risk assessment and treatment. J Endocrinol Invest. 2019;42(10):1149–64. https://doi.org/10.1007/s40618-019-01041-6.
18. Reid IR, Horne AM, Mihov B, Stewart A, Garratt E, Wong S, Wiessing KR, Bolland MJ, Bastin S, Gamble GD. Fracture prevention with Zoledronate in older women with osteopenia. N Engl J Med. 2018;379(25):2407–16. https://doi.org/10.1056/NEJMoa1808082.
19. Black DM, Reid IR, Boonen S, Bucci-Rechtweg C, Cauley JA, Cosman F, Cummings SR, Hue TF, Lippuner K, Lakatos P, Leung PC, Man Z, Martinez RL, Tan M, Ruzycky ME, Su G, Eastell R. The effect of 3 versus 6 years of zoledronic acid treatment of osteoporosis: a randomized extension to the HORIZON-Pivotal Fracture Trial (PFT). J Bone Miner Res. 2012;27(2):243–54. https://doi.org/10.1002/jbmr.1494.
20. Black DM, Reid IR, Cauley JA, Cosman F, Leung PC, Lakatos P, Lippuner K, Cummings SR, Hue TF, Mukhopadhyay A, Tan M, Aftring RP, Eastell R. The effect of 6 versus 9 years of zoledronic acid treatment in osteoporosis: a randomized second extension to the HORIZON-Pivotal Fracture Trial (PFT). J Bone Miner Res. 2015;30(5):934–44. https://doi.org/10.1002/jbmr.2442.
21. Crandall CJ, Newberry SJ, Diamant A, Lim YW, Gellad WF, Booth MJ, Motala A, Shekelle PG. Comparative effectiveness of pharmacologic treatments to prevent fractures: an updated systematic review. Ann Intern Med. 2014;161(10):711–23. https://doi.org/10.7326/m14-0317.
22. Tadrous M, Wong L, Mamdani MM, Juurlink DN, Krahn MD, Levesque LE, Cadarette SM. Comparative gastrointestinal safety of bisphosphonates in primary osteoporosis: a network meta-analysis. Osteoporos Int. 2014;25(4):1225–35. https://doi.org/10.1007/s00198-013-2576-2.
23. Andrici J, Tio M, Eslick GD. Meta-analysis: oral bisphosphonates and the risk of oesophageal cancer. Aliment Pharmacol Ther. 2012;36(8):708–16. https://doi.org/10.1111/apt.12041.
24. Sun K, Liu JM, Sun HX, Lu N, Ning G. Bisphosphonate treatment and risk of esophageal cancer: a meta-analysis of observational studies. Osteoporos Int. 2013;24(1):279–86. https://doi.org/10.1007/s00198-012-2158-8.
25. Maraka S, Kennel KA. Bisphosphonates for the prevention and treatment of osteoporosis. BMJ. 2015;351:h3783. https://doi.org/10.1136/bmj.h3783.
26. Marx RE. Pamidronate (Aredia) and zoledronate (Zometa) induced avascular necrosis of the jaws: a growing epidemic. J Oral Maxillofac Surg. 2003;61(9):1115–7. https://doi.org/10.1016/s0278-2391(03)00720-1.
27. Lo JC, O'Ryan FS, Gordon NP, Yang J, Hui RL, Martin D, Hutchinson M, Lathon PV, Sanchez G, Silver P, Chandra M, McCloskey CA, Staffa JA, Willy M, Selby JV, Go AS. Prevalence of osteonecrosis of the jaw in patients with oral bisphosphonate exposure. J Oral Maxillofac Surgery. 2010;68(2):243–53. https://doi.org/10.1016/j.joms.2009.03.050.
28. Khan AA, Morrison A, Hanley DA, Felsenberg D, McCauley LK, O'Ryan F, Reid IR, Ruggiero SL, Taguchi A, Tetradis S, Watts NB, Brandi ML, Peters E, Guise T, Eastell R, Cheung AM, Morin SN, Masri B, Cooper C, Morgan SL, Obermayer-Pietsch B, Langdahl BL, Al Dabagh R, Davison KS, Kendler DL, Sandor GK, Josse RG, Bhandari M, El Rabbany M, Pierroz DD, Sulimani R, Saunders DP, Brown JP, Compston J. Diagnosis and management of osteonecrosis of the jaw: a systematic review and international consensus. J Bone Miner Res. 2015;30(1):3–23. https://doi.org/10.1002/jbmr.2405.
29. Black DM, Delmas PD, Eastell R, Reid IR, Boonen S, Cauley JA, Cosman F, Lakatos P, Leung PC, Man Z, Mautalen C, Mesenbrink P, Hu H, Caminis J, Tong K, Rosario-Jansen T, Krasnow J, Hue TF, Sellmeyer D, Eriksen EF, Cummings SR. Once-yearly zoledronic acid for treatment of postmenopausal osteoporosis. N Engl J Med. 2007;356(18):1809–22. https://doi.org/10.1056/NEJMoa067312.
30. Choi WS, Lee JI, Yoon HJ, Min CK, Lee SH. Medication-related osteonecrosis of the jaw: a preliminary retrospective study of 130 patients with multiple myeloma. Maxillofac Plastic Reconstr Surg. 2017;39(1):1. https://doi.org/10.1186/s40902-016-0099-4.

31. Mohan PC, Howe TS, Koh JS, Png MA. Radiographic features of multifocal endosteal thickening of the femur in patients on long-term bisphosphonate therapy. Eur Radiol. 2013;23(1):222–7. https://doi.org/10.1007/s00330-012-2587-y.
32. Gedmintas L, Solomon DH, Kim SC. Bisphosphonates and risk of subtrochanteric, femoral shaft, and atypical femur fracture: a systematic review and meta-analysis. J Bone Miner Res. 2013;28(8):1729–37. https://doi.org/10.1002/jbmr.1893.
33. Dell RM, Adams AL, Greene DF, Funahashi TT, Silverman SL, Eisemon EO, Zhou H, Burchette RJ, Ott SM. Incidence of atypical nontraumatic diaphyseal fractures of the femur. J Bone Miner Res. 2012;27(12):2544–50. https://doi.org/10.1002/jbmr.1719.
34. Miller PD. The kidney and bisphosphonates. Bone. 2011;49(1):77–81. https://doi.org/10.1016/j.bone.2010.12.024.
35. Reid IR, Gamble GD, Mesenbrink P, Lakatos P, Black DM. Characterization of and risk factors for the acute-phase response after zoledronic acid. J Clin Endocrinol Metab. 2010;95(9):4380–7. https://doi.org/10.1210/jc.2010-0597.
36. Cummings SR, San Martin J, McClung MR, Siris ES, Eastell R, Reid IR, Delmas P, Zoog HB, Austin M, Wang A, Kutilek S, Adami S, Zanchetta J, Libanati C, Siddhanti S, Christiansen C. Denosumab for prevention of fractures in postmenopausal women with osteoporosis. N Engl J Med. 2009;361(8):756–65. https://doi.org/10.1056/NEJMoa0809493.
37. Bone HG, Wagman RB, Brandi ML, Brown JP, Chapurlat R, Cummings SR, Czerwinski E, Fahrleitner-Pammer A, Kendler DL, Lippuner K, Reginster JY, Roux C, Malouf J, Bradley MN, Daizadeh NS, Wang A, Dakin P, Pannacciulli N, Dempster DW, Papapoulos S. 10 years of denosumab treatment in postmenopausal women with osteoporosis: results from the phase 3 randomised FREEDOM trial and open-label extension. Lancet Diabetes Endocrinol. 2017;5(7):513–23. https://doi.org/10.1016/s2213-8587(17)30138-9.
38. Cummings SR, Ferrari S, Eastell R, Gilchrist N, Jensen JB, McClung M, Roux C, Törring O, Valter I, Wang AT, Brown JP. Vertebral fractures after discontinuation of Denosumab: a post hoc analysis of the randomized placebo-controlled FREEDOM trial and its extension. J Bone Miner Res. 2018;33(2):190–8. https://doi.org/10.1002/jbmr.3337.
39. Anastasilakis AD, Polyzos SA, Makras P, Aubry-Rozier B, Kaouri S, Lamy O. Clinical features of 24 patients with rebound-associated vertebral fractures after Denosumab discontinuation: systematic review and additional cases. J Bone Miner Res. 2017;32(6):1291–6. https://doi.org/10.1002/jbmr.3110.
40. McClung MR, Wagman RB, Miller PD, Wang A, Lewiecki EM. Observations following discontinuation of long-term denosumab therapy. Osteoporos Int. 2017;28(5):1723–32. https://doi.org/10.1007/s00198-017-3919-1.
41. Bone HG, Hosking D, Devogelaer JP, Tucci JR, Emkey RD, Tonino RP, Rodriguez-Portales JA, Downs RW, Gupta J, Santora AC, Liberman UA. Ten years' experience with alendronate for osteoporosis in postmenopausal women. N Engl J Med. 2004;350(12):1189–99. https://doi.org/10.1056/NEJMoa030897.
42. Deeks ED. Denosumab: a review in postmenopausal osteoporosis. Drugs Aging. 2018;35(2):163–73. https://doi.org/10.1007/s40266-018-0525-7.
43. Donneau AF, Reginster JY. Cardiovascular safety of strontium ranelate: real-life assessment in clinical practice. Osteoporos Int. 2014;25(2):397–8. https://doi.org/10.1007/s00198-013-2583-3.
44. Khosla S, Burr D, Cauley J, Dempster DW, Ebeling PR, Felsenberg D, Gagel RF, Gilsanz V, Guise T, Koka S, McCauley LK, McGowan J, McKee MD, Mohla S, Pendrys DG, Raisz LG, Ruggiero SL, Shafer DM, Shum L, Silverman SL, Van Poznak CH, Watts N, Woo SB, Shane E. Bisphosphonate-associated osteonecrosis of the jaw: report of a task force of the American Society for Bone and Mineral Research. J Bone Miner Res. 2007;22(10):1479–91. https://doi.org/10.1359/jbmr.0707onj.
45. Reginster JY, Seeman E, De Vernejoul MC, Adami S, Compston J, Phenekos C, Devogelaer JP, Curiel MD, Sawicki A, Goemaere S, Sorensen OH, Felsenberg D, Meunier PJ. Strontium ranelate reduces the risk of nonvertebral fractures in postmenopausal women with osteopo-

rosis: TREATMENT of Peripheral Osteoporosis (TROPOS) study. J Clin Endocrinol Metab. 2005;90(5):2816–22. https://doi.org/10.1210/jc.2004-1774.

46. Ettinger B, Black DM, Mitlak BH, Knickerbocker RK, Nickelsen T, Genant HK, Christiansen C, Delmas PD, Zanchetta JR, Stakkestad J, Gluer CC, Krueger K, Cohen FJ, Eckert S, Ensrud KE, Avioli LV, Lips P, Cummings SR. Reduction of vertebral fracture risk in postmenopausal women with osteoporosis treated with raloxifene: results from a 3-year randomized clinical trial. Multiple Outcomes of Raloxifene Evaluation (MORE) Investigators. JAMA. 1999;282(7):637–45. https://doi.org/10.1001/jama.282.7.637.
47. Camacho PM, Petak SM, Binkley N, Clarke BL, Harris ST, Hurley DL, Kleerekoper M, Lewiecki EM, Miller PD, Narula HS, Pessah-Pollack R, Tangpricha V, Wimalawansa SJ, Watts NB. American Association of Clinical Endocrinologists and American College of Endocrinology clinical practice guidelines for the diagnosis and treatment of postmenopausal osteoporosis—2016. Endocrine Practice. 2016;22(Suppl 4):1–42. https://doi.org/10.4158/ep161435.gl.
48. Delmas PD, Ensrud KE, Adachi JD, Harper KD, Sarkar S, Gennari C, Reginster JY, Pols HA, Recker RR, Harris ST, Wu W, Genant HK, Black DM, Eastell R. Efficacy of raloxifene on vertebral fracture risk reduction in postmenopausal women with osteoporosis: four-year results from a randomized clinical trial. J Clin Endocrinol Metab. 2002;87(8):3609–17. https://doi.org/10.1210/jcem.87.8.8750.
49. Tu KN, Lie JD, Wan CKV, Cameron M, Austel AG, Nguyen JK, Van K, Hyun D. Osteoporosis: a review of treatment options. P&T. 2018;43(2):92–104.
50. Rossouw JE, Anderson GL, Prentice RL, LaCroix AZ, Kooperberg C, Stefanick ML, Jackson RD, Beresford SA, Howard BV, Johnson KC, Kotchen JM, Ockene J. Risks and benefits of estrogen plus progestin in healthy postmenopausal women: principal results from the Women's Health Initiative randomized controlled trial. JAMA. 2002;288(3):321–33. https://doi.org/10.1001/jama.288.3.321.
51. Silverman SL, Adachi JD, Dennison E. Bisphosphonate drug holidays: we reap what we sow. Osteoporos Int. 2016;27(3):849–52. https://doi.org/10.1007/s00198-015-3453-y.
52. Dennison EM, Cooper C, Kanis JA, Bruyere O, Silverman S, McCloskey E, Abrahamsen B, Prieto-Alhambra D, Ferrari S. Fracture risk following intermission of osteoporosis therapy. Osteoporos Int. 2019;30(9):1733–43. https://doi.org/10.1007/s00198-019-05002-w.
53. Shane E, Burr D, Ebeling PR, Abrahamsen B, Adler RA, Brown TD, Cheung AM, Cosman F, Curtis JR, Dell R, Dempster D, Einhorn TA, Genant HK, Geusens P, Klaushofer K, Koval K, Lane JM, McKiernan F, McKinney R, Ng A, Nieves J, O'Keefe R, Papapoulos S, Sen HT, van der Meulen MC, Weinstein RS, Whyte M. Atypical subtrochanteric and diaphyseal femoral fractures: report of a task force of the American Society for Bone and Mineral Research. J Bone Miner Res. 2010;25(11):2267–94. https://doi.org/10.1002/jbmr.253.
54. Adler RA, El-Hajj Fuleihan G, Bauer DC, Camacho PM, Clarke BL, Clines GA, Compston JE, Drake MT, Edwards BJ, Favus MJ, Greenspan SL, McKinney R Jr, Pignolo RJ, Sellmeyer DE. Managing osteoporosis in patients on long-term bisphosphonate treatment: report of a task force of the American Society for Bone and Mineral Research. J Bone Miner Res. 2016;31(1):16–35. https://doi.org/10.1002/jbmr.2708.
55. Compston J, Cooper A, Cooper C, Gittoes N, Gregson C, Harvey N, Hope S, Kanis JA, McCloskey EV, Poole KES, Reid DM, Selby P, Thompson F, Thurston A, Vine N. UK clinical guideline for the prevention and treatment of osteoporosis. Arch Osteoporos. 2017;12(1):43. https://doi.org/10.1007/s11657-017-0324-5.
56. Watts NB, Chines A, Olszynski WP, McKeever CD, McClung MR, Zhou X, Grauer A. Fracture risk remains reduced one year after discontinuation of risedronate. Osteoporos Int. 2008;19(3):365–72. https://doi.org/10.1007/s00198-007-0460-7.

Chapter 6
Anabolic and Emerging Therapies

Jean Zhang and Elaine Dennison

Introduction

Pharmacological therapy for osteoporosis can be divided into two categories of drugs: those decreasing resorption by inhibiting osteoclast activities, and those that increase bone formation by promoting osteoblast activities. Anabolic therapy falls into the latter category. The most well-known anabolic therapy is teriparatide, which was first approved by US Food and Drug Administration (FDA) in late 2002, and shortly followed by approval by European Medicines Agency (EMA) in the summer of 2003. There are a number of anabolic targets including parathyroid hormone (PTH), growth hormone (GH), insulin-like growth factor (IGF) 1, strontium, fluoride, bone morphogenetic protein (BMP)-2, BMP-7 (also called osteogenic protein-1 [OP-1]), basic fibroblast growth factors (bFGFs) and vascular endothelial growth factor (VEGF). In this chapter we will discuss existing anabolic and emerging therapies (Fig. 6.1).

Parathyroid Hormone

In skeletal tissue, PTH primarily binds to PTH-1 receptor (PTH1R), a G-protein-coupled receptor which is expressed in mesenchymal stem cells, osteoblasts and osteocytes. PTH stimulates bone formation through several mechanisms; it stimulates the conversion of mesenchymal stem cells and bone lining cells into osteoblasts, and inhibits apoptosis of osteoblasts. PTH has been shown to be involved with

J. Zhang
MRC Lifecourse Epidemiology Centre, Southampton, UK
e-mail: jz@mrc.soton.ac.uk

E. Dennison (✉)
MRC Lifecourse Epidemiology Centre, University of Southampton, Southampton, UK
e-mail: emd@mrc.soton.ac.uk

E. Dennison (ed.), *Osteoporosis Treatment*, https://doi.org/10.1007/978-3-030-78128-6_6

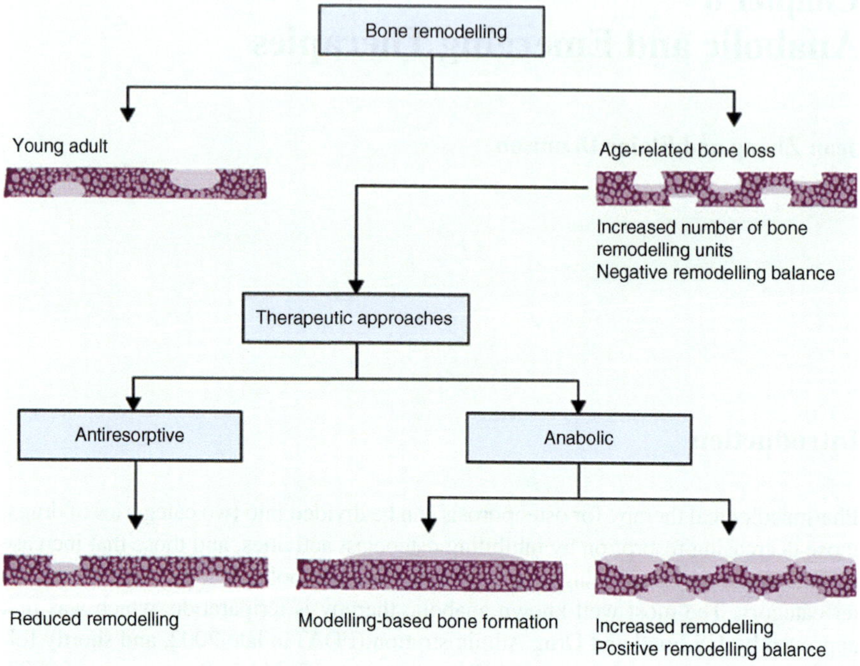

Fig. 6.1 Therapeutic approaches to anti-osteoporosis medication. (Reproduced with permission from [1])

numerous growth factors, transcription factors, and regulatory genes in the process of osteogenesis [2]. In primary and secondary hyperparathyroidism, high bone turnover has been observed with consequent decreased bone mass resulting in osteoporosis [3]. However intermittent injection of PTH peptides in humans [4, 5] have resulted in an increase in bone mass. Hence while the predominate residual effect of intermittent injections of PTH is anabolic, catabolic actions also occur. The presence of PTH increases the rate of bone turnover, and bone markers in clinical studies show an early stimulation of bone formation followed by increased bone resorption [5].

Clinical Efficacy of Teriparatide

Teriparatide is a recombinant human PTH containing the 1–34 amino acid terminal fragment of PTH and it is primarily administered as a 20 μg daily subcutaneous injection into the abdomen or thigh for 18–24 months [6, 7]. Teriparatide, and alongside other anabolic therapies are not usually the first line treatment for osteoporosis, with anti-resorptive treatment been the most commonly used first line therapy for osteoporosis management.

A number of trials involving human participants have been conducted to investigate the effects of PTH on bone density outcome [8–12], and fractures [13].

The Fracture Prevention Trial showed that treatment of postmenopausal osteoporosis with PTH (1–34) increased vertebral, femoral, and total-body BMD; and decreased the risk of vertebral and non-vertebral fractures [9]. This randomised controlled trial allocated 1637 postmenopausal women with prior vertebral fractures to receive 20 or 40 μg of PTH (1–34) or placebo, administered subcutaneously daily, alongside daily supplements of 1000 mg of calcium and 400–1200 IU of vitamin D. An increase of BMD at follow up, median duration of observation 21 months, was observed at lumbar spine, total hip, neck of femur, and trochanter, relative to placebo for both doses of PTH [9]. Risk of vertebral fractures was similarly reduced, with a 65% relative risk reduction in the PTH (1–34) 20 μg group and a 69% relative risk reduction in the PTH (1–34) 40 μg group in comparison to placebo [9]. The incidence of total non-vertebral fractures was also reduced in the treated group [9]. There were no significant differences in serious adverse effects between the three groups though a higher rate of hypercalcaemia was observed in the 40 μg dosage PTH group. The study was terminated early due to concern regarding development of osteosarcomas in Fischer rats in a concurrent study [14], although in this report no cases of osteosarcoma was recorded.

In other work, a number of other clinical trials have demonstrated evidence of fracture reduction with the use of teriparatide. A meta-analysis combined randomised controlled trials (RCTs) with the use of teriparatide in patients with osteoporosis, demonstrating efficacy against hip fracture [OR 0.44 (0.22–0.87)] in patients treated with teriparatide compared with controls [15]. In a network meta-analysis that focused on the clinical effectiveness of teriparatide for the prevention of osteoporotic fragility fractures, researchers showed that those treated with teriparatide had significant benefit compared to placebo [16] while a second meta-analysis demonstrated significant anti-fracture efficacy for both non-vertebral and vertebral fractures, though fracture reduction was not significant at the hip [17].

The Vertebral Fracture Treatment Comparisons in Osteoporotic Women (VERO) study, compared teriparatide to risedronate in ≥45 years old women with ≥2 moderate or ≥1 severe vertebral fracture and a BMD T-score of ≤−1.50, in a head to head, double-blinded and double-dummy trial [18]. The primary outcome measure was the diagnosis of new radiographic vertebral fractures at 24 months, which occurred in 5.4% of women in the teriparatide group compared to 12.0% in the risedronate group. 4.8% of patients in the teriparatide group and 9.8% of those in the risedronate group sustained clinical fractures with a hazard ratio (HR) of 0.48, 95% CI 0.32–0.74; the study also found a smaller percentage of non-vertebral fragility fractures occurred in the teriparatide group compared to the risedronate group, although the HR did not reach statistical significance.

Bone turnover marker response to the initiation of teriparatide follows a consistent pattern with an increase of bone formation serum markers up to 12 months [19] with evidence of dampening of such effect at 18–36 months [20]. Bone resorption serum markers have a delayed increase with the peak and decline towards baseline occurring after 12 months of teriparatide [20]. A rapid increase in spinal BMD is also noted within the first 6 months of initiation of teriparatide [13] whereas rise in hip BMD is often slower taking up to 12 months [21]. Finally, in the Denosumab and Teriparatide

(DATA) Study, a randomised open label study, participants received 20 μg teriparatide daily or 60 mg denosumab every 6 months, or both [19]. At 12 months, lumbar spine BMD increased more in the combination group than in the teriparatide, or denosumab groups; femoral-neck BMD also increased more in the combination group than in the teriparatide, and denosumab groups, and as well as total hip BMD.

Side Effects

Low incidences of hypercalcaemia occurring up to within 24 hours of injection have been noted in clinical trials [9], and a post hoc analysis noted a higher incidence of hypercalcaemia in patients with moderate renal impairment [22]. In a postmarketing surveillance study, the incidence of those with hypercalcaemia (serum calcium >11 mg/dL) treated with teriparatide was <1% [23]. Hence while higher levels of urinary calcium excretion have been noted in participants injected with teriparatide compared to placebo, the magnitude of increase is modest and the most common adverse events noted in clinical trials include nausea, headache, arthralgia, and fatigue [21, 24].

The carcinogenic effect observed in Fischer rats was also observed in Sprague-Dawley rats [25], and both rat models demonstrated the development of bone tumours were dose- and duration-dependent. The development of osteosarcoma was not observed in studies involving non-human primates with exposure to teriparatide or PTH (1–84) for up to 18 months of treatment and 36 months of observations [26, 27]. Studies involving human participants with both PTH (1–34) and PTH (1–84) have not reported cases of developing skeletal malignancies [9, 28]; national registries of PTH have also been reassuring regarding osteosarcoma risk in these patients [29–31].

Fracture Healing

It has been suggested that PTH may enhance fracture but clinical studies have not been unanimous [32, 33]. The European Calcified Tissue Society recently published a systemic review evaluating the effects teriparatide has on healing of atypical femur fractures (AFF), and while they did not find robust evidence in support of using teriparatide for fracture healing, observational data did suggest the use of teriparatide may result in faster healing of surgically treated AFFs [34].

Practical Considerations

As previously mentioned teriparatide and other anabolic agents are largely second line therapy choice in osteoporosis management, and participants are likely to have had previous exposure to other anti-osteoporotic therapy. Participants who have received previous anti-resorptives have been noted to have a slower response to subsequent treatment with teriparatide [35, 36]. There is some evidence suggestive of a slight differing effect on BMD gain dependent on the type of anti-resorptive used; participants with previous exposure to risedronate then treated with teriparatide have been showed to have greater spinal BMD gain compared to those with treated with alendronate initially [35]. Those treated with raloxifene then switched onto teriparatide have been shown to have higher spinal and hip BMD gain than those exposed to alendronate previously [36]. Results from the European Forseto® (EUROFOS) Study showed previous exposure and duration of anti-resorptive therapy did not affect the BMD response at any skeletal site to starting teriparatide [21]. Another management approach investigated is the continuation of anti-resorptives with the addition of teriparatide, such as addition of teriparatide to such drugs have largely demonstrated the addition of teriparatide resulted in greater spinal BMD gain compared those remaining on anti-resorptive alone [37–39]. Cosman and colleagues explored the use of teriparatide in a cyclic regime for 48 months, with 3 months on and 3 months off, compared with the approved regime of daily treatment for 24 months in both treatment naïve and alendronate treated women [40], generally favouring the usual therapeutic regime.

Abaloparatide

Abaloparatide is a human PTH related peptide containing 34-amino acid peptide of N-terminal residues (PTHrP (1–34)); it is a selective activator of the PTH1R. It is administered as an 80 μg daily subcutaneous injection for a duration up to 2 years [41]. Abaloparatide achieved FDA approval in 2017 for the treatment of postmenopausal women with osteoporosis at high risk for fracture; however, it was rejected by EMA in 2018, on the grounds of lack of effectiveness at preventing non-vertebral fractures in postmenopausal women and the safety concern with regards to the medication's effects on the heart, such as increases in heart rate and palpitations [42].

Clinical Efficacy of Abaloparatide

Leder and colleague carried out a phase 2, multi-national, double-blinded, placebo controlled trial in osteoporotic postmenopausal women that compared varying doses of abaloparatide or 20 μg teriparatide [43], demonstrating BMD rises in all treated groups relative to placebo. A year later, a larger phase 3 double-blinded RCT, $n = 2463$, the Abaloparatide Comparator Trial in Vertebral Endpoints (ACTIVE) published their results [44]. Postmenopausal women were randomised to 18 months of daily subcutaneous injections of placebo; 80 μg abaloparatide; or open-label 20 μg teriparatide. Of 2463 recruited women, 1901 (77%) completed the study, the primary outcome was the presence of new morphometric vertebral fractures which occurred in

0.58% of participants in the abaloparatide group and in 4.22% of those in the placebo group, leading to RR: 0.14 (95% CI, 0.05–0.39), $p < .001$. In the secondary outcomes, the BMD at total hip, femoral neck and lumbar spine all significantly increased at 18 months from baseline compared to the placebo group. However, for the occurrence of non-vertebral fracture in the abaloparatide group was 2.7%, compared with 4.7% in the placebo group, and this only just reach statistical significance.

Participants from the ACTIVE study were then recruited into an extension study, the ACTIVExtend study, which incorporated further treatment with 24 months of alendronate [45]. The BMD gained sustained in the ACTIVE study was not only maintained but also appear to be further increased during the ACTIVExtend study [46]. Those in the abaloparatide/alendronate group demonstrated significant reduced risks of vertebral, non-vertebral, clinical, and major osteoporotic fractures [45]. In further analysis, greater reductions in relative risk for new vertebral, non-vertebral, clinical, and major osteoporotic fractures were noted in patients in the abaloparatide/alendronate group compared to those in the placebo/alendronate group, with subgroup analysis showing no differential effects.

Bone formation makers increase significantly with abaloparatide 40 and 80-µg therapy with a significant linear dose response. In the ACTIVE study, P1NP significantly peaked at month 1, and by 3 months P1NP level began to decrease in the abaloparatide group, however the P1NP level remained significant higher compared to placebo at 3, 6 and 12 months despite the relative decrease [44]. The bone resorption marker, CTX had been shown to have a slower response, increasing from 12 weeks onwards. In terms of BMD response, abaloparatide follows a similar pattern to that of teriparatide [44, 45].

The clinical efficacy of abaloparatide in fracture risk reduction has been evaluated in a network meta-analysis, which included data from 22 studies including osteoporotic postmenopausal women who were eligible for intervention for either primary or secondary prevention [47]. Abaloparatide was found to have the greatest treatment effect relative to placebo in the vertebral fracture network (RR = 0.13; 95% CrI 0.04–0.34), the non-vertebral fracture network (RR = 0.50; 95% CrI 0.28–0.85), and also the wrist fracture network (RR = 0.39; CrI 0.15–0.90).

Side Effects

In both the phase 2 and ACTIVE studies, the proportion of participants reporting treatment-emergent adverse events (TEAEs) were similar across the various groups. More study discontinuation occurred in the abaloparatide group than other groups due to adverse events, common adverse effects leading to discontinuation include nausea, dizziness, headache, and palpitations [43, 44] The safety profile of abaloparatide has been further analysed in post analysis using the data from the ACTIVE study. One of particular interest is the cardiovascular safety of abaloparatide in postmenopausal women, given this was one of the contributory factors that lead to a rejection by the EMA. In this post hoc analysis [48], abaloparatide was associated with transient increase in heart rate compared to teriparatide and placebo, and a slightly higher decrease in blood pressure 1-h post-treatment compared to teriparatide and placebo. A higher percentage of participants in the abaloparatide group discontinued with the study due to TEAEs potentially linked with HR and BP changes, 3.3, 1.3 and 0.6% in the abaloparatide, teriparatide and placebo groups, respectively. Encouragingly the proportion of participants with serious cardiac adverse events were similar across the groups. Analysis shows the time to first incidence of major adverse cardiovascular events (MACEs) and heart failure (HF) was significantly longer for abaloparatide compared to placebo, during the ACTIVE period: abaloparatide versus placebo, HR 0.30 (95% CI: 0.10, 0.91), $p = 0.02$, abaloparatide versus teriparatide HR 0.85 (0.23, 3.15, $p = 0.80$; during the ACTIVExtend period: abaloparatide/alendronate versus placebo/alendronate HR 0.58 (0.28, 1.15), $p = 0.11$. The analysis of time to first incidence of MACE did not show any significant differences the groups.

Sclerostin

Sclerostin is a monomeric glycoprotein encoded by the Sost gene which potently inhibits bone formation. The absence of this protein can result in medical conditions such as high bone mass phenotype, sclerosteosis and Van Buchem disease [49]. Sclerostin, an antagonist of Wnt signalling, is primarily expressed by osteocytes, and the expression progressively increase as osteocytes mature [50].

Promising results from preclinical studies using rodent and primates models, studying the effects of anti-sclerostin monoclonal antibodies have shown positive skeletal effects such as an increase in bone formation at trabecular, endocortical and periosteal surfaces [51–53]. A significant threefold increase in osteoblastic surface and osteoid surface were seen alongside with a 65% increase in mineralising surface in 6-month-old ovariectomised rats treated with sclerostin antibody [54]. Another study group using mouse model administered with sclerostin antibody demonstrated the conversion of quiescent lining cells to active osteoblasts [55], which poses the possibility of modelling-based bone formation as the driving force. In bone formation, two mechanisms exist, firstly remodelling-based, which is coupled with bone resorption, and secondly modelling-based which occurs directly on quiescent surfaces. The use of sclerostin antibodies in animal models have been shown to not only increase bone formation but also reduce parameters of bone resorption leading to an increase in BMD [51, 52, 56]. Observation of uncoupling of bone resorption which is commonly seen in osteoblast-mediated bone formation and osteoclast-mediated bone resorption during remodelling-based bone formation have been noted [51, 52, 57]. In ovariectomised rats treated with 5 weeks of sclerostin antibody, an increase of 69% in trabecular bone volume was observed as well as an increase in total bone forming surface in comparison with the controls [58]. This anabolic response was mainly modelling-based formation driven [58]. In human trials, a decrease in bone resorption markers have been seen [57, 59], however this response varies in animal models [60].

Romosozumab

Romosozumab is a humanised anti-sclerostin monoclonal antibody. It was initially rejected by the FDA before securing an approval for the treatment of osteoporosis in 2019 and later on in the same year approval from EMA was gained, with continuous monitoring of its safety data through the real world data. Romosozumab is administered at a dose of 210 mg, subcutaneously once every month for 12 doses in the abdomen or thigh.

Clinical Efficacy of Romosozumab

McClung and colleagues conducted an international, phase 2, dose-ranging study assessing efficacy and safety to romosozumab treatment in 419 osteoporotic postmenopausal women [59]. Participants were randomly allocated to receive subcutaneous romosozumab monthly (at a dose of 70 mg, 140 mg, or 210 mg) or every 3 months (140 mg or 210 mg), subcutaneous placebo, or an open-label active comparator: oral alendronate (70 mg weekly) or subcutaneous teriparatide (20 μg daily), for a duration of 12 months. The primary outcome was the percentage change in BMD at 12 months, for all romosozumab groups, regardless of dosing or frequency intervals the spinal BMD gain was significantly higher compared to placebo. Similar patterns were seen in comparison with teriparatide. The monthly 140 mg and 210 mg group had significantly higher percentage of spinal BMD gain compared to alendronate group. The largest gain was observed with the monthly 210 mg romosozumab dosing group at 12 months (11.3% at lumbar spine, 4.1% at total hip, 3.7% at femoral neck), and the increases with this dosing were significantly greater than compared to alendronate and teriparatide groups.

Two pivotal phases 3 trials were then subsequently published. The Fracture study in postmenopausal women with osteoporosis (FRAME) trail was a phase 3, international, randomised, double-blind, placebo-controlled study that recruited 7180 postmenopausal women with osteoporosis [61]. The participants were randomly assigned to either monthly 210 mg romosozumab or placebo injections for 12 months (double-blind period), then followed by 12 months of 6 monthly denosumab injections for all (open-label period). At 12 months, the use of romosozumab was significantly associated with a lower fracture risk for new vertebral fractures and new clinical fractures compared to the placebo group, with a non-significant reduction in new non-vertebral fracture in the romosozumab group. At 24 months, following transition to denosumab for all groups, the rates of vertebral fractures were significantly lower in the romosozumab group than the placebo group.

A year later, the active-controlled fracture study in postmenopausal women with osteoporosis at high risk of fracture (ARCH) trial was released. The ARCH trial was a phase 3 international, randomised, double-blind, alendronate-controlled study involving 4093 osteoporotic, postmenopausal women with at least one vertebral fracture or proximal femur fracture [62] who received either monthly 210 mg romosozumab injection or weekly oral 70 mg alendronate for 12 months (double blind period), followed by all participants receiving weekly oral 70 mg alendronate for further 12 months (open-label period). The primary endpoints demonstrated that at 24 months the use of romosozumab followed by alendronate resulted in lower incidence of new vertebral fracture, 6.2%, than in the alendronate alone group, 11.9%, giving a 48% risk reduction, and a lower incidence of clinical fractures in the romosozumab/alendronate group, 9.7%, compared to alendronate alone group, 13%, resulting in a 27% risk reduction. Secondary outcomes in this trial included the incidence of non-vertebral fractures at 24 months, 8.7% in the romosozumab/alendronate group compared 10.6% in alendronate along group, giving a 19% risk reduction.

A further phase 3 study was conducted in evaluating the efficacy and safety of romosozumab in osteoporotic men. The placebo-controlled study evaluating the efficacy and safety of romosozumab in treating men with osteoporosis (BRIDGE) study is an international, randomised, double-blind, placebo-controlled study of 245 men aged 55–90 years with osteoporosis and a history of fragility fracture (excluding hip fracture) or vertebral fracture [63]. The participants were randomly allocated in a 2:1 fashion to either monthly 210 mg romosozumab injection or monthly placebo injection for 12 months. The primary outcome in this trial was the percentage change of spinal BMD at 12 months from baseline, which was significantly higher in the romosozumab group (12.1%) compared to placebo (1.2%). Secondary outcomes included percentage change from baseline in total hip and femoral neck BMD at 12 months, which also showed significant higher BMD gains from baseline compared to placebo.

The rapid BMD gain observed in the first year of treatment with romosozumab followed by maintaining of the BMD gain with the use of denosumab may be an attractive option for clinicians. As previously discussed in this chapter, previous exposure to anti-resorptives such as bisphosphates can blunt or delay the effect exerted by teriparatide, another anabolic agent. STRUCTURE (an open-label study to evaluate the effect of treatment with romosozumab or teriparatide in postmenopausal women) study was a phase 3, international, randomised, open-label, active-controlled, parallel-group trial conducted to investigate the effect of romosozumab versus teriparatide in 436 osteoporotic postmenopausal women with previous bisphosphonate treatment, demonstrating superior gains in the romosozumab group [64]. The STRUCTURE trial also showed there were significant greater areal BMD gains at lumbar spine and femoral neck in the romosozumab group compared to teriparatide group at 6 and 12 months. The significant total hip BMD gain observed in the STRUCTURE trial highlights a potential target opportunity in the management of osteoporosis in those with previous exposure to bisphosphates, given the perceived delayed effect in hip BMD gain with teriparatide.

From meta-analyses, romosozumab has been associated with greater increases of BMD at lumbar spine, femoral neck, and total hip compared with placebo and significantly lower risks of new vertebral, non-vertebral, and hip fractures compared with other therapies such as alendronate and teriparatide [65, 66]. In one meta-analysis, the authors attempted to look at the risk of adjudicated cardiovascular serious events and deaths, which was increased with the use of 210 mg romosozumab compared to placebo. However only 2 studies were included, and the results did not reach statistical significance [66]. Regardless, it is important to be mindful of the potential cardiovascular risk, which will be discussed in further detail in the side effect section below.

Side Effects

The percentage of participants reporting adverse events and serious adverse events were largely similar across all the groups in the clinical trials of this agent. However, in both the ARCH and BRIDGE trials, higher numbers of adjudicated cardiovascular serious adverse event were observed during the period of treatment with romosozumab compared to placebo/alendronate groups [62, 63]. Therefore, resulting in clinical practice, romosozumab is not recommended for postmenopausal women with previous cardiovascular history or high cardiovascular risks. A very low number of osteonecrosis of the jaw (ONJ) and AFF were reported in the FRAME and ARCH trials [61, 62]. Binding antibodies and antibodies with in vitro neutralising activity were detected in very low percentages of participants with no apparent loss of efficacy.

Emerging Therapies

In this section, some of the promising emerging therapies and potential therapeutic targets in the management of osteoporosis will be discussed.

Biosimilars

A biosimilar is a biological medicine with high similarities to another already approved biological medicine, i.e.: the reference medicine, in terms of its structure, biological activity and efficacy, safety and immunogenicity profile [48, 67]. A number of such therapies have already been released, with more anticipated [68, 69].

Cathepsin K Inhibitor

Cathepsin K is a lysosomal cysteine protease found primarily in osteoclasts, and as a protease, its major role involves in degradation of bone via collagen e.g.: type I collagen and human cortical bone collagen breakdown [70]. Data from "knock out" animal models i.e.: deficiency of cathepsin K gene showed the development of skeletal hypermineralisation and phenotypically mimic some aspects of the human disease pycnodysostosis in that bone biopsies from those with pycnodysostosis show evidence of increased bone mass, decreased bone remodelling, and severely decreased dynamic parameters of bone formation [70]. It became evident functional cathepsin K is important for balanced bone turnover. A number of cathepsin K inhibitors have reached the phase II/II trial stage, but unfortunately to date, no Cathepsin K inhibitor has gained approval for clinical use. Balicatib, was investigated in a phase I study. However, the trial had to be stopped prematurely due to dermatological adverse effect, the development of morphea-like skin hardening [71, 72]. ONO-5334, reached phase 2 clinical trial stage, and its efficacy and safety was assessed in an international, 12-month, randomised, double-blind, placebo- and active-controlled parallel-group study [73]. Despite early encouraging outcomes, ONO-5334 was not advanced onto a phase 3 trial.

The most progressed cathepsin K inhibitor was odanacatib; encouraging evidence from phase 2 clinical trials showed progressive lumbar spine, total hip and femoral neck BMD gains in postmenopausal women but a higher incidence of a composite of cardiovascular death, myocardial infarction or stroke, new onset atrial fibrillation and stroke alone have been observed in treatment groups leading to the research programme being abandoned. The underlying mechanism or mechanisms for the relationship between cathepsin K inhibitor and increased cardiovascular risks remain unclear, but it is unlikely cathepsin K inhibitors will become part of osteoporosis management in the near future [74–78].

Other Promising Therapies

Blosozumab is another potential therapeutics in the same class of category as romosozumab. It is a humanised immunoglobulin G4 monoclonal antibody against sclerostin. A multiple dosing phase 2 trial found the use of Blosozumab was associated with statistically significant dose-related increase BMD at lumbar, femoral neck and total hip sites [79]. The frequencies of adverse events were similar across all groups except for mild injection site reactions were reported more frequently in the blosozumab groups than placebo. Thirty-five percent of participants developed anti-blosozumab antibodies after exposure, with some suggestions this may blunt efficacy.

Conclusion

While fewer anabolic therapies have been available to clinicians to date, with many potential therapies failing late in clinical testing due to safety concerns, recent advances have led to significant new opportunities in the management of osteoporosis.

References

1. Compston JE, McClung MR, Leslie WD. Osteoporosis. Lancet. 2019;393(10169):364–76.
2. Langub MC, Monier-Faugere MC, Qi Q, et al. Parathyroid hormone/parathyroid hormone-related peptide type 1 receptor in human bone. J Bone Miner Res. 2001;16(3):448–56.
3. Silva BC, Costa AG, Cusano NE, et al. Catabolic and anabolic actions of parathyroid hormone on the skeleton. J Endocrinol Invest. 2011;34(10):801–10.
4. Dempster DW, Cosman F, Parisien M, et al. Anabolic actions of parathyroid hormone on bone. Endocr Rev. 1993;14(6):690–709.
5. Compston JE. Skeletal actions of intermittent parathyroid hormone: effects on bone remodelling and structure. Bone. 2007;40(6):1447–52.
6. Administration FaD. Forteo (teriparatide) injection. 2020. https://www.accessdata.fda.gov/drugsatfda_docs/label/2020/021318s053lbl.pdf.
7. Agency EM. Forsteo (teriparatide). 2020. https://www.ema.europa.eu/en/medicines/human/EPAR/forsteo.
8. Dempster DW, Cosman F, Kurland ES, et al. Effects of daily treatment with parathyroid hormone on bone microarchitecture and turnover in patients with osteoporosis: a paired biopsy study. J Bone Miner Res. 2001;16(10):1846–53.
9. Neer RM, Arnaud CD, Zanchetta JR, et al. Effect of parathyroid hormone (1-34) on fractures and Bone mineral density in postmenopausal women with osteoporosis. N Engl J Med. 2001;344(19):1434–41.
10. Hodsman AB, Kisiel M, Adachi JD, et al. Histomorphometric evidence for increased bone turnover without change in cortical thickness or porosity after 2 years of cyclical hPTH(1-34) therapy in women with severe osteoporosis. Bone. 2000;27(2):311–8.
11. Kurland ES, Cosman F, McMahon DJ, et al. Parathyroid hormone as a therapy for idiopathic osteoporosis in men: effects on bone mineral density and bone markers. J Clin Endocrinol Metab. 2000;85(9):3069–76.
12. Fujita T, Inoue T, Morii H, et al. Effect of an intermittent weekly dose of human parathyroid hormone (1-34) on osteoporosis: a randomized double-masked prospective study using three dose levels. Osteoporos Int. 1999;9(4):296–306.
13. Lindsay R, Nieves J, Formica C, et al. Randomised controlled study of effect of parathyroid hormone on vertebral-bone mass and fracture incidence among postmenopausal women on oestrogen with osteoporosis. Lancet. 1997;350(9077):550–5.
14. Vahle JL, Long GG, Sandusky G, et al. Bone neoplasms in F344 rats given teriparatide [rhPTH(1-34)] are dependent on duration of treatment and dose. Toxicol Pathol. 2004;32(4):426–38.
15. Díez-Pérez A, Marin F, Eriksen EF, et al. Effects of teriparatide on hip and upper limb fractures in patients with osteoporosis: a systematic review and meta-analysis. Bone. 2019;120:1–8.
16. Simpson EL, Martyn-St James M, Hamilton J, et al. Clinical effectiveness of denosumab, raloxifene, romosozumab, and teriparatide for the prevention of osteoporotic fragility fractures: a systematic review and network meta-analysis. Bone. 2020;130:115081.
17. Barrionuevo P, Kapoor E, Asi N, et al. Efficacy of pharmacological therapies for the prevention of fractures in postmenopausal women: a network meta-analysis. J Clin Endocrinol Metabol. 2019;104(5):1623–30.
18. Kendler DL, Marin F, Zerbini CAF, et al. Effects of teriparatide and risedronate on new fractures in post-menopausal women with severe osteoporosis (VERO): a multicentre, double-blind, double-dummy, randomised controlled trial. Lancet. 2018;391(10117):230–40.
19. Tsai JN, Uihlein AV, Lee H, et al. Teriparatide and denosumab, alone or combined, in women with postmenopausal osteoporosis: the DATA study randomised trial. Lancet. 2013;382(9886):50–6.
20. Leder BZ, Tsai JN, Uihlein AV, et al. Two years of Denosumab and teriparatide administration in postmenopausal women with osteoporosis (the DATA extension study): a randomized controlled trial. J Clin Endocrinol Metab. 2014;99(5):1694–700.

21. Boonen S, Marin F, Obermayer-Pietsch B, et al. Effects of previous antiresorptive therapy on the bone mineral density response to two years of teriparatide treatment in postmenopausal women with osteoporosis. J Clin Endocrinol Metab. 2008;93(3):852–60.
22. Miller PD, Schwartz EN, Chen P, et al. Teriparatide in postmenopausal women with osteoporosis and mild or moderate renal impairment. Osteoporos Int. 2007;18(1):59–68.
23. Gold DT, Pantos BS, Masica DN, et al. Initial experience with teriparatide in the United States. Curr Med Res Opin. 2006;22(4):703–8.
24. Obermayer-Pietsch BM, Marin F, McCloskey EV, et al. Effects of two years of daily teriparatide treatment on BMD in postmenopausal women with severe osteoporosis with and without prior antiresorptive treatment. J Bone Miner Res. 2008;23(10):1591–600.
25. Watanabe A, Yoneyama S, Nakajima M, et al. Osteosarcoma in Sprague-Dawley rats after long-term treatment with teriparatide (human parathyroid hormone (1-34)). J Toxicol Sci. 2012;37(3):617–29.
26. Vahle JL, Zuehlke U, Schmidt A, et al. Lack of Bone neoplasms and persistence of bone efficacy in cynomolgus macaques after long-term treatment with teriparatide [rhPTH(1-34)]. J Bone Miner Res. 2008;23(12):2033–9.
27. Fox J, Miller MA, Newman MK, et al. Treatment of skeletally mature ovariectomized rhesus monkeys with PTH(1-84) for 16 months increases bone formation and density and improves trabecular architecture and biomechanical properties at the lumbar spine. J Bone Miner Res. 2007;22(2):260–73.
28. Greenspan SL, Bone HG, Ettinger MP, et al. Effect of recombinant human parathyroid hormone (1-84) on vertebral fracture and bone mineral density in postmenopausal women with osteoporosis: a randomized trial. Ann Intern Med. 2007;146(5):326–39.
29. Andrews EB, Gilsenan AW, Midkiff K, et al. The US postmarketing surveillance study of adult osteosarcoma and teriparatide: study design and findings from the first 7 years. J Bone Miner Res. 2012;27(12):2429–37.
30. Gilsenan A, Harding A, Kellier-Steele N, et al. The Forteo patient registry linkage to multiple state cancer registries: study design and results from the first 8 years. Osteoporos Int. 2018;29(10):2335–43.
31. Gilsenan A, MK, Harris D, Kellier-Steele N, Andrews EA, editors. Results from a fifteen-year postmarketing drug safety surveillance studyof adult osteosarcoma and teriparatide in the US. North American Association of Central Cancer Registries Annual Conference, Vancouver, British Columbia, Canada; 2019.
32. Shi Z, Zhou H, Pan B, et al. Effectiveness of teriparatide on fracture healing: a systematic review and meta-analysis. PLoS One. 2016;11(12):e0168691.
33. Lou S, Lv H, Wang G, et al. The effect of teriparatide on fracture healing of osteoporotic patients: a meta-analysis of randomized controlled trials. Biomed Res Int. 2016;2016:6040379.
34. van de Laarschot DM, McKenna MJ, Abrahamsen B, et al. Medical management of patients after atypical femur fractures: a systematic review and recommendations from the European Calcified Tissue Society. J Clin Endocrinol Metab. 2020;105(5):1682–99.
35. Miller PD, Delmas PD, Lindsay R, et al. Early responsiveness of women with osteoporosis to teriparatide after therapy with alendronate or risedronate. J Clin Endocrinol Metab. 2008;93(10):3785–93.
36. Ettinger B, San Martin J, Crans G, Pavo I. Differential effects of teriparatide on BMD after treatment with raloxifene or alendronate. J Bone Miner Res. 2004;19(5):745–51.
37. Cosman F, Nieves J, Zion M, et al. Daily and cyclic parathyroid hormone in women receiving alendronate. N Engl J Med. 2005;353(6):566–75.
38. Cosman F, Eriksen EF, Recknor C, et al. Effects of intravenous zoledronic acid plus subcutaneous teriparatide [rhPTH(1-34)] in postmenopausal osteoporosis. J Bone Miner Res. 2011;26(3):503–11.
39. Cosman F, Nieves JW, Zion M, et al. Effect of prior and ongoing raloxifene therapy on response to PTH and maintenance of BMD after PTH therapy. Osteoporos Int. 2008;19(4):529–35.

40. Cosman F, Nieves JW, Roimisher C, et al. Administration of teriparatide for four years cyclically compared to two years daily in treatment Naïve and alendronate treated women. Bone. 2019;120:246–53.
41. Administration UFaD. TYMLOS™ (abaloparatide) injection. 2017. https://www.accessdata.fda.gov/drugsatfda_docs/label/2017/208743lbl.pdf.
42. Agency EM. Eladynos, abaloparatide. 2018. https://www.ema.europa.eu/en/medicines/human/EPAR/eladynos.
43. Leder BZ, O'Dea LS, Zanchetta JR, et al. Effects of abaloparatide, a human parathyroid hormone-related peptide analog, on bone mineral density in postmenopausal women with osteoporosis. J Clin Endocrinol Metab. 2015;100(2):697–706.
44. Miller PD, Hattersley G, Riis BJ, et al. Effect of Abaloparatide vs placebo on new vertebral fractures in postmenopausal women with osteoporosis: a randomized clinical trial. JAMA. 2016;316(7):722–33.
45. Bone HG, Cosman F, Miller PD, et al. ACTIVExtend: 24 months of alendronate after 18 months of Abaloparatide or placebo for postmenopausal osteoporosis. J Clin Endocrinol Metab. 2018;103(8):2949–57.
46. Leder BZ, Zapalowski C, Hu MY, et al. Fracture and bone mineral density response by baseline risk in patients treated with Abaloparatide followed by alendronate: results from the phase 3 ACTIVExtend trial. J Bone Miner Res. 2019;34(12):2213–9.
47. Reginster JY, Bianic F, Campbell R, et al. Abaloparatide for risk reduction of nonvertebral and vertebral fractures in postmenopausal women with osteoporosis: a network meta-analysis. Osteoporos Int. 2019;30(7):1465–73.
48. Cosman F, Peterson LR, Towler DA, et al. Cardiovascular safety of abaloparatide in postmenopausal women with osteoporosis: analysis From the ACTIVE phase 3 trial. J Clin Endocrinol Metab. 2020;105(11):3384–95.
49. Baron R, Kneissel M. WNT signaling in bone homeostasis and disease: from human mutations to treatments. Nat Med. 2013;19(2):179–92.
50. Poole KE, van Bezooijen RL, Loveridge N, et al. Sclerostin is a delayed secreted product of osteocytes that inhibits bone formation. FASEB J. 2005;19(13):1842–4.
51. Li X, Ominsky MS, Warmington KS, et al. Sclerostin antibody treatment increases bone formation, bone mass, and bone strength in a rat model of postmenopausal osteoporosis. J Bone Miner Res. 2009;24(4):578–88.
52. Ominsky MS, Vlasseros F, Jolette J, et al. Two doses of sclerostin antibody in cynomolgus monkeys increases bone formation, bone mineral density, and bone strength. J Bone Miner Res. 2010;25(5):948–59.
53. Ke HZ, Richards WG, Li X, Ominsky MS. Sclerostin and Dickkopf-1 as therapeutic targets in bone diseases. Endocr Rev. 2012;33(5):747–83.
54. Nioi P, Taylor S, Hu R, et al. Transcriptional profiling of laser capture microdissected subpopulations of the osteoblast lineage provides insight into the early response to Sclerostin antibody in rats. J Bone Miner Res. 2015;30(8):1457–67.
55. Kim SW, Lu Y, Williams EA, et al. Sclerostin antibody administration converts bone lining cells into active osteoblasts. J Bone Miner Res. 2017;32(5):892–901.
56. Li X, Ominsky MS, Villasenor KS, et al. Sclerostin antibody reverses bone loss by increasing bone formation and decreasing bone resorption in a rat model of male osteoporosis. Endocrinology. 2018;159(1):260–71.
57. Padhi D, Jang G, Stouch B, et al. Single-dose, placebo-controlled, randomized study of AMG 785, a sclerostin monoclonal antibody. J Bone Miner Res. 2011;26(1):19–26.
58. Ominsky MS, Niu QT, Li C, et al. Tissue-level mechanisms responsible for the increase in bone formation and bone volume by sclerostin antibody. J Bone Miner Res. 2014;29(6):1424–30.
59. McClung MR, Grauer A, Boonen S, et al. Romosozumab in postmenopausal women with low bone mineral density. N Engl J Med. 2014;370(5):412–20.
60. Ominsky MS, Boyce RW, Li X, Ke HZ. Effects of sclerostin antibodies in animal models of osteoporosis. Bone. 2017;96:63–75.

61. Cosman F, Crittenden DB, Adachi JD, et al. Romosozumab treatment in postmenopausal women with osteoporosis. N Engl J Med. 2016;375(16):1532–43.
62. Saag KG, Petersen J, Brandi ML, et al. Romosozumab or alendronate for fracture prevention in women with osteoporosis. N Engl J Med. 2017;377(15):1417–27.
63. Lewiecki EM, Blicharski T, Goemaere S, et al. A phase III randomized placebo-controlled trial to evaluate efficacy and safety of Romosozumab in men with osteoporosis. J Clin Endocrinol Metabol. 2018;103(9):3183–93.
64. Langdahl BL, Libanati C, Crittenden DB, et al. Romosozumab (sclerostin monoclonal antibody) versus teriparatide in postmenopausal women with osteoporosis transitioning from oral bisphosphonate therapy: a randomised, open-label, phase 3 trial. Lancet. 2017;390(10102):1585–94.
65. Liu Y, Cao Y, Zhang S, et al. Romosozumab treatment in postmenopausal women with osteoporosis: a meta-analysis of randomized controlled trials. Climacteric. 2018;21(2):189–95.
66. Kaveh S, Hosseinifard H, Ghadimi N, et al. Efficacy and safety of Romosozumab in treatment for low bone mineral density: a systematic review and meta-analysis. Clin Rheumatol. 2020;39(11):3261–76.
67. Agency EM. Biosimilars in the EU: Information guide for healthcare professionals. 2017 [updated 29/10/2019]. https://www.ema.europa.eu/en/documents/leaflet/biosimilars-eu-information-guide-healthcare-professionals_en.pdf.
68. Takács I, Jókai E, Kováts DE, Aradi I. The first biosimilar approved for the treatment of osteoporosis: results of a comparative pharmacokinetic/pharmacodynamic study. Osteoporos Int. 2019;30(3):675–83.
69. Hagino H, Narita R, Yokoyama Y, et al. A multicenter, randomized, rater-blinded, parallel-group, phase 3 study to compare the efficacy, safety, and immunogenicity of biosimilar RGB-10 and reference once-daily teriparatide in patients with osteoporosis. Osteoporos Int. 2019;30(10):2027–37.
70. Drake MT, Clarke BL, Oursler MJ, Khosla S. Cathepsin K inhibitors for osteoporosis: biology, potential clinical utility, and lessons learned. Endocr Rev. 2017;38(4):325–50.
71. Adami S, Supronik J, Hala T, et al. Effect of one year treatment with the cathepsin-K inhibitor, balicatib, on bone mineral density (BMD) in postmenopausal women with osteopenia/osteoporosis. 2006. S24-S p.
72. Peroni A, Zini A, Braga V, et al. Drug-induced morphea: report of a case induced by balicatib and review of the literature. J Am Acad Dermatol. 2008;59(1):125–9.
73. Eastell R, Nagase S, Ohyama M, et al. Safety and efficacy of the cathepsin K inhibitor ONO-5334 in postmenopausal osteoporosis: the OCEAN study. J Bone Miner Res. 2011;26(6):1303–12.
74. Eisman JA, Bone HG, Hosking DJ, et al. Odanacatib in the treatment of postmenopausal women with low bone mineral density: three-year continued therapy and resolution of effect. J Bone Miner Res. 2011;26(2):242–51.
75. Bone HG, McClung MR, Roux C, et al. Odanacatib, a cathepsin-K inhibitor for osteoporosis: a two-year study in postmenopausal women with low bone density. J Bone Miner Res. 2010;25(5):937–47.
76. Brixen K, Chapurlat R, Cheung AM, et al. Bone density, turnover, and estimated strength in postmenopausal women treated with odanacatib: a randomized trial. J Clin Endocrinol Metab. 2013;98(2):571–80.
77. Bone HG, Dempster DW, Eisman JA, et al. Odanacatib for the treatment of postmenopausal osteoporosis: development history and design and participant characteristics of LOFT, the long-term odanacatib fracture trial. Osteoporos Int. 2015;26(2):699–712.
78. McClung MR, O'Donoghue ML, Papapoulos SE, et al. Odanacatib for the treatment of postmenopausal osteoporosis: results of the LOFT multicentre, randomised, double-blind, placebo-controlled trial and LOFT extension study. Lancet Diabetes Endocrinol. 2019;7(12):899–911.
79. Recker RR, Benson CT, Matsumoto T, et al. A randomized, double-blind phase 2 clinical trial of blosozumab, a sclerostin antibody, in postmenopausal women with low bone mineral density. J Bone Miner Res. 2015;30(2):216–24.

Chapter 7
The Osteoporosis Treatment Gap

Elizabeth M. Curtis, Cyrus Cooper, and Nicholas C. Harvey

Introduction

Osteoporosis has evolved over recent decades from being viewed as an inevitable consequence of ageing to becoming a recognised disease, with a diagnostic definition, validated methods of assessment, and a wide range of highly effective medications [1, 2]. However, it is apparent that despite these advances, the care of people with osteoporosis is still far from optimal worldwide: indeed most men and women at high fracture risk do not receive treatment [3]. This is true even in patients who have sustained a fragility fracture, with, in many cases, fewer than 20% actually receiving therapies to reduce the risk of fracture in the year following the fracture

E. M. Curtis (✉)
MRC Lifecourse Epidemiology Centre, University of Southampton, Southampton General Hospital, Southampton, UK

Rheumatology Department, University Hospitals Southampton NHS Foundation Trust, Southampton, UK
e-mail: bc@mrc.soton.ac.uk

C. Cooper
MRC Lifecourse Epidemiology Centre, University of Southampton, Southampton General Hospital, Southampton, UK

NIHR Oxford Biomedical Research Unit, University of Oxford, Oxford, UK

NIHR Southampton Biomedical Research Centre, University of Southampton and University Hospitals Southampton NHS Foundation Trust, Southampton, UK
e-mail: cc@mrc.soton.ac.uk

N. C. Harvey
MRC Lifecourse Epidemiology Centre, University of Southampton, Southampton General Hospital, Southampton, UK

NIHR Southampton Biomedical Research Centre, University of Southampton and University Hospitals Southampton NHS Foundation Trust, Southampton, UK
e-mail: nch@mrc.soton.ac.uk

E. Dennison (ed.), *Osteoporosis Treatment*, https://doi.org/10.1007/978-3-030-78128-6_7

[4, 5]. Rates of treatment are particularly poor for older women and those living in long-term care. Large gaps in service provision exist; indeed the use of fracture risk assessment tools (such as FRAX®) varies 1000-fold worldwide. This variability is far greater than the 30-fold variation in crude, or ten-fold variation in age-standardised, hip fracture incidence globally [6, 7]. Global variation in availability of internet access, lack of national assessment guidelines for osteoporosis in many countries, and the presence of alternative assessment algorithms only partially explain these differences [6].

Whilst the under-assessment and treatment of those at very high risk of further fracture is of great concern, even more alarming is the apparent downward trend in treatment with anti-osteoporosis medications after hip fracture, which has been demonstrated both in the USA, European and UK populations [8, 9]. There are many potential causes for this trend, including the elevation of concerns regarding rare but serious anti-resorptive drug-related side effects such as atypical femoral fractures and osteonecrosis of the jaw, and the recent changes to treatment reimbursement in the US [3]. In this chapter, we present an overview of the reasons for suboptimal osteoporosis care, or "treatment gaps", at all levels, and discuss possible remedial approaches.

The Osteoporosis Treatment Gap

A Minority of Patients at High Fracture Risk Receive Appropriate Assessment and Treatment

It is widely recognised that disparities exist between the population at high fracture risk, or who have experienced a low trauma fracture, and the number who receive appropriate osteoporosis assessment and treatment [3]. As an example, in the UK, analysis of the Clinical Practice Research Datalink (CPRD) has demonstrated inadequacies in both primary and secondary fracture prevention. Initial improvements in prescription rates were encouraging; following a hip fracture in the UK, the probability of anti-osteoporosis drug prescription increased from just 7% in 2000, to 46% in 2010 [10], with older patients (≥75 years of age) particularly benefiting from this trend. At any given point in time, the cumulative incidence of anti-osteoporosis therapy was greater in women (8% in 2000, 51% in 2010) than in men (4% in 2000, 34% in 2010). Given this steady increase in the awareness of the need for anti-osteoporosis drugs over a 10 year period, a continued trend in increased prescribing would have made perfect sense. However, despite fewer than 50% of hip fracture patients receiving treatment, from around 2011, a plateau and a possible decrease in prescriptions has occurred in the UK [11]. Local trends in prescribing anti-osteoporosis therapies appeared to persist over time, with substantial geographic heterogeneity within the UK, for example, in the North East of the UK the odds ratio for anti-osteoporosis medication following a hip fracture was 1.29 (95% CI:

0.89, 1.87) and in the South Central region 0.56 (95% CI: 0.43, 0.73), the North West being the referent. Over the subsequent 5-years of follow-up, these geographic trends persisted indicating systematic differences in provision of osteoporosis care [12].

The Treatment Gap in Osteoporosis Is a Worldwide Problem

Such patterns in secondary fracture prevention are present in many countries. A prospective observational study of over 60,000 older women recruited from primary care practices in ten countries across US, Europe and Australia (the GLOW study), demonstrated that over 80% of women with a fragility fracture did not receive osteoporosis treatment [13]. In another international prospective study of 1795 patients who sustained a low trauma hip fractures in ten countries (Australia, Austria, Estonia, France, Italy, Lithuania, Mexico, Russia, Spain, and the UK), just 27% were prescribed anti-osteoporosis therapy after the hip fracture [14].

Trends in prescribing (incorporating both primary and secondary prevention) are consistent with these findings. Figure 7.1 shows that anti-osteoporosis medication prescription rates in the UK rose from 2.3 to 169.7 prescriptions per 10,000 person-years amongst women from 1990 to 2006. However, following this rise, prescription rates plateaued and then decreased by 12% from 2009 to 2012 (Fig. 7.1).

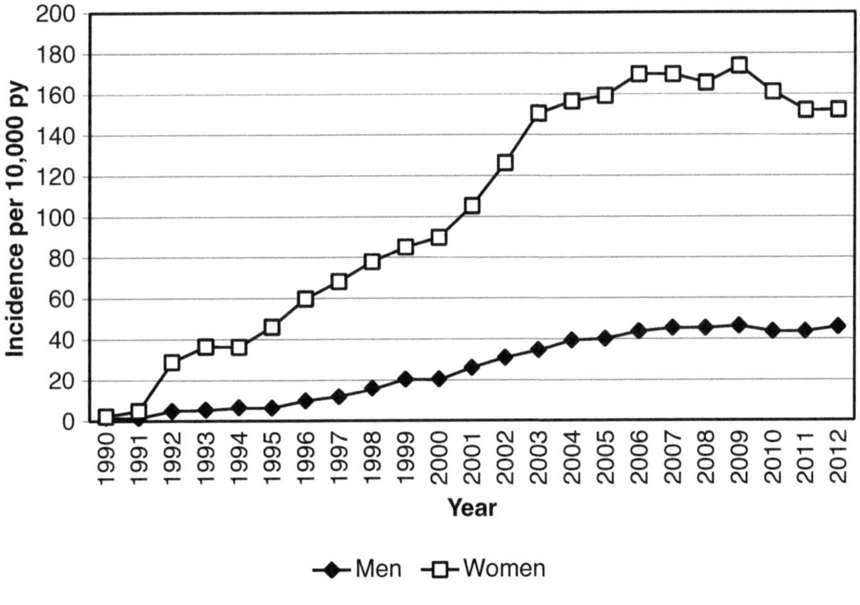

Fig. 7.1 Antiosteoporosis medication prescription incidence from 1990–2012 in the UK population aged 50 years or over, reproduced with permission from [15]

In men, prescription rates rose less steeply from 1990 to 2007 and then plateaued from 2008 onwards, with marked differences in prescription of anti-osteoporosis medications according to ethnicity and geographic location in both sexes [15].

Treatment uptake for osteoporosis similarly increased in Europe up to 2008, thereafter plateaued, and in more recent years has fallen [16]. Within Europe, there is marked inter-country variation in the treatment of individuals at high risk of osteoporotic fracture [16]. The percentage of patients at high fracture risk (defined using FRAX®) who were not treated (the "treatment gap") varied from just 25% in Spain to 95% in Bulgaria. It was estimated that, within the EU in 2010, out of the 21.3 million men and women who exceeded FRAX "high risk" level, 12.3 million (58%) were untreated [14, 16–19]. Similar findings have been documented in a more recent study of six European countries (Fig. 7.2) [20]. These estimates are conservative, since treatment will have been given to an unknown proportion of low risk women [21], though have been supported by findings from Spanish studies using individual-level data from primary care prescription databases from over 1.5 million participants [22]. In Danish registry studies, osteoporosis medication use plateaued in 2014 and declined thereafter. Interestingly, hip fracture rates also declined between 2005 and 2015 by 30%, but only 20% (at most) of the observed reduction could be attributed to treatment. The authors concluded that the magnitude of anti-osteoporosis therapy use was insufficient to make a meaningful impact on the fracture burden within Danish society and represented a missed opportunity for reducing hip fracture rates [23].

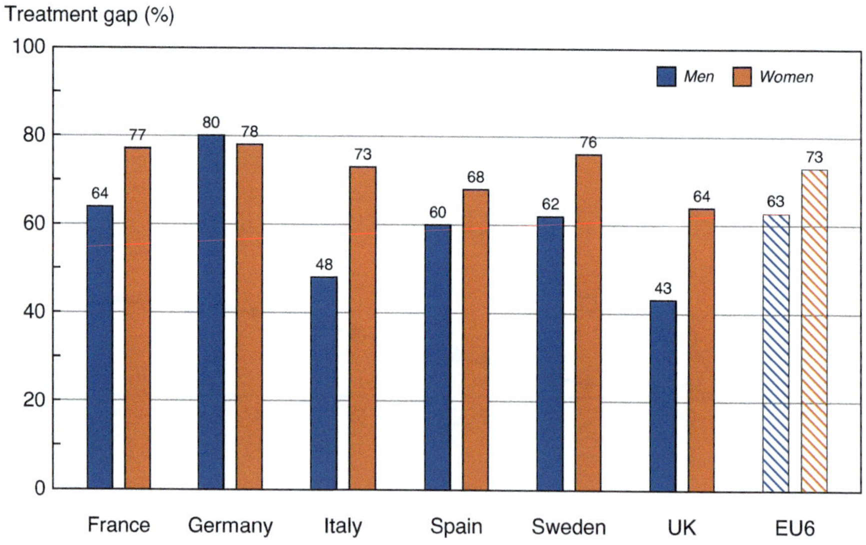

Fig. 7.2 The treatment gap in six European countries in 2017. The figure shows the percentage of women at high fracture risk who do not receive antiosteoporosis treatment. (Reproduced with permission from [20])

Similar findings have emerged from a large retrospective analysis using U.S. administrative insurance claims data of almost 100,000 men and women aged over 50 years who were hospitalized for hip fracture [8]. The study examined the uptake of osteoporosis medication within a year of hospital discharge; the estimated probability of receiving osteoporosis medication within this time period was 28.5% but showed a significant decline over a 10-year interval, from 40.2% in 2002 to 20.5% in 2011 [8]. Findings from the US Medical Expenditure Panel Survey are supportive of this, demonstrating a marked reduction in the prevalence of bisphosphonate use from 2007 onwards, particularly among women [24].

Reasons for the Treatment Gap in Osteoporosis

Awareness of the Condition and Perception of Benefit/ Risk Balance

As shown by the studies cited above, anti-resorptive treatment rates both in primary and secondary fracture prevention increased until 5–10 years ago. The clinical situation was bolstered by policy and risk assessment advances, including the use of FRAX® and other risk calculators, [25, 26] guidance on intervention [17, 19, 27], combined with the availability of cheaper, generic bisphosphonates. In spite of this outwardly prospering field, treatment rates have sadly declined in recent years, both in those at high risk of fracture and in those who have suffered a fracture, despite the huge expansion of the at-risk population [28].

Many factors appear to contribute to this phenomenon. One such reason is that strategies at a national and international level have not been implemented sufficiently to impact primary and secondary prevention. For patients and clinicians alike, the idea of managing a future "risk" makes primary fracture prevention more difficult, rather than treating a disease event which has already impacted the patient. Musculoskeletal diseases in general are viewed by policymakers and patients alike as a of lesser importance than outcomes such as cancers and heart disease [3], despite the fact that the musculoskeletal disease has been shown to be a leading course of disability worldwide by the Global Burden of Disease initiative [29]. Indeed the disability associated with fragility fractures in the population is comparable to that imposed by lung cancer, chronic obstructive pulmonary disease and ischaemic stroke (Fig. 7.3) [20].

In the case of osteoporosis, there is a stark mismatch between the perceived and actual severity of the condition. Many do not recognise that, for example, a hip fracture is associated with a 20% associated reduced survival compared with non-fracture peers and, as such, is a devastating life event [1]. Contrast this with a parallel event such as an acute myocardial infarction: it is unimaginable that it would be acceptable in the developed world for less than 50% of such cardiac patients to receive risk-reducing therapies such as aspirin and other antiplatelet agents,

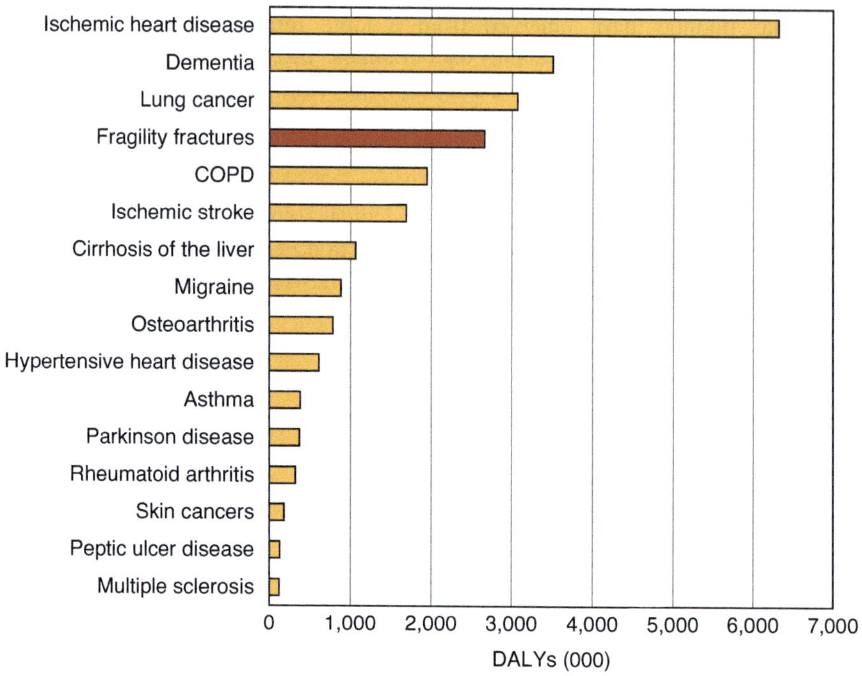

Fig. 7.3 Disability adjusted life years by disease in six European countries covering 17 selected non-communicable diseases. (Reproduced with permission from [20])

antihypertensives and statins [30]. A large international cohort of older women, GLOW, clearly documents this risk misperception, in which many underestimated their own fracture risk in comparison to their peers [31].

Physicians' perceptions of osteoporosis and efficacy of treatments have been further confused by harmful and inaccurate conclusions about the treatment of osteoporosis in high impact journals [32, 33]. Despite overwhelming evidence (as stated by international and national societies such as the International Osteoporosis Foundation and the American Society for Bone and Mineral Research), clear damage has been done [34].

Concerns about Rare but Serious Side-Effects Have Been Overemphasized

There are abundant data showing that alarming reports about osteoporosis medication in the media have been followed by a reduction in use of these medications, despite evidence that the benefits of treatment clearly outweigh the risks for the vast majority of users [35]. In order to better understand patients' concerns regarding medication safety, one study used data from the Medical Expenditure Panel Survey and National Inpatient Sample in the US to examine relationships between medication use, internet searches for alendronate 2006–2010, and safety concerns reported in the media [24]. Clear spikes of internet search activity were observed to correspond to events such as a 2006 lawsuit filed against Merck (for Fosamax allegedly causing osteonecrosis of the jaw (ONJ)), an ABC World News feature in 2010 on the associations between Fosamax and atypical femoral fractures (AFFs), and various other reports in the media serious but rare side effects, set in parallel with the regression in bisphosphonate use by more than 50% between 2008 and 2012. The Australian Longitudinal Study on Women's Health findings were in keeping with the findings from the US; anti-osteoporosis medication use grew over the period 2000 to 2007 but then shrank from 2007 to 2010. In Australia, interventions to remedy this, including the relaxation of the indications for bone density testing and a subsidy for anti-osteoporosis medications had little effect; the most marked declines in prescriptions coincided with negative press for antiresorptive therapy such as a 2007 major report on ONJ [36].

In absolute terms, the serious long-term adverse side-effects of bisphosphonates are very rare (with incidences ranging from 1/100,000 to 1/10,000 per year) [37]. However, the approach to risk/benefit communication has largely been on the side of declaring risk, amongst the media (as demonstrated above), physicians and policymakers. The substantial impact of the underlying condition on morbidity and increased mortality, with fracture risk markedly decreased by anti-osteoporosis medications, appears often forgotten in these discussions. For example, UK National Institute for Health and Care Excellence (NICE) recently issued guidance on multimorbidity [38], and targeted bisphosphonates for review after 3 years treatment despite the evidence for their longer term efficacy and safety being of greater reliability than the other treatments considered for 3 year review.

In a recent review of the benefits versus risks for BP therapy [39], the benefits for fracture reduction for short-term therapy for 3–5 years was shown to far outweigh any risks of AFFs. Using the set of assumptions about AFF risk with best evidence [relative risk of 1.7 for any BP use [40]], the study states that treating 10,000 osteoporotic women for 3 years would lead to the prevention of 1000 fractures (including 110 hip fractures) whilst causing only 0.08 AFFs. Put another way, for one AFF associated with 3 years of BP treatment, 1200 fractures (including about 130 hip and 850 vertebral fractures) would be prevented [41].

In longer term users, the concerns regarding the rare side effects of AFFs and ONJ are compounded by studies suggesting that longer therapy duration increases these risks. This has led to the widely held opinion that all patients on long-term treatment with bisphosphonates or denosumab should be offered a treatment holiday: however the existing evidence does not entirely support this. For example, following denosumab discontinuation rapid bone loss has been described, with around a 5% incidence of vertebral fractures [42], indicating that treatment holidays on denosumab should not be offered without replacing with another anti-osteoporosis therapy. In terms of long term bisphosphonate use, reassuringly, a Danish study has demonstrated that users of alendronate, even after 10 years of use, have a lasting reduction in fracture risk compared with matched controls, and that the number of hip fractures prevented is still substantially greater than the number of subtrochanteric femoral fractures occurring [43]. A new systematic review led by the International Osteoporosis Foundation has concluded that drug holidays should only be considered in patients at low fracture risk [44]. Thus, it is evident that the osteoporosis field needs to vastly improve its approach to communicating the balance of treatment risks and benefits, and to work towards countering poorly evidenced stories in the media, as and when they occur.

Global Shortfall in Policies Addressing Bone Health

Osteoporosis, when compared with other non-communicable diseases, has rarely attracted justifiable levels of attention from governments, policy makers and healthcare providers. National policies on access to, and reimbursement of measurement of bone density with dual-energy x-ray absorptiometry (DXA) will have a great impact on the assessment and treatment of this disease. Various regional audits have been published by the International Osteoporosis Foundation (IOF) (https://www.iofbonehealth.org/regional-audits) covering Latin America, the European Union, Eastern Europe, the Middle East, Africa, Central Asia, and Asia Pacific. These have demonstrated large variations in terms of the epidemiology, financial and societal costs and burden of osteoporosis e.g. in the Asia Pacific region, whilst Hong Kong, Japan, Republic of Korea, Singapore, Australia and New Zealand, had 12–24 DXA machines per million of population, India, Pakistan, China, Indonesia, Philippines, Sri Lanka and Vietnam were severely under-resourced, having less than 1 DXA machine per million of population. The audits demonstrated that insurance or healthcare policies in many countries did not reimburse BMD testing and osteoporosis treatment which served as a barrier to osteoporosis care access. Similar inequalities were seen in Europe, where it was calculated that 11 DXA machines per million of population were needed for adequate osteoporosis care provision. Only 16 European countries fell into this category of "adequate" provision, and 9 countries were considered to have "very inadequate" provision with fewer than 8.4 DXA units per million (the UK, Luxembourg, Czech Republic, Hungary, Bulgaria, Latvia, Lithuania, Poland and Romania) [45]. In addition, reimbursement for DXA scanning was extremely variable between EU member states; with reimbursement only offered if the BMD demonstrated osteoporosis in certain countries (Bulgaria and Switzerland), only if BMD was measured after a fracture (Germany), or only if the patient was referred by a specialist (Poland).

Whilst no official IOF audit is available for North America, treatment reimbursement also varies greatly, depending on each patient's health insurance. The evolution of healthcare reform in the USA from a "fee for service" system to a system which supports improved disease prevention and care coordination, with financial incentives to encourage healthcare professionals or systems to improve patient outcomes ought to improve osteoporosis detection and treatment. However, the number of DXA providers has fallen following a major drop in reimbursement in this area, resulting in over one million fewer DXA scans performed per year in women aged 50–64 in recent years [46], a change which coincides with a plateau in the secular decline (up until 2012) in age and sex adjusted hip fracture rates [47].

Approaches to Close the Osteoporosis Treatment Gap

Identification, Assessment and Treatment of Individuals Who Experience an Osteoporotic Fracture

As described by the evidence detailed above, fragility fractures represent a huge burden on societies worldwide. Patient perception of fracture risk is often underestimated, as osteoporosis is a silent condition until a fracture happens [48, 49]. Therefore, primary prevention is usually reliant on health care practitioners who need to have the time and incentive to assess fracture risk and explain the purpose of treatment to their patients. Consequently, secondary prevention, in which patients are identified for treatment on the basis of a previous low trauma fracture, is the approach usually taken.

Several methods have been explored to enable fracture risk assessment and initiation of appropriate treatment – some based upon staff, others on IT and others upon a combination of the two. The multi-disciplinary Fracture Liaison Service (FLS) is one of the most successful of these systems [50, 51], incorporating rheumatologists, orthogeriatricians, other physicians, clinical nurse specialists and allied health professionals and is described in detail later in this book in the chapter on secondary fracture prevention [52]. "Capture the Fracture®", an initiative of the International Osteoporosis Foundation (http://www.capturethefracture.org/) is "a global campaign to facilitate the implementation of coordinated, multi-disciplinary models of care for secondary fracture prevention." [53, 54]. This scheme has helped to document the huge variation in the quality, scope and availability of secondary prevention facilities, not only within, but also between countries. The Capture the Fracture initiative aims to raise the quality and coverage of these services, and has been shown to be both clinically valuable and cost-effective [55]. A global call to action is now underway, bringing together international societies with the aim of closing the osteoporosis care gap and reversing the ongoing decline in anti-osteoporosis medications after fracture [56].

Vertebral fracture case finding is an additive approach to secondary fracture prevention, as many such events go undetected—it has been shown that around 12% of postmenopausal women with osteoporosis have one or more vertebral deformities, but fewer than one in three of these individuals come to clinical attention [57]. Primary care-based screening strategies [58], and history taking methods distinguishing "vertebral fracture-type back pain" from other types of back pain may assist their detection [59]. Different methods for radiological assessment of vertebral fractures exist, including radiographs, CT scans and vertebral fracture software in DXA. The automated detection of prevalent vertebral fracture on CT scans using artificial intelligence technologies will be another avenue for secondary fracture prevention [60, 61].

Primary Prevention: Avoiding a First Fracture

In osteoporosis, there is ongoing debate regarding the benefits of a widespread systematic screening approach, leading to higher treatment rates (with its associated cost and side-effect risk), and a case-finding approach focused on those at highest individual risk (with its associated issue of under-treatment). Whilst DXA-based osteoporosis screening is officially a standard policy in the US (at age 65 years in women, age 70 in men, and in individuals over 50 years who have suffered a fracture as an adult) [62], in the majority of countries population screening is not judged to be cost-effective. Primary prevention is therefore generally focused on case-finding strategies, reliant on the physician identifying clinical risk factors [17–19, 63].

In the UK, a randomised controlled trial across seven centres was recently undertaken (the UK SCOOP study), examining both the clinical and cost-effectiveness of screening older women in primary care for primary fracture prevention, as described in detail in Chap. 2. The screening intervention was shown to lead to reduction in hip fracture risk by 28% [64, 65]. Additionally, over the 5-year follow-up, screening led to greater use of osteoporosis medications compared with the usual care arm, particularly in those screened participants found to be at high risk of fracture (73% vs 2% using osteoporosis medications), Fig. 7.4. Importantly, relative adherence to treatment was also 70% greater in these participants after 5 years [66]. Those at highest baseline fracture risk appeared to benefit most from screening (as would be

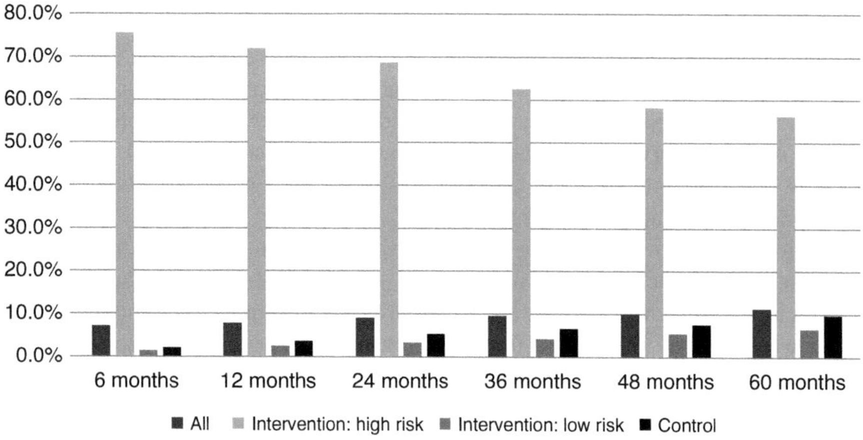

Fig. 7.4 Anti-osteoporosis medication use over the duration of the SCOOP trial by randomisation group (screening [intervention] vs usual care [control]). (Reproduced with permission from [66])

expected, since these were the individuals targeted for treatment) [67], and importantly, was shown to be cost-effective (the cost per quality adjusted life year (QALY) gained was £2772 compared with the control arm) [68] with long term cost effectiveness also demonstrated [69]. The finding that women who were identified by FRAX as moderate or high risk of fracture benefited most from a screening programme was supported by the Danish Risk Stratified Osteoporosis Strategy Evaluation (ROSE) study, though this study found no overall effect on fracture incidence of a screening strategy [70]. A lesser effect was observed in a further study in the Netherlands [71] and a recent meta-analysis of the three trials suggested that screening late to a 20% decrease in hip fracture risk [72]. A recent evidence report and systematic review for the US Preventive Services Task Force concluded that screening to prevent osteoporosis in women may reduce hip fractures [73].

Once a patient has been identified as requiring fracture risk assessment, the threshold at which treatment should be given will vary according to factors such as healthcare provision, willingness to pay and cost of medications [7]. The majority of guidelines internationally use FRAX® as the measure of fracture risk, but 38 of the 120 guidelines identified in a recent systematic review gave no direction on translating FRAX probabilities into a treatment decision [26]. Threshold setting is as much a philosophical as scientific process, which decides whether a level should be fixed, or age dependent, and calibrated to the specific country. Given the marked variation in fracture rates between countries, this latter consideration seems mandatory, and the benefits and caveats associated with fixed or age-dependent thresholds are presented in detail in [26]. In the UK, FRAX is linked to the age-dependent (up to the age of 70 years) thresholds of the National Osteoporosis Guideline Group (NOGG) [19], with the threshold predicated on the probability of future fracture conferred by a prior fracture. This approach has been shown to be cost effective in the UK, and Is the basis for 22 guidelines internationally [26], but contrasts markedly with that of the UK National Institute of Health and Care Excellence (NICE). In the 2017 technology appraisal of bisphosphonates [74], a pure health economic approach, in the context of a very common disease and extremely inexpensive therapies, led to a 1% risk of major osteoporotic fracture over 10 years as the threshold above which these medications were considered cost-effective. Unfortunately this was often interpreted as payers as an intervention threshold, a situation which if permitted to continue would have resulted in many adults at low risk of fracture being inappropriately treated [75], but which was later resolved by referral to NOGG guidance for clinical, rather than health economic thresholds [76]. Most recently, in a development of the IOF-ESCEO European Guidelines [27], the concept of a stratified approach to treatment based on fracture risk has been introduced such that those individuals at very high fracture risk might be considered for anabolic therapy first line [77]. This approach recognises the substantially raised risk of a further fracture within the first 2 years after an index fracture [78, 79] and the greater magnitude and faster time course of action of anabolic agents compared with antiresorptives. Such innovations in the approach to treatment should ensure that the most appropriate therapy is targeted to each individual based on their particular risk profile, and also that measures such as bone densitometry are used most efficiently (Fig. 7.5).

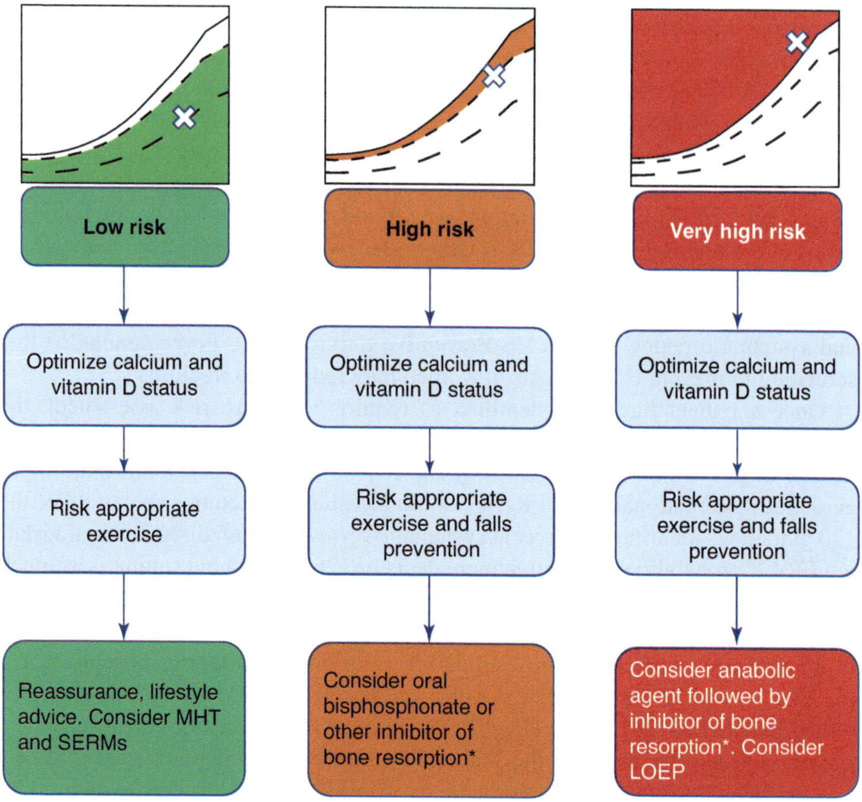

Fig. 7.5 Treatment options at different levels of baseline fracture risk. Reproduced with permission from [77]. Note that risk categories do not specifically correspond to age or menopause status. *LOEP* local osteoenhancement procedure

Conclusion

Recent decades have seen a dramatic transformation in osteoporosis, from having been viewed historically as an inescapable consequence of ageing, to now being recognised as an established chronic non-communicable disease, with diagnostic criteria, validated methods of risk assessment and an enviable range of therapeutic medications. Despite this backdrop, however, there is evidence from the UK, US and continental Europe that treatment rates have declined substantially in the last 5 years. With ageing populations and overstretched health services, osteoporosis may often fall off the list of priorities for both clinicians and patients. The rare but serious adverse effects of antiresorptive therapies have become a disproportionately (and an inappropriately) major concern, amplified by sensationalised media reports, which have usually been inadequately countered by the clinical academic community [5]. These fears and the resulting reduced prescribing have been exacerbated by reductions in reimbursement in the US, mirrored in new guidance. It is apparent that many patients, doctors and dentists and patients now appear more concerned by the rare but serious side effects of antiresorptives than they are of the osteoporosis and fragility fractures [5].

The clear imperative to urgently tackle this issue has been recognised by key organisations such as the International Osteoporosis Foundation and the American Society for Bone and Mineral Research, leading to the publication of recommendations and roadmaps to address the critical care gap in osteoporosis treatment [56, 80, 81]. Improved public awareness and public health strategies to improve bone health from a young age will also contribute to prevention of osteoporosis in future generations. Given the rapid ageing of the global population and the importance of good musculoskeletal health in old age, we must come together to ensure that during the coming decade, 2020–2030, hailed by the WHO and others as the "Decade of Healthy Ageing", bone health and fracture prevention become the priority they so urgently need to be.

References

1. Harvey N, Dennison E, Cooper C. Osteoporosis: impact on health and economics. Nat Rev Rheumatol. 2010;6(2):99–105.
2. Curtis EM, Moon RJ, Dennison EM, Harvey NC, Cooper C. Recent advances in the pathogenesis and treatment of osteoporosis. Clin Med. 2016;16(4):360–4. https://doi.org/10.7861/clinmedicine.16-4-360.
3. Harvey NC, McCloskey EV, Mitchell PJ, Dawson-Hughes B, Pierroz DD, Reginster JY, et al. Mind the (treatment) gap: a global perspective on current and future strategies for prevention of fragility fractures. Osteoporos Int. 2017;28(5):1507–29. https://doi.org/10.1007/s00198-016-3894-y.
4. Giangregorio L, Papaioannou A, Cranney A, Zytaruk N, Adachi JD. Fragility fractures and the osteoporosis care gap: an international phenomenon. Semin Arthritis Rheum. 2006;35(5):293–305. https://doi.org/10.1016/j.semarthrit.2005.11.001.
5. Kanis JA, Svedbom A, Harvey N, McCloskey EV. The osteoporosis treatment gap. J Bone Miner Res. 2014;29(9):1926–8. https://doi.org/10.1002/jbmr.2301.
6. Kanis JA, Johansson H, Oden A, Cooper C, McCloskey EV. Worldwide uptake of FRAX. Arch Osteoporos. 2014;9(1):166. https://doi.org/10.1007/s11657-013-0166-8.
7. Kanis JA, Oden A, McCloskey EV, Johansson H, Wahl DA, Cooper C. A systematic review of hip fracture incidence and probability of fracture worldwide. Osteoporos Int. 2012;23(9):2239–56. https://doi.org/10.1007/s00198-012-1964-3.
8. Solomon DH, Johnston SS, Boytsov NN, McMorrow D, Lane JM, Krohn KD. Osteoporosis medication use after hip fracture in U.S. patients between 2002 and 2011. J Bone Miner Res. 2014;29(9):1929–37. https://doi.org/10.1002/jbmr.2202.
9. van der Velde RY, Wyers CE, Teesselink E, Geusens PP, van den Bergh JP, de Vries F, et al. Trends in oral anti-osteoporosis drug prescription in the United Kingdom between 1990 and 2012: variation by age, sex, geographic location and ethnicity. Bone. 2016;94:50–5. https://doi.org/10.1016/j.bone.2016.10.013.
10. Klop C, Welsing PM, Cooper C, Harvey NC, Elders PJ, Bijlsma JW, et al. Mortality in British hip fracture patients, 2000-2010: a population-based retrospective cohort study. Bone. 2014;66:171–7. https://doi.org/10.1016/j.bone.2014.06.011.
11. Hawley S, Leal J, Delmestri A, Prieto-Alhambra D, Arden NK, Cooper C, et al. Anti-osteoporosis medication prescriptions and incidence of subsequent fracture among primary

hip fracture patients in England and Wales: an interrupted time-series analysis. J Bone Miner Res. 2016;31(11):2008–15. https://doi.org/10.1002/jbmr.2882.
12. Shah A, Prieto-Alhambra D, Hawley S, Delmestri A, Lippett J, Cooper C, et al. Geographic variation in secondary fracture prevention after a hip fracture during 1999-2013: a UK study. Osteoporos Int. 2017;28(1):169–78. https://doi.org/10.1007/s00198-016-3811-4.
13. Greenspan SL, Wyman A, Hooven FH, Adami S, Gehlbach S, Anderson FA Jr, et al. Predictors of treatment with osteoporosis medications after recent fragility fractures in a multinational cohort of postmenopausal women. J Am Geriatr Soc. 2012;60(3):455–61. https://doi.org/10.1111/j.1532-5415.2011.03854.x.
14. Svedbom A, Hernlund E, Ivergard M, Compston J, Cooper C, Stenmark J, et al. Osteoporosis in the European Union: a compendium of country-specific reports. Arch Osteoporos. 2013;8(1–2):137. https://doi.org/10.1007/s11657-013-0137-0.
15. van der Velde RY, Wyers CE, Teesselink E, Geusens PP, van den Bergh JP, de Vries F, et al. Trends in oral anti-osteoporosis drug prescription in the United Kingdom between 1990 and 2012: variation by age, sex, geographic location and ethnicity. Bone. 2017;94:50–5. https://doi.org/10.1016/j.bone.2016.10.013.
16. Hernlund E, Svedbom A, Ivergard M, Compston J, Cooper C, Stenmark J, et al. Osteoporosis in the European Union: medical management, epidemiology and economic burden: a report prepared in collaboration with the International Osteoporosis Foundation (IOF) and the European Federation of Pharmaceutical Industry Associations (EFPIA). Arch Osteoporos. 2013;8(1–2):136. https://doi.org/10.1007/s11657-013-0136-1.
17. Kanis JA, McCloskey EV, Johansson H, Cooper C, Rizzoli R, Reginster JY. European guidance for the diagnosis and management of osteoporosis in postmenopausal women. Osteoporos Int. 2013;24(1):23–57. https://doi.org/10.1007/s00198-012-2074-y.
18. Lekamwasam S, Adachi JD, Agnusdei D, Bilezikian J, Boonen S, Borgstrom F, et al. A framework for the development of guidelines for the management of glucocorticoid-induced osteoporosis. Osteoporos Int. 2012;23(9):2257–76. https://doi.org/10.1007/s00198-012-1958-1.
19. Compston J, Cooper A, Cooper C, Gittoes N, Gregson C, Harvey N, et al. UK clinical guideline for the prevention and treatment of osteoporosis. Arch Osteoporos. 2017;12(1):43. https://doi.org/10.1007/s11657-017-0324-5.
20. Borgström F, Karlsson L, Ortsäter G, Norton N, Halbout P, Cooper C, et al. Fragility fractures in Europe: burden, management and opportunities. Arch Osteoporos. 2020;15(1):59. https://doi.org/10.1007/s11657-020-0706-y.
21. Diez-Perez A, Hooven FH, Adachi JD, Adami S, Anderson FA, Boonen S, et al. Regional differences in treatment for osteoporosis. The Global Longitudinal Study of Osteoporosis in Women (GLOW). Bone. 2011;49(3):493–8. https://doi.org/10.1016/j.bone.2011.05.007.
22. Martin-Merino E, Huerta-Alvarez C, Prieto-Alhambra D, Alvarez-Gutierrez A, Montero-Corominas D. Secular trends of use of anti-osteoporotic treatments in Spain: a population-based cohort study including over 1.5 million people and more than 12 years of follow-up. Bone. 2017;105:292–8. https://doi.org/10.1016/j.bone.2017.08.031.
23. Abrahamsen B, Skjodt MK, Vestergaard P. Hip fracture rates and time trends in use of anti-osteoporosis medications in Denmark for the period 2005 to 2015: missed opportunities in fracture prevention. Bone. 2019;120:476–81. https://doi.org/10.1016/j.bone.2018.12.016.
24. Jha S, Wang Z, Laucis N, Bhattacharyya T. Trends in media reports, oral bisphosphonate prescriptions, and hip fractures 1996-2012: an ecological analysis. J Bone Miner Res. 2015;30(12):2179–87. https://doi.org/10.1002/jbmr.2565.
25. Kanis JA, Hans D, Cooper C, Baim S, Bilezikian JP, Binkley N, et al. Interpretation and use of FRAX in clinical practice. Osteoporos Int. 2011;22(9):2395–411.
26. Kanis JA, Harvey NC, Cooper C, Johansson H, Oden A, McCloskey EV. A systematic review of intervention thresholds based on FRAX: a report prepared for the National Osteoporosis Guideline Group and the International Osteoporosis Foundation. Arch Osteoporos. 2016;11(1):25. https://doi.org/10.1007/s11657-016-0278-z.

27. Kanis JA, Cooper C, Rizzoli R, Reginster JY. European guidance for the diagnosis and management of osteoporosis in postmenopausal women. Osteoporos Int. 2019;30(1):3–44. https://doi.org/10.1007/s00198-018-4704-5.
28. Oden A, McCloskey EV, Kanis JA, Harvey NC, Johansson H. Burden of high fracture probability worldwide: secular increases 2010-2040. Osteoporos Int. 2015;26(9):2243–8. https://doi.org/10.1007/s00198-015-3154-6.
29. Global Burden of Disease Study 2013 Collaborators. Global, regional, and national incidence, prevalence, and years lived with disability for 301 acute and chronic diseases and injuries in 188 countries, 1990–2013: a systematic analysis for the Global Burden of Disease Study 2013. Lancet. 2015;386(9995):743–800. https://doi.org/10.1016/s0140-6736(15)60692-4.
30. Austin PC, Tu JV, Ko DT, Alter DA. Factors associated with the use of evidence-based therapies after discharge among elderly patients with myocardial infarction. CMAJ. 2008;179(9):901–8. https://doi.org/10.1503/cmaj.080295.
31. Siris ES, Gehlbach S, Adachi JD, Boonen S, Chapurlat RD, Compston JE, et al. Failure to perceive increased risk of fracture in women 55 years and older: the Global Longitudinal Study of Osteoporosis in Women (GLOW). Osteoporos Int. 2011;22(1):27–35. https://doi.org/10.1007/s00198-010-1211-8.
32. Järvinen TL, Michaëlsson K, Jokihaara J, Collins GS, Perry TL, Mintzes B, et al. Overdiagnosis of bone fragility in the quest to prevent hip fracture. BMJ. 2015;350:h2088. https://doi.org/10.1136/bmj.h2088.
33. Järvinen TLN, Michaëlsson K, Aspenberg P, Sievänen H. Osteoporosis: the emperor has no clothes. J Intern Med. 2015;277(6):662–73. https://doi.org/10.1111/joim.12366.
34. Compston J. Overdiagnosis of osteoporosis: fact or fallacy? Osteoporos Int. 2015;26(8):2051–4. https://doi.org/10.1007/s00198-015-3220-0.
35. Cipriani C, Pepe J, Minisola S, Lewiecki EM. Adverse effects of media reports on the treatment of osteoporosis. J Endocrinol Invest. 2018;41(12):1359–64. https://doi.org/10.1007/s40618-018-0898-9.
36. Peeters G, Tett SE, Duncan EL, Mishra GD, Dobson AJ. Osteoporosis medication dispensing for older Australian women from 2002 to 2010: influences of publications, guidelines, marketing activities and policy. Pharmacoepidemiol Drug Saf. 2014;23(12):1303–11. https://doi.org/10.1002/pds.3703.
37. Adler RA, El-Hajj Fuleihan G, Bauer DC, Camacho PM, Clarke BL, Clines GA, et al. Managing osteoporosis in patients on long-term bisphosphonate treatment: report of a task force of the American Society for Bone and Mineral Research. J Bone Miner Res. 2016;31(1):16–35. https://doi.org/10.1002/jbmr.2708.
38. Farmer C, Fenu E, O'Flynn N, Guthrie B. Clinical assessment and management of multimorbidity: summary of NICE guidance. BMJ. 2016;354:i4843. https://doi.org/10.1136/bmj.i4843.
39. Black DM, Rosen CJ. Clinical practice. Postmenopausal osteoporosis. N Engl J Med. 2016;374(3):254–62. https://doi.org/10.1056/NEJMcp1513724.
40. Gedmintas L, Solomon DH, Kim SC. Bisphosphonates and risk of subtrochanteric, femoral shaft, and atypical femur fracture: a systematic review and meta-analysis. J Bone Miner Res. 2013;28(8):1729–37. https://doi.org/10.1002/jbmr.1893.
41. Black DM, Abrahamsen B, Bouxsein ML, Einhorn T, Napoli N. Atypical femur fractures: review of epidemiology, relationship to bisphosphonates, prevention, and clinical management. Endocr Rev. 2019;40(2):333–68. https://doi.org/10.1210/er.2018-00001.
42. Brown JP, Roux C, Törring O, Ho P-R, Beck Jensen J-E, Gilchrist N, et al. Discontinuation of denosumab and associated fracture incidence: analysis from the fracture reduction evaluation of denosumab in osteoporosis every 6 months (FREEDOM) trial. J Bone Miner Res. 2013;28(4):746–52. https://doi.org/10.1002/jbmr.1808.
43. Abrahamsen B, Eiken P, Prieto-Alhambra D, Eastell R. Risk of hip, subtrochanteric, and femoral shaft fractures among mid and long term users of alendronate: nationwide cohort and nested case-control study. BMJ. 2016;353:i3365. https://doi.org/10.1136/bmj.i3365.

44. Dennison EM, Cooper C, Kanis JA, Bruyere O, Silverman S, McCloskey E, et al. Fracture risk following intermission of osteoporosis therapy. Osteoporos Int. 2019;30(9):1733–43. https://doi.org/10.1007/s00198-019-05002-w.
45. Kanis JA, Borgstrom F, Compston J, Dreinhofer K, Nolte E, Jonsson L, et al. SCOPE: a scorecard for osteoporosis in Europe. Arch Osteoporos. 2013;8:144. https://doi.org/10.1007/s11657-013-0144-1.
46. Overman RA, Farley JF, Curtis JR, Zhang J, Gourlay ML, Deal CL. DXA utilization between 2006 and 2012 in commercially insured younger postmenopausal women. J Clin Densitom. 2015;18(2):145–9. https://doi.org/10.1016/j.jocd.2015.01.005.
47. Lewiecki EM, Adler RA, Curtis J, Gagel RF, Saag KG, Singer A et al. Hip fractures and declining DXA testing: at a breaking point? J Bone Miner Res. 2016.
48. Grover ML, Edwards FD, Chang YH, Cook CB, Behrens MC, Dueck AC. Fracture risk perception study: patient self-perceptions of bone health often disagree with calculated fracture risk. Womens Health Issues. 2014;24(1):e69–75. https://doi.org/10.1016/j.whi.2013.11.007.
49. Gregson CL, Dennison EM, Compston JE, Adami S, Adachi JD, Anderson FA Jr, et al. Disease-specific perception of fracture risk and incident fracture rates: GLOW cohort study. Osteoporos Int. 2014;25(1):85–95. https://doi.org/10.1007/s00198-013-2438-y.
50. Eisman JA, Bogoch ER, Dell R, Harrington JT, McKinney RE Jr, McLellan A, et al. Making the first fracture the last fracture: ASBMR task force report on secondary fracture prevention. J Bone Miner Res. 2012;27(10):2039–46. https://doi.org/10.1002/jbmr.1698.
51. Mitchell PJ. Best practices in secondary fracture prevention: fracture liaison services. Curr Osteoporos Rep. 2013;11(1):52–60. https://doi.org/10.1007/s11914-012-0130-3.
52. Drew S, Judge A, Cooper C, Javaid MK, Farmer A, Gooberman-Hill R. Secondary prevention of fractures after hip fracture: a qualitative study of effective service delivery. Osteoporos Int. 2016;27(5):1719–27. https://doi.org/10.1007/s00198-015-3452-z.
53. Akesson K, Marsh D, Mitchell PJ, McLellan AR, Stenmark J, Pierroz DD, et al. Capture the fracture: a best practice framework and global campaign to break the fragility fracture cycle. Osteoporos Int. 2013;24(8):2135–52. https://doi.org/10.1007/s00198-013-2348-z.
54. Javaid MK, Kyer C, Mitchell PJ, Chana J, Moss C, Edwards MH, et al. Effective secondary fracture prevention: implementation of a global benchmarking of clinical quality using the IOF capture the fracture(R) best practice framework tool. Osteoporos Int. 2015;26(11):2573–8. https://doi.org/10.1007/s00198-015-3192-0.
55. Mitchell P, Akesson K, Chandran M, Cooper C, Ganda K, Schneider M. Implementation of models of care for secondary osteoporotic fracture prevention and orthogeriatric models of care for osteoporotic hip fracture. Best Pract Res Clin Rheumatol. 2016;30(3):536–58. https://doi.org/10.1016/j.berh.2016.09.008.
56. Conley RB, Adib G, Adler RA, Åkesson KE, Alexander IM, Amenta KC, et al. Secondary fracture prevention: consensus clinical recommendations from a multistakeholder coalition. J Bone Miner Res. 2020;35(1):36–52. https://doi.org/10.1002/jbmr.3877.
57. Cooper C, Atkinson EJ, O'Fallon WM, Melton LJ. Incidence of clinically diagnosed vertebral fractures: a population-based study in Rochester, Minnesota, 1985-1989. J Bone Miner Res. 1992;7(2):221–7.
58. Clark EM, Gould V, Morrison L, Ades AE, Dieppe P, Tobias JH. Randomized controlled trial of a primary care-based screening program to identify older women with prevalent osteoporotic vertebral fractures: Cohort for Skeletal Health in Bristol and Avon (COSHIBA). J Bone Miner Res. 2012;27(3):664–71. https://doi.org/10.1002/jbmr.1478.
59. Clark EM, Gooberman-Hill R, Peters TJ. Using self-reports of pain and other variables to distinguish between older women with back pain due to vertebral fractures and those with back pain due to degenerative changes. Osteoporos Int. 2016;27(4):1459–67. https://doi.org/10.1007/s00198-015-3397-2.
60. Oei L, Koromani F, Breda SJ, Schousboe JT, Clark EM, van Meurs JB, et al. Osteoporotic vertebral fracture prevalence varies widely between qualitative and quantitative radiological

assessment methods: the Rotterdam study. J Bone Miner Res. 2018;33(4):560–8. https://doi.org/10.1002/jbmr.3220.

61. Muehlematter UJ, Mannil M, Becker AS, Vokinger KN, Finkenstaedt T, Osterhoff G, et al. Vertebral body insufficiency fractures: detection of vertebrae at risk on standard CT images using texture analysis and machine learning. Eur Radiol. 2019;29(5):2207–17. https://doi.org/10.1007/s00330-018-5846-8.
62. Cosman F, de Beur SJ, LeBoff MS, Lewiecki EM, Tanner B, Randall S, et al. Clinician's guide to prevention and treatment of osteoporosis. Osteoporos Int. 2014;25(10):2359–81. https://doi.org/10.1007/s00198-014-2794-2.
63. Lekamwasam S, Adachi JD, Agnusdei D, Bilezikian J, Boonen S, Borgstrom F, et al. An appendix to the 2012 IOF-ECTS guidelines for the management of glucocorticoid-induced osteoporosis. Arch Osteoporos. 2012;7(1–2):25–30. https://doi.org/10.1007/s11657-012-0070-7.
64. Shepstone L, Fordham R, Lenaghan E, Harvey I, Cooper C, Gittoes N, et al. A pragmatic randomised controlled trial of the effectiveness and cost-effectiveness of screening older women for the prevention of fractures: rationale, design and methods for the SCOOP study. Osteoporos Int. 2012;23(10):2507–15. https://doi.org/10.1007/s00198-011-1876-7.
65. Shepstone L, Lenaghan E, Cooper C, Clarke S, Fong-Soe-Khioe R, Fordham R, et al. Screening in the community to reduce fractures in older women (SCOOP): a randomised controlled trial. Lancet. 2018;391(10122):741–7. https://doi.org/10.1016/s0140-6736(17)32640-5.
66. Parsons CM, Harvey N, Shepstone L, Kanis JA, Lenaghan E, Clarke S, et al. Systematic screening using FRAX(®) leads to increased use of, and adherence to, anti-osteoporosis medications: an analysis of the UK SCOOP trial. Osteoporos Int. 2020;31(1):67–75. https://doi.org/10.1007/s00198-019-05142-z.
67. McCloskey E, Johansson H, Harvey NC, Shepstone L, Lenaghan E, Fordham R, et al. Management of patients with high baseline hip fracture risk by FRAX reduces hip fractures-a post hoc analysis of the SCOOP study. J Bone Miner Res. 2018;33(6):1020–6. https://doi.org/10.1002/jbmr.3411.
68. Turner DA, Khioe RFS, Shepstone L, Lenaghan E, Cooper C, Gittoes N, et al. The cost-effectiveness of screening in the community to reduce osteoporotic fractures in older women in the UK: economic evaluation of the SCOOP study. J Bone Miner Res. 2018;33(5):845–51. https://doi.org/10.1002/jbmr.3381.
69. Söreskog E, Borgström F, Shepstone L, Clarke S, Cooper C, Harvey I, et al. Long-term cost-effectiveness of screening for fracture risk in a UK primary care setting: the SCOOP study. Osteoporos Int. 2020;31(8):1499–506. https://doi.org/10.1007/s00198-020-05372-6.
70. Rubin KH, Rothmann MJ, Holmberg T, Hoiberg M, Moller S, Barkmann R, et al. Effectiveness of a two-step population-based osteoporosis screening program using FRAX: the randomized Risk-stratified Osteoporosis Strategy Evaluation (ROSE) study. Osteoporos Int. 2018;29(3):567–78. https://doi.org/10.1007/s00198-017-4326-3.
71. Merlijn T, Swart KM, van Schoor NM, Heymans MW, van der Zwaard BC, van der Heijden AA, et al. The effect of a screening and treatment program for the prevention of fractures in older women: a randomized pragmatic trial. J Bone Miner Res. 2019;34(11):1993–2000. https://doi.org/10.1002/jbmr.3815.
72. Merlijn T, Swart KMA, van der Horst HE, Netelenbos JC, Elders PJM. Fracture prevention by screening for high fracture risk: a systematic review and meta-analysis. Osteoporos Int. 2020;31(2):251–7. https://doi.org/10.1007/s00198-019-05226-w.
73. Viswanathan M, Reddy S, Berkman N, Cullen K, Middleton JC, Nicholson WK, et al. Screening to prevent osteoporotic fractures: updated evidence report and systematic review for the US preventive services task ForceUSPSTF evidence report: screening to prevent osteoporotic FracturesUSPSTF evidence report: screening to prevent osteoporotic fractures. JAMA. 2018;319(24):2532–51. https://doi.org/10.1001/jama.2018.6537.
74. NICE. TA464: bisphosphonates for treating osteoporosis. London: National Institute for Health and Care Excellence; 2017.

75. Harvey NC, McCloskey E, Kanis J, Compston J, Cooper C. Bisphosphonates in osteoporosis: NICE and easy? Lancet. 2017;390(10109):2243–4.
76. Harvey NC, McCloskey E, Kanis JA, Compston J, Cooper C. Cost-effective but clinically inappropriate: new NICE intervention thresholds in osteoporosis (technology appraisal 464). Osteoporos Int. 2018;29(7):1511–3. https://doi.org/10.1007/s00198-018-4505-x.
77. Kanis JA, Harvey NC, McCloskey E, Bruyere O, Veronese N, Lorentzon M, et al. Algorithm for the management of patients at low, high and very high risk of osteoporotic fractures. Osteoporos Int. 2020;31(1):1–12. https://doi.org/10.1007/s00198-019-05176-3.
78. Kanis JA, Johansson H, Oden A, Harvey NC, Gudnason V, Sanders KM, et al. Characteristics of recurrent fractures. Osteoporos Int. 2018;29(8):1747–57. https://doi.org/10.1007/s00198-018-4502-0.
79. Kanis JA, Johansson H, Harvey NC, Gudnason V, Sigurdsson G, Siggeirsdottir K, et al. Adjusting conventional FRAX estimates of fracture probability according to the recency of sentinel fractures. Osteoporos Int. 2020;31(10):1817–28. https://doi.org/10.1007/s00198-020-05517-7.
80. Khosla S, Hofbauer LC. Osteoporosis treatment: recent developments and ongoing challenges. Lancet Diabetes Endocrinol. 2017;5(11):898–907. https://doi.org/10.1016/S2213-8587(17)30188-2.
81. Harvey NC, McCloskey E. Gaps and solutions in bone health: a global framework for improvement. 2016.

Chapter 8
Effective Risk Communication and Improving Adherence

Charlotte Beaudart, Nannan Li, Mickael Hiligsmann, and Stuart Silverman

Introduction

Despite the substantial human, economic and societal burden of osteoporotic fractures and the availability of effective and safe osteoporosis medications, osteoporosis remains largely underdiagnosed and undertreated. The treatment gap, discussed in detail in the previous chapter and defined as the percentage of eligible individuals not receiving treatment with osteoporosis medication in the largest five countries of the European Union plus Sweden, was estimated to be 73% for women and 63% for men in 2017 [1]. In addition, adherence to osteoporosis medications remains poor and suboptimal, with numerous patients not appropriately taking their medicines or discontinuing therapies earlier [2].

The decision by an individual patient to take an osteoporosis medication or engage in healthy lifestyle behaviours (e.g. taking calcium, vitamin D and taking regular exercise), depends on the patient's understanding of their individual fracture risk, their understanding of the risks and benefits of taking action and the risks of not taking action, and the barriers to implementing an action plan. Patients at risk for fractures who do not take actions to reduce risk may not be

C. Beaudart · N. Li · M. Hiligsmann
Department of Health Services Research, CAPHRI Care and Public Health Research Institute, Maastricht University, Maastricht, the Netherlands
e-mail: c.beaudart@uliege.be; n.li@maastrichtuniversity.nl; m.hiligsmann@maastrichtuniversity.nl

S. Silverman (✉)
Cedars-Sinai Medical Center, Los Angeles, CA, USA

OMC Clinical Research Center, Beverly Hills, CA, USA
e-mail: stuarts@bhillsra.com

E. Dennison (ed.), *Osteoporosis Treatment*, https://doi.org/10.1007/978-3-030-78128-6_8

recognizing their own vulnerability ro fracture. Once individuals do understand that they are at risk of future fracture and that they wish to consider taking medication or change behaviour, they need to overcome whatever barriers exist and then initiate that behaviour or medication (i.e. primary adherence). They will need to take the medication as prescribed by the health care professional (i.e. implementation or compliance). They will need to continue taking the medication or maintain lifestyle change for the long term (i.e. secondary adherence or persistence). If they are taking medication, they may stop or change medications due to perceived or experienced risks and/or perceived lack of efficacy or simply decide they do not wish to take medication. They may simply choose not to persist with lifestyle changes.

In this chapter we will start by understanding factors involved in adherence or persistence to medication and behaviours and then try to understand the complexities of the communication of risk to an individual.

Adherence to Osteoporotic Medication

Definition of Medication Adherence

Adherence to medication is a crucial part of patient care and necessary for reaching clinical goals [3] while non-adherence leads to poor clinical outcomes, higher morbidity and death rates, and unnecessary healthcare expenditure. A World Health Organisation (WHO) report underlines the fact that adherence to chronic treatments is often as low as 50% [4]. Poor or non-adherence to medication therefore remains a major problem in most chronic diseases, including osteoporosis [2].

Medication adherence has been defined in several ways. The WHO defined adherence in 2001 as "the degree to which the person's behaviour corresponds with the agreed recommendations from a health care provider [5]." In 2012, a collaboration of European research groups in the field of medication adherence funded by the European Commission suggested the ABC taxonomy for describing and defining adherence to medications, which consisted of three components: (a) initiation, (b) implementation and (c) discontinuation [6]. Initiation occurs when the patient takes the first dose of a prescribed medication, discontinuation marks the end of therapy, when the next dose to be taken is omitted and no more doses are taken thereafter, and implementation is the extent to which a patient's actual dosing corresponds to the prescribed dosing regimen, from initiation until the last dose. Medication persistence is further defined as the length of time between initiation and the last dose, which immediately precedes discontinuation [6].This definition is in agreement with the definition of the Group for the Respect of Ethics Excellence in Science in osteoporosis [7], with the exception that implementation has replaced compliance, and initiation is preferred over primary adherence [2].

Measures of Adherence

Quantification of adherence is crucial to provide researchers, clinicians, and patients with meaningful metrics and further to estimate the effectiveness of prescribed therapies. Different methods are available to quantify medication adherence, consisting of direct and indirect methods. A description of the methods of adherence measurements including advantages and disadvantages can be found in Table 8.1.

Direct methods include measurements of the drug (or a metabolite) concentration in body fluids [8]. Although it may be considered as being an adequate and precise method, some variables should be taken into account, including drug metabolism, individual variation in the pharmacokinetics of the drug, drug-drug interactions and drug-food interactions, which may interfere with the accuracy of the

Table 8.1 Measures of adherence [8]

Methods of measurement	Parameter measured	Advantages	Disadvantages
Direct			
Measurement of drug/metabolite levels	Concentration of the drug/metabolite	Accurate; Objective, proving the ingestion of the drug	Costly; Invasive; Inter individual differences
Indirect			
Self-reporting	A value that is interpreted in regards to a pre-established cut-off point	Easy to use; Inexpensive	Overestimate adherence; Subjective, influenced by recall or reporting bias
Pill counts	Number of doses missed	Simple Mostly used in clinical trials	No evidence of ingested medication
Electronic databases	Medication possession ration (MPR); Proportion of days covered (PDC)	Easy to use; Inexpensive; Non-invasive, patients not aware that they are being monitored; Especially specific to identify non-adherent patients	Evidence of the drug being dispensed but not ingested
Electronic monitoring devices	Overall percentage of doses taken; Dosing regime	Objective; Additional information on degree of adherence; One of the most accurate methods	The patient is aware of the evaluation; No actual evidence that the medication is being ingested

method. In addition, direct methods are difficult to use in practice by reason of being costly and time-consuming, and could be viewed as invasive by some patients. Therefore, various indirect methods are more commonly currently used to measure medication adherence, including self-report, pill count, electronic monitoring and the use of prescription and refill databases.

Self-reporting such as by diaries or retrospective questionnaires, is the simplest method for measuring adherence. It may be useful for assessing very recent drug use [9], however, it tends to overestimate adherence over a long time period, in comparison to direct methods, since the patients may be influenced by recall or reporting bias due to selective disclosure of non-adherence information by the patient [8].

Pill count is a straightforward method which calculates the number of doses that have been taken between appointments and compares it with the total number of doses that the patient has received. An adherence ratio is then calculated. It can assess an average adherence, but does not give specific information about daily adherence or patterns of adherence [9].

Electronic monitoring devices, such as Medication Event Monitoring System (MEMS) are devices incorporated in the container that stores the dosing history of the patient's prescribed medication. It is commonly used in clinical trials though is more difficult to use in real-life settings and has been proven to be highly accurate in several studies. It may be used as a reference standard for validating other adherence methods [8].

Electronic databases are based on the assumption that prescription refilling patterns coincide with medication taking behaviour. Prescription refill data have the capacity to provide rough adherence estimations since they offer information on the possession of medication and not proof on actual intake of medicine, and in some cases could give overestimations. They gives the opportunity to assess non-adherence in a large population over an extensive period of time, including multi-drug non-adherence. However, they do not give information on individual patients' rates of adherence [8].

The overall measurement/calculation of adherence is commonly conducted using Medication Possession Ratio (MPR) and Proportion of Days Covered (PDC). MPR is usually defined as the sum of all days of medication supply received during a given time [7]. PDC is the number of days when the drug was available divided by the number of days in the study period [8]. A cut-off point is commonly advised (at least 80% adherent), which categorizes the patients as being adherent and non-adherent [10, 11].

Generally, electronic databases are the appropriate method to measure initiation and discontinuation of therapy while electronic monitoring is the preferred method for implementation, although they could be difficult to set up in real-life settings. The use of self-reports or pill counts could be alternative methods [2].

Adherence to Osteoporotic Medications: State of the Art

Osteoporosis medications have been shown to be effective in fracture risk reduction [12], however, as a chronic disease, non-adherence to pharmacological treatment in osteoporosis is a well-recognized problem [13] and reported in several studies. As discussed previously, bisphosphonates are the first line drugs for osteoporosis. In line with treatment initiation rates in other diseases [14], about 20–30% of patients do not initiate a treatment after a prescription for oral bisphosphonates [15] even when there is no cost to the patient of the medication. In addition, patients on bisphosphonates frequently miss doses [14]. Furthermore, multiple large observational studies from countries with different health systems have reported low rates of long-term adherence with oral bisphosphonates (daily or weekly) [14]. In a recent review [16] including 89 studies published up to April 2018, the mean persistence of oral bisphosphonates for 6 months, 1 year and 2 years ranged from 34.8% to 71.3%, 17.7% to 74.8% and 12.9% to 72.0%, respectively. Although a number of studies reported high levels of persistence and adherence, patient persistence and adherence with oral bisphosphonates was poor and reduced notably over time. In a Belgian study [17], the rate of persistence was estimated at 39.5% for postmenopausal women at 1 year (without a gap of more than 5 weeks in treatment), while 48.1% of patients had a 12-month MPR ≥80% (patients as being adherent).

Apart from bisphosphonates, other osteoporosis medications are also commonly used. A recent systematic review and meta-analysis reported substantial heterogeneity in reports of persistence and adherence rates with parenteral osteoporosis therapies [18]. Twenty nine studies examined persistence to teriparatide, with persistence rates of 10–87% (median 55%) at 1 year and 10–69% (median 29.5%) at 2 years. A 2-year Japanese observational study [19] showed that once-daily teriparatide adherence and persistence rates were higher among patients who enrolled in a patient support program than among those who did not (54.2 vs. 48.3%). Although we expect greater persistence with treatment injected by a health care practitioner (e.g., denosumab), persistence remains suboptimal after 24 months. Median persistence rates of 46% were estimated at 2 years for denosumab [18].

Low adherence to osteoporotic medications is thus well recognized, and has been shown to reduce the potential benefits of osteoporosis therapy leading to increased risk of fractures and representing a substantial clinical and economic burden. Understanding the determinants of patient non-adherence and the potential effects of adherence-enhancing interventions are therefore crucial.

Determinants of Non-adherence

Adherence is a complex multidimensional phenomenon; profiles of non-adherence differ from patient to patient. Some patients never initiate a treatment, while others delay initiation of therapy. There are patients who frequently miss doses, and multi-week drug holiday periods have also been observed [20]. Several patients discontinue treatment earlier than prescribed and many patients are noted to have undergone multiple episodes of starting and stopping drugs [2].

The WHO has classified factors for non-adherence of medication into five main categories: socio-economic factors, health care team and system related factors, condition-related factors, therapy-related factors, and patient-related factors [21]. Kardas et al. [22] conducted an umbrella review up to December 2009 on the déterminants of patient adherence on the basis of a recently agreed European consensus taxonomy and terminology. Fifty one reviews were identified covering 771 individual factor items, of which most were determinants of implementation, and only 47 determinants of persistence with medication.

In the field of osteoporosis, Yeam et al. [23] performed a systematic review up to January 2018 and identified 24 factors with 139 sub-factors that influence patients' adherence to anti-osteoporotic therapy from 124 relevant studies. These factors were then grouped into categories as per the WHO recommendation [21]. Condition-related factors that were associated with poorer medication adherence included, among others, polypharmacy. Patients who had never taken a prescription medication also demonstrated poorer global adherence [15]. A history of falls was associated with higher medication adherence. Patient-related factors which were associated with poorer medication adherence included older age and misconceptions about osteoporosis, while therapy-related factors included higher dosing frequency and medication side effects. Both perceived and experienced side effects are reasons for non-adherence, and patients are easily influenced by information from social media or searching online. One study reported that rare yet serious harmful events through prescription of bisphosphonates have received wide coverage in the media and have resulted in perceived risks by the public that may be out of proportion to the absolute risks, leading patients to not fill or refill prescriptions for these drugs [24]. Health system-based factors associated with poorer medication adherence included care under different medical specialties and lack of patient education. Socio-economic-related factors associated with poorer medication adherence included current smoker and lack of medical insurance coverage. In general, patient-related factors were the most commonly studied domain across all studies, followed by therapy-related domains (e.g. convenience of administration, frequency of administration) and condition-related domains.

Additionally, patient perceptions and preferences with osteoporosis medications were also shown to impact adherence behaviour [25] and discontinuation rates [26]. A review investigated the preferences of patients for osteoporosis drug reporting that osteoporotic patients have preferences for medications and their attributes, in particular for less-frequent dosing regimens [27]. Furthermore, another study [28] reported that the low rate of osteoporosis medication initiation may stem from participants having difficulty trusting the content of the video vignettes included in the intervention, since these educational materials were not endorsed by a source familiar to the patient (e.g. their treating physician). As medication non-adherence is affected by multiple determinants, suitable measurement and multifaceted interventions may be effective to enhance patient adherence to medication.

Consequences of Poor Adherence to Osteoporosis Medications

Poor adherence to osteoporosis medications has substantial clinical and economic consequences. Multiple studies have been conducted to investigate the impact of osteoporosis treatment adherence on fracture risk. Siris et al. [29] undertook a meta-analysis that indicated that adhérence and persistence with osteoporosis medications are suboptimal, resulting in increased rates of fragility fractures. Similarly, Ross et al. [30] conducted a meta-analysis and reported that fracture risk increases by approximately 30% with non-adherence and by 30% to 40% with non-persistence. Imaz et al. [31] assessed the impact of adherence to oral bisphosphonates on fracture rate and provided a pooled 46% increased fracture risk in non-compliant patients compared with compliant patients. The increased fracture risk was higher for clinical vertebral fractures than non-vertebral and hip fractures. In addition, another study [32] indicated that among patients who received teriparatide, low-MPR was a significant risk factor for any fracture (OR = 1.64; $p < 0.01$), vertebral fracture (OR = 2.56; $p = 0.001$), and non-vertebral fracture (OR = 1.44; $p = 0.013$). Furthermore, persistence to generic formulations has been shown to be poorer than for branded formulations for some osteoporosis medications [33, 34].

These clinical consequences also lead to economic consequences. For example, an Irish study [35] indicated that poor adherence with osteoporosis medications resulted in around a 50% reduction in the potential benefits observed in clinical trials and a doubling of the cost per quality-adjusted life-years (QALY) gained from these medications. Similar results have been observed in other studies [36, 37]. Therefore, poor adherence and failure to persist with osteoporosis medications results not only in deteriorating health outcomes, but also in a decreased cost-effectiveness of pharmacotherapy [35]. The integration of medication adherence into pharmacoeconomic analyses has therefore been recommended in several studies [38, 39]. A recent published osteoporosis-specific guideline for the design and conduct of an economic evaluation in osteoporosis has suggested the use of real-world medication adherence in an alternative scenario, as well as sensitivity analyses varying adherence levels [37].

Interventions to Improve Adherence to Osteoporosis Medications

In recent years, several interventions and programs have been developed to improve medication adherence for osteoporosis (see Table 8.2). Hiligsmann et al. [40] systematically reviewed studies that evaluated interventions to improve medication adherence in osteoporosis. A total of 20 studies were included. The most frequent intervention was education, followed by monitoring/supervision, suggested drug regimens, drug regimens and patient support, pharmacist intervention, and electronic prescription. In 2019, Cornelissen et al. [41] updated the previous review including recently published relevant studies up to December 2018. Interventions

Table 8.2 Interventions identified through previous systematic reviews

	Hiligsmann et al. [38]	Cornelissen et al. [41]
Time period	January 1999–June 2012	July 2012–December 2018
Total studies included	20	15
Types of interventions	Education (n = 11) Monitoring/supervision (n = 4) Drug regimens (n = 2) Drug regimens and patient support (n = 1) Pharmacist intervention (n = 1) Electronic prescription (n = 1)	Education (n = 9) Drug regimen (n = 3) Monitoring and supervision (n = 2) Interdisciplinary collaboration (n = 1)
Studies with positive effects (improved medication adherence)	Education (n = 4) Drug regimens (n = 2) Drug regimens and patient support (n = 1) Pharmacist intervention (n = 1) Electronic prescription (n = 1)	Education (n = 2) Monitoring and supervision (n = 1)

were classified as patient education, suggested drug regimens, monitoring and supervision, and interdisciplinary collaboration, with mixed results on medication adherence and persistence, though more positive effects were observed for multi-component interventions with active patient involvement, counselling and shared decision-making.

Specially, ***patient education*** is the most frequent intervention considered in both reviews [38, 39], which can be classified into different forms including group educational sessions (consisted of meetings with 4–6 patients and a psychologist), provision of education material (providing booklets or flyers with information or providing DVDs with visual information), the use of a decision aid, and motivational interviewing. In some cases, education was combined with counselling. The method of administration and the intensity of patient counselling varied from offering patients advice and recommendation concerning the educational material [42] up to four telephonic follow-up calls combined with four group sessions in 12 months [43]. One study [44] combining patient education, counselling, blood tests, BMD test prescription, and follow-up phone calls reported an increase in adherence between 40 (minimal) and 53% (intensive) in the intervention groups, compared with 19% in usual care. In another study [45], an education program was combined with a referral to an endocrinologist by a nurse reporting significant improvement of implementation rates compared with usual care. In addition, a coordinator-based screening program was conducted in a study by Beaton et al. [42], reporting significant improvements in BMD testing and treatment initiation after the initiation of this program. Hence the initiation of patient education can improve patients' interaction/communication with doctors/coordinators and, therefore, their knowledge of osteoporosis and perception of future fracture risk.

Special ***drug regimen implementation*** is an important determinant of non-adherence, in particular for bisphosphonates. Several studies indicated that a flexible dosing regimen was associated with improved adherence. One study [46] reported that compared to common oral bisphosphonates, prescription of gastro-resistant (GR) risedronate tablets with less strict administration requirements was associated with improved persistence. Another study [47] indicated that a significant difference between the flexible and fixed regimens was seen in persistence in favour of the flexible regimen. In addition, longer dosing regimen (such as 6-month subcutaneous injection of denosumab or yearly intravenous injection of zoledronic acid) may improve adherence, although adherence levels have also been disappointing and far from optimal [2].

Monitoring and supervision such as phone calls and counselling may also improve medication adherence. One study [48] suggested that implementation of telephone monitoring (medical secretaries contacted the patients every 2 months by telephone) in the routine medical management of osteoporosis could contribute to a reduction of complications associated with treatment discontinuation compared with patients without telephone follow-up (67% vs. 30%,). In another study [49], the MeMo program consisted of initial structured counselling (regarding administration, effectiveness, and possible side-effects) and continuous actively monitoring after 2 weeks (focused on patients' first experiences with adverse effects and drug administration problems), and every 3 months, where pharmacists actively searched for patients who should have redeemed a new prescription for their osteoporosis medication. Compared with patients in usual care, non-adherence and discontinuation with osteoporosis medication were decreased for patients who participated in this program. Monitoring and supervision could enhance communication between patients and caregivers and further motivate patients to maintain good adherence to the treatment.

Fracture liaison services (FLSs) represent an ***interdisciplinary collaboration*** program which connects different physicians (institutional health care professionals (HCPs) with primary care physicians (PCPs) in outpatient settings) and facilitate communication between them and patients for secondary fracture prevention. A systematic review and meta-analysis [50] indicated that compared with patients receiving usual care (or those in the control arm), patients receiving care from an FLS program had higher treatment initiation (38.0% vs 17.2%) and greater adherence (57.0% vs 34.1%), significant FLS-associated with improvements in treatment (95% CI 0.16–0.25) and adherence (95% CI 0.13–0.31). In addition, multiple studies have also reported that FLSs have a potential to improve treatment initiation [51, 52]. The FLS is described in detail in the next chapter.

Shared decision-making offers a structured way to incorporate evidence as well as patient values and preferences into medical decision making [53], and has been increasingly recommended in several recent guidelines for its potential of improving treatment initiation and medication adherence. Decision aids are frequently used to facilitate elements in shared decision making. In one study patients received a standard brochure, or a decision aid (a tailored pictographic 10-year fracture risk estimate, absolute risk reduction with bisphosphonates, side effects, and out-of-pocket cost) [54] with the group receiving the decision aid having higher adherence to medication. In addition, patients receiving the decision aid were 1.8 times more likely to correctly identify their 10-year fracture risk and 2.7 times more likely to identify their estimated risk reduction with bisphosphonates.

As discussed earlier in this book, Bone turnover marker response has been used as an intervention for improving treatment adherence [38, 55]. Low response may be detected shortly after treatment has been started and may indicate low adherence, low bioavailability, interactions with other drugs, or the presence of secondary osteoporosis [56]. The IOF and European Calcified Tissue Society Working Group has suggested monitoring the adherence of bisphosphonates by measuring Serum PINP (procollagen type I N-terminal propeptide) and CTX (collagen type I C-terminal telopeptide) at baseline and 3 months after starting therapy to check for a decrease above the least significant change (decrease of more than 38% for PINP and 56% for CTX). If a significant decrease is observed, the treatment should continue, but if no decrease occurs, the clinician should reassess to identify any problems with the treatment, specifically the possibility of low adherence [57]. In addition, a positive message that highlights a good bone turnover marker response can be associated with a significant improvement in persistence [55].

Interventions discussed above could facilitate interaction/communication between patients and doctors, and therefore help patients improve their knowledge of osteoporosis and understand risks and benefits, which would further improve the quality of clinical decisions and motivate patients to maintain good adherence to osteoporotic-medications. Because well understood communication from healthcare professionals is the foundation of a patient's appropriate understanding of risks, we will now review recommendations and existing tools for effective communication of general health-related risks as well as effective communication of osteoporosis fracture risk.

Effective Risk Communication to Improve Osteoporosis Management

General Health Risk Communication

Bias in Patients-Doctors' Health Communication

Effective communication between a healthcare professional and patient is an important aspect of patient-centred care. Appropriate communication of health-related risks is essential to help patients make the best-informed health-related decisions that are in concordance with their personal values, experiences, and preferences. However, informing patients about their risk of developing a disease, the risk reduction or benefits associated with a drug intake or risk of side-effects associated with a treatment remains challenging. Different factors could (partially) explain difficulties encountered by patients in understanding information provided by their clinicians.

The perception by the patient of the risk that doctors communicate to them is based on the patient's understanding of the medical information provided to them. Patients usually do not understand the complete information provided by healthcare professionals but take the gist or essential message of the medical information. This gist is also influenced by the source of the information (e.g. physician, pharmacist, social media or media coverage). The information is also influenced by several different types of biases which patients often unconsciously use in their medical decision-making:

- ***Immediacy bias:*** A new or novel risk may be perceived differently [58]. If information was heard recently or easily remembered, it may be judged more likely to be true. A good example of this is the side effect osteonecrosis of the jaw (ONJ). Although exceptionally rare, when covered by the media in reports, patients fill fewer osteoporosis medications [15].
- ***Catastrophic bias:*** A side effect may be more easily remembered and feared if it is sensational or catastrophic. A jawbone dying (ONJ) or hip breaking spontaneously (atypical femoral fracture; AFF) is more likely to be remembered than an upset stomach from an oral bisphosphonate.
- ***Optimism bias:*** People view risks as riskier for other people than themselves [59]. Post-menopausal women at increased risk of fracture tend to underestimate their risk of fracture [60].
- ***Pessimism bias:*** Some individuals overestimate their risk of side effects. They feel that side effects always happen to them when they take a medicine, no matter how low the risk.
- ***Categorical bias:*** Patients, when they hear of a risk, may simply consider the medicine as safe or dangerous. After they learned of the risk of ONJ and AFF, some patients first considered all bisphosphonate drugs as dangerous, then considered all osteoporosis medications as dangerous.

The way clinicians communicate about risk is therefore of primary importance. Rules, recommendations, and guidance for successful risk communication between clinicians and patients have been developed.

General Recommendations for an Effective Communication of Risks

In the report of the science of patient input program of the Medical Device Innovation Consortium (MDIC) published in September 2020 and entitled "*Best practices for communicating benefits, risks and uncertainty for medical devices*' [61], a comprehensive assessment of benefits and risks communication is provided. After providing an overview of the opportunities for communicating benefits, risks and uncertainty information throughout clinical research, direct-to consumer advertising, social media channels, patient decision aids, etc. and defining key concepts of benefits, risks, harm, patient preference, risk tolerance and uncertainty attitudes, authors presented evidence-based key factors and available tools for making an optimal communication. Among other [62–64], authors presented guidelines from the Food and Drug Administration (FDA) published in 2016 [65]. Within its *Guidance to Industry ``Patient Preference Information – Voluntary Submission, Review in Premarket Approval Applications, Humanitarian Device Exemption Applications, and De Novo Requests, and Inclusion in Decision Summaries and Device Labeling"*, the FDA concluded that no single format of risk communication from healthcare professionals to patients is universally superior to another format but developed the following overall recommendations:

1. Avoid solely verbal descriptions of uncertainty. Patients may interpret what "low" and "high" risks are differently;
2. Avoid fractions, decimals, and different denominators when presenting risks of multiple treatments. These are relatively difficult for cognitive processing and rely on numeracy skills;
3. If possible, describe the benefits and risks in absolute scales (e.g. 1 in 100) instead of relative terms, which better inform the actual benefits and risks;
4. If possible, use multiple formats simultaneously (e.g., verbal frequency, percent, and icon array/pictograph). Relative understanding of these formats varies from patient to patient. Moreover, one format may make the other formats easier to understand;
5. If possible, describe uncertainty in both positive and negative framing(e.g., 20% chance of adverse events or 80% chance of no adverse events) to avoid cognitive bias. Indeed, the way health care professionals frame the risk (e.g. 'Is a treatment 90% effective or 10% ineffective?') may influence whether the patient accepts the information.
6. Pre-test the communication format. Since patient populations vary, pre-testing the chosen format can improve the comprehension of the format by the study population of interest.

Since patients may immediately forget the information that doctors present to them [66], or simply choose to ignore this information, it is important to keep messages about risk simple. Simplified language (e.g. avoidance of clinical or statistical jargon, use of simple and well-structured sentences), is recommended so people with low literacy can read and understand the information [64]. A range of terms are commonly used in day-to-day life to describe risk. For example, risk may be categorised as "low", "moderate", "high" or "very high". A systematic review performed in 2014 [67], compared the use of numbers to the use of words in communicating risks. Results indicated that verbal descriptors including "common", "uncommon" and "rare" lead to an overestimation of the probability of adverse effects compared to numerical information. Interpretation of these terms varies widely from person to person and therefore authors have suggested using examples (i.e. comparison of medical risks to common nonmedical risks such as a risk of a traffic accident) or analogies to illustrate the meaning of such terms [68]. Another recent study pointed to a very considerable variation in the numerical translation of verbal probability by both patients and clinicians suggesting that verbal probability expression should not be used in isolation for communication between doctors and patients [69].

Nevertheless, "adding" a verbal description to a numeric data may be useful to better frame the information so a participant understands the risk.

Another important aspect in risk communication is the valence (negativity or positivity) of words used by clinicians. When talking about risk, it is possible to present either benefits or risks, or to communicate using positive/gain terms or using negative/loss terms. To illustrate that, researchers found that presenting adverse event information before benefits (compared to benefits before adverse events) lowers the likelihood that subjects will perceive that the benefits outweigh the risks of a proposed new medication [70]. Warning patients of risks such as side-effects has also been shown to increase the incidence of these side-effects, (through the nocebo effect) while positively framing risk information did not [71].

It is also important for the clinician to build a trust-based relationship with patients. If patients have trust in their healthcare provider, they are more likely to understand and accept the information [72]. Nevertheless, it has been shown that information about risk sometimes needs to be heard and confirmed by other persons (e.g. a spouse, a child, a caregiver, or a friend) who may or may not be present before being accepted. Healthcare professionals should therefore try to understand the role of others in risk communication, particularly social media in decision making but also the perspective of peers, family, and friends.

Communication of Numeric Data

It has been shown that numerous patient-related factors such as advanced age [73] or low literacy [74] may impair understanding of evidence-based information such as numerical concepts. Lipkus et al. [75] showed that many patients cannot perform basic numeric tasks. Even among highly educated people, they found that 16% incorrectly answered a simple question about risk magnitude (e.g. Which represents the larger risk: 1%, 5% or 10%)?). Highly numerate people are likely to pay more attention to numbers, better understand them, and ultimately use them more often in decisions. Lower numeracy has also been shown to be associated with overestimation of risk probabilities, being more susceptible to being influenced by factors other than numerical data (e.g., framing, mood states, feedback from others), and greater denominator neglect [76]. Denominator neglect is a classical bias met in ratio concepts understanding. People often pay too much attention to the number of times an event happens (numerator) without paying attention to the overall number of opportunities for it to happen (denominator). For example in a perfect example of denominator neglect Yamagishi et al. [77] showed in one study that people rated the likelihood of a cancer killing 1286 out of 10,000 people (i.e. 12.86%) as higher than 24.14 out of 100 people (i.e. 24.14%).

Communication of risks can be presented to the patient under different more or less complex numeric formats. First, it is recommended that clinicians present as simple frequencies rather than a percentage. Indeed, this format has been shown to be preferred by patients and improves understanding [62, 64, 78–81]. Second, it has been shown that numerical likelihoods presented as 1-in-X (e.g. 1 in 25) are processed fasted and are perceived as conveying larger likelihoods than the x-in-100 (e.g. 4 in 100) and percentage formats (e.g. 4%) [82, 83]. Pighin and al [84]. suggested that the 1-in-X format may increase the ability to identify oneself as affected with the possible outcome. Third, there is also a general agreement that decimals (e.g. likelihood of 0.03) should not be used in risk communicates as they may lead to misunderstanding [85]. Fourth, it has been shown that the concept of number need to treat (NNT) may not be readily understood by patients and should be avoided in doctor-patient communication [62, 64, 79, 86]. Fifth, when presenting frequencies information, healthcare professionals should keep the dominator constant to reduce effort and increase comprehension of individuals (e.g. always keep the denominator as 1000 and avoid presenting one time the risk as x of 50 and a second time the risk as x of 1000).

Careful attention to information presentation allows everyone, including less numerate people, to better integrate numbers and use them more effectively in decision making. One solution could be to test the presentation of numeric information with target audiences whenever possible and adapt it as many times it is necessary to increase the comprehensibility and usability of the information; future research in this area is needed.

Communication Using Visual Aid Presentations

Presenting information visually as well as numerically may improve understanding [87–90] though interpretation of graphics have been shown to be dependent upon instructions provided [91] as visual displays can still misrepresent information.

It has been suggested that type and formatting of graphics seems to influence comprehension and behaviour (Fig. 8.1). Some studies have suggested that the formats that are perceived most accurately and easily by patients are bar graphs (Fig. 8.1c) and pictographs (Fig. 8.1c) [92, 93]. while areal presentations (e.g. pie charts (Fig. 8.1a)) seems less effective [94]. Pictographs (Fig. 8.1c)can be a useful way to highlight the number of people affected, or not affected, by a medical treatment [95]. In this type of graph, an icon display of symbols or figures shows the entire population at risk (the denominator) and highlighted icons show those in whom an event occurred (the numerator). Icon arrays may be an effective method for eliminating denominator neglect [96]. The performance of icon array however depends on the numerator size. When the outcome is less than 100/1000, for example, pictographs are better understood than bar charts. However, for more even outcomes (e.g. higher than 100/1000), icon array arrangement may be complicated and bar charts seems to work better [97]. Depending on the aim of the communication, pictograms, or pictures to illustrate the risk, can also be used (Fig. 8.1g). A recent study [98] explored the impact of different type of pictures (anatomical pictures, photos, cartoons and drawings) on health information perception. This study however failed to show the superiority of any type of picture in understanding risk. Finally, it also appears that the combination of different graphic risk presentations formats seems preferable to a single presentation. In a preference study [99] that

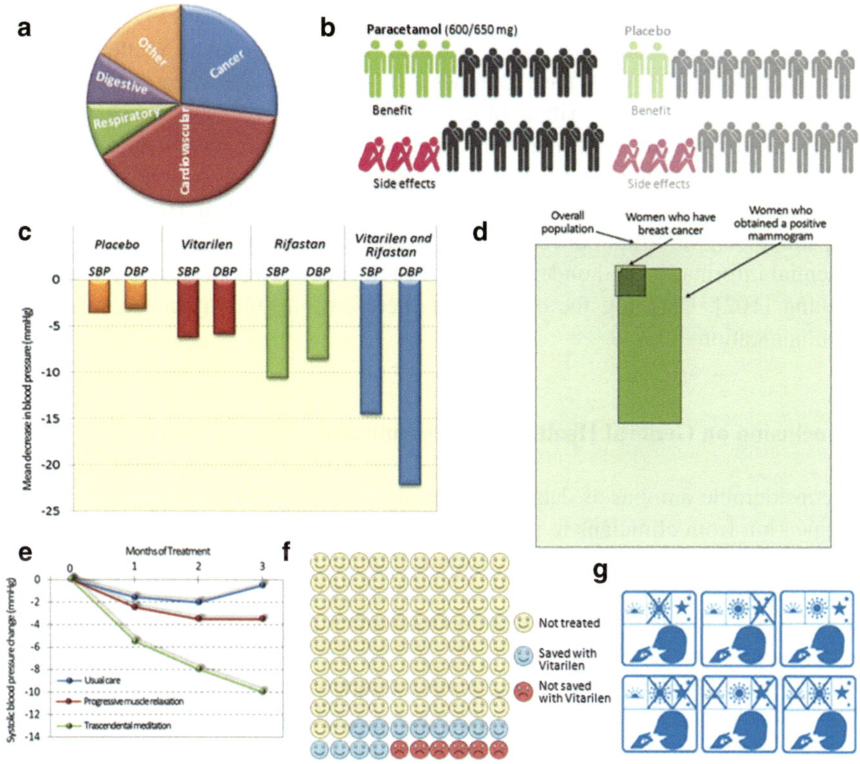

Fig. 8.1 Examples of visual aids (Figure issued from Garcia-Retamero et al. [89], used with permission). (**a**) A pie chart reporting the proportion of deaths by cause of death. (**b**) Icon arrays representing benefits and side effects of a medical treatment and a placebo. (**c**) A bar chart comparing the efficacy of two medical treatments (DBP = diastolic blood pressure; SBP = systolic blood pressure). (**d**) A visual grid to help infer the predictive value of mammography screening. (**e**) A line plot comparing the efficacy of several therapies. (**f**) Icon arrays to communicate treatment–risk reduction. (**g**) Pictograms reporting dosage, timing, and action information about prescribed medications

compared six types of graphical representations, an augmented bar chart combined with a flow diagram seemed to be the most preferred combined format of risk communication.

Communication Using Leaflets

In 2006, a study reviewing 50 leaflets of the most prescribed medicines in England and Wales highlighted substantial variation in the methods used to communicate risk to patients [100], and in which only 8% of leaflets provided any form of numerical indication of risk. Communication using patient information leaflets have shown variable results in regards to its efficacy. In a study including 1000 health practitioners, only a small minority of responders correctly stated the meaning of terms that are used to describe the risk presented in a communication leaflet [101]. Another study reported that patients who are provided with supplementary written information in the form of leaflets have a higher level of knowledge when compared with patients who received no written information [101].

It is also important to keep in mind that less information may be more effective. When designing leaflets or education materials, there is a natural tendency to present a lot of information to be sure not to miss any important data. However, presenting too much information can distract patients, prevent them focusing on the essential information and understanding the information that is needed for decision making [102]. Catching the essential is therefore one important feature in risk communication.

Conclusion on General Health Risk Communication

A considerable amount of data highlights the importance of well-build risk communication from clinicians to patients using adequate support tools. Different factors may improve the quality of communication between healthcare professionals and patients: the way the information is presented from clinicians, the capacity of the clinicians to adapt their language to the patient they have in from of them, the relationship between clinicians and patients, the way the information is understood by patients, the self-perception and understanding of their own disease, their perspective in regards of their own health, their health literacy, their numeracy, their own emotions and experiences, etc. The globality of these rules could be applied for communicating risk in various pathologies, including communication of fractures risk for osteoporosis population.

Risk Communication in the Context of Osteoporosis Medication

Importance of Risk Communication Is Osteoporosis

Adequate risk communication is especially important in a disease like osteoporosis where fracture risk, treatments effects and risk of side-effects represent key information for an informed decision [103]. Current data reveals care gaps and limited communication about fracture risks between therapists and patients [104, 105]. Osteoporosis patients are often dissatisfied with the information they received from health professionals. Studies also report difficulties of patients in interpreting the diagnosis of osteoporosis, the risk of fracture and the way they have to manage their disease in everyday life [104]. Moreover, poor quality of written materials available to communicate information about prevention and treatment of osteoporosis is also often observed, which limits informed decision making [106]. From a clinical and public health point of view, there is a huge need for a patient's understanding of the risk of fractures and their consequences. Research also shows that patients often do not consider themselves at risk of fracture, even if they have suffered a previous fracture, which is an important aspect to consider by clinicians in fracture risk communication [107]. It is not always necessary for doctors to calculate fracture risk and some may even consider fracture risk assessment as not necessary for certain categories of patients. Indeed, most countries accept the presence of a previous fracture or a very low BMD as being evidence of need for treatment alone without fracture risk assessment [108]. Nevertheless, even with those patients, the communication of fracture risk may be a good opportunity to involve the patients in the understanding and management of their own disease and also to motivate patients to be more adherent to treatment. Indeed, fractures in both men and women often precedes a cascade of declining mobility, physical activity, muscle strength, quality of life and balance contributing to the loss of independence in daily activities that could further lead to institutionalization, as well as falls and fall-related injuries including fractures and increased mortality risk [109–111].

Even if clinical indicators, performance measures, and educational tools to better understand and identify fracture risk are now available, realizing the full benefits of these advances is not always easy.

Key Elements for Optimal Communication of Fractures Risk

For effective fractures risk communication, healthcare professionals need to consider what is important to communicate to patients, what are the patient's needs (e.g. health and biopsychosocial needs) and what is the best way to communicate this information [112, 113]. Optimal fracture risk communication should ideally involve not only patients but also primary care physicians (PCPs). PCPs are often the first line in this risk communication since they have an important role in the care of osteoporosis patients. Healthcare professionals should be able to verify that patients understand the conversation and feel free to ask questions and express their concerns. The teach-back method could also be interesting to assess patients' understanding of their fracture risk [114, 115]. Key components of risk communication also include important communications skills with the use of terminology that is appropriate for the patient's level of health care education. Moreover, clinicians that are best equipped to communicate risks and benefits are those that are familiar with the medical evidence, are statistically literate, have clinical experience with osteoporosis and its treatment options, and able to translate complex information to a form that is understood by the patient.

Communication can be achieved using written or electronic educational material such as clinical tools (e.g., brochures, graphs, videos, models) or visual graphs that underline the fracture risks (e.g. icon array, bar graph, etc.) [116]. Much more than risk numbers are needed, and, ideally, fracture risk tools should be integrated into bone densitometry reporting or placed into comprehensive, user-friendly, decision aids [117]. In the context of osteoporosis and risk of fractures, output from a fracture tool should ideally provide information in several different ways not all patients receive and digest information about treatment in the same way.

Communication of Fractures Risk Using Letters and Educational Brochures

The most investigated tool to communicate about fracture risk consists of an individual letter with patient's fracture risk and an educational brochure mailed or posted rapidly after a DXA scan [118–125]. This is considered as a rapid, low-cost, direct-to-patient risk of fracture communication tool. Pre-post interventional pilot studies [122, 123] have demonstrated that a personalized letter and an information brochure as a technique of risk communication improved osteoporosis knowledge, feelings of susceptibility regarding osteoporosis as well as the understanding of DXA results. However, this method of communication, tested through different randomized controlled trials [118–120, 125], using usual care as control, has failed to demonstrate the positive impact of this communication tool on change in bone health behaviour of participants (e.g. treatment initiation, calcium and vitamin D intake, enhancing preventive measures against risk of fractures, etc.). It is possible that many patients do not understand the written fracture risk information. Moreover, educational materials such as brochures about osteoporosis or internet websites are often inadequate in their display of evidence-based information and risk communication. Quality of understanding may therefore be limited using this written communication approach. Direct-to consumer conversation may improve disease-state and risk awareness. Counselling and decisions aids has been shown to be more effective [119]. Decision aids should nevertheless be accurate, unbiased, and effective at communicating the desired information.

Communication of Fractures Risk Using Pictures

The communication of fracture risk can be accompanied with a visual representation to allow a better patient's understanding and interpretation. In 2014, Edmonds et al. [126] provided preferences of 142 patients suffering from osteoporosis for four different visual deceptions of fracture risk (Fig. 8.2):

1. "Faces array" (Fig. 8.2(1)), which is a pictogram comprising 100 faces. In the example provided in Fig. 8.2, 79 were smiling and 21 were coloured red and frowning, depicting a 21% risk of breaking a bone in the next 10 days.
2. "Arrow" (Fig. 8.2(2)), which is a horizontally oriented arrow-shaped, directional graph that integrates a red, yellow and green coloured "stoplight" system to indicate risk. Low risk is associated with green, moderate is associated with yellow and high risk is associated with red. All parts of the arrow are of equal widths.
3. "Stoplight" (Fig. 8.2(4)), which is an illustration that integrates stoplight colours using a rectangular depiction that does not imply a progression (unlike the arrow presentation) and is scaled to 100 risk.
4. "Bar" (Fig. 8.2(3)) which is an illustration employing a graduated stoplight colour system but is oriented vertically, similar to thermometers tools.

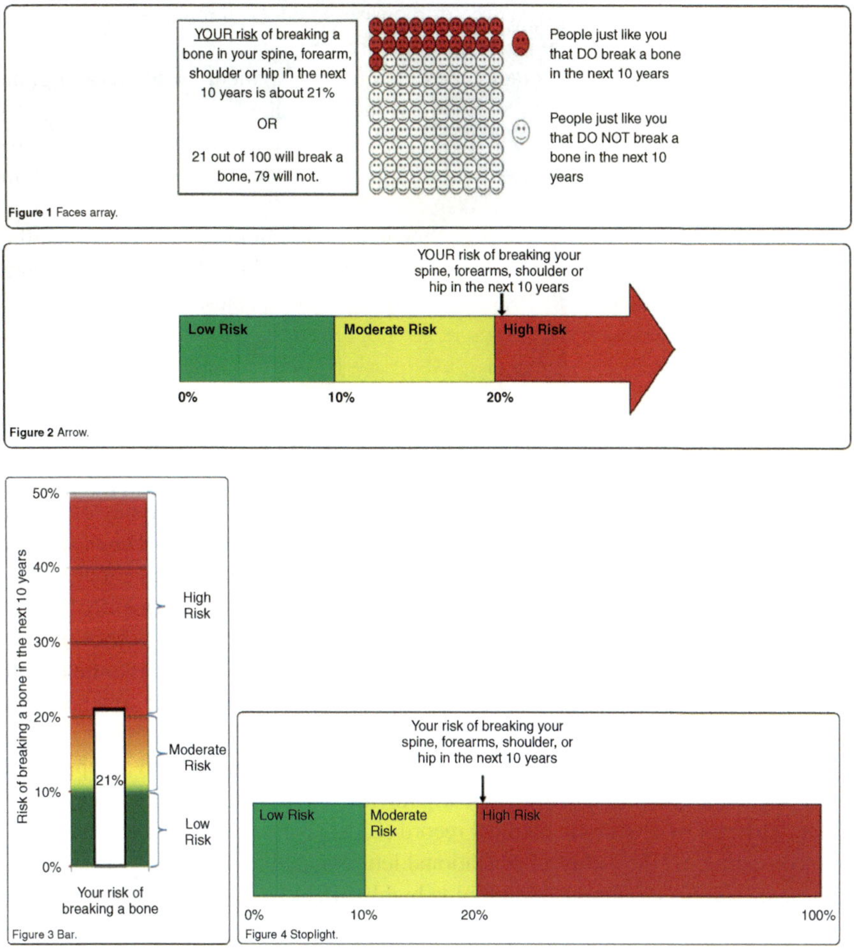

Fig. 8.2 Four risk depictions (Figure issued from Edmonds et al. [126], used with permission)

Of the four risk depictions investigated, the bar graph was the most preferred (selected by 37% of the participants) compared to stoplight (selected by 24%), faces (selected by 22%) or arrow (selected by 17%). The stoplight colour system was regarded as the most "clear," "clean," and "easy to read". Finally, the majority of subjects rated the pictogram as the most difficult to understand as this format does not allow people to quickly ascertain their individual risk category.

Up to now, no study has been able to rate the effectiveness of these visual presentations on patient's intentions of taking medication to prevent fractures [54, 127]. It has not been proven that one technique is superior to another to initiate treatment of patients. Moreover, sometimes the concept of "high risk" for future fracture, even when using a visual graph highlighting the "high risk" segment, can be confusing and can have varying levels of meaning to patients. Many patients believe that "high risk" has little relevance to their personal circumstances [104].

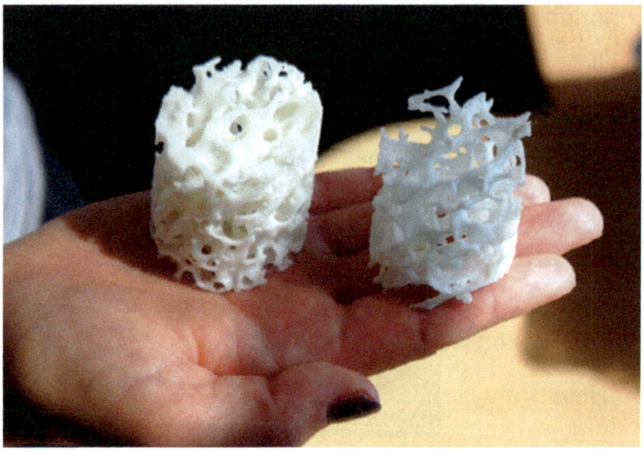

Fig. 8.3 3-D printed models used as intervention (Figure issued from Stephens et al. [128], used with permission)

New Techniques to Communicate Fractures Risk in Osteoporosis

Communication of fracture risk can also be achieved using other types of visual presentations. In 2016, Stephens et al. [128] tested the efficacy of a 3-D bone model (Fig. 8.3) to communicate fracture risk. In this study, patients received either a standard physician interview following their DXA or an interview augmented by the presentation of a 3-D bone model. This communication technique was shown to be effective in modifying cognitive and emotional representations relevant to treatment initiation among people with osteoporosis, which might facilitate commencement of treatment.

A study by Feldstein et al. [129] compared two interventions with a population receiving either patient-specific clinical guideline advice to the primary care provider delivered by electronic medical record (EMR) message or a second intervention consisting of EMR plus an educational letter mailed to the patient. The results indicated that this communication tool is highly effective at increasing the proportion of patients who receive a BMD measurement or an osteoporosis medication. No added value of the letter mailed to the patient was however noticed.

Conclusion on Fractures Risk Communication

Several risk algorithms have been developed and are available for the assessment of individuals' risk of fractures. The FRAX® tool, for example, allows us to estimate the risk of fracture over 10 years. Developing online tools to convert output of those fracture risk algorithms into friendly and visual presentation could facilitate professionals communicating with patients about fracture risk, either at time if visit or later, by mail or email. Using available and effective educational materials in daily practice to communicate in a highly efficient manner about risk could be an important step in enhancing patient education, self-management of the disease, acceptation of treatment and, ultimately, adherence to treatment. Nevertheless, further studies are needed to offer a more comprehensive approach of optimal communication about fractures and osteoporosis risks. Cultural differences between patients, that may impact communication comprehension, are often not considered in studies and further investigation of the impact of these cultural differences on the understanding of health information and fractures risks could be valuable.

Recommendations for Clinical Practice and Conclusion

Key Recommendations

1. Healthcare professionals need to optimize the doctor- patient relationship, in order to increase patients' trust in the healthcare provider and team.
2. Healthcare professionals need to better understand the individual perspective of the patient in front of them in terms of the patient's perceived risks and benefits for therapy. They need to be good listeners as patients are now more likely to suggest their own treatment plan.
3. Healthcare professionals need to understand the patient's self-perception of fracture risk.
4. Healthcare professionals need to understand the role of biases in decision-making by their patients.
5. Healthcare professionals need to optimise their communication with patients (e.g. framing effects). To do this they need to understand their patient's level of health literacy and numeracy.
6. Healthcare professionals need to better understand the role of other factors, particularly social media in decision making, but also the perspective of peers, family and friends.
7. Healthcare professionals need to understand cultural differences between patients (e.g. are decisions made only by the patient or by patient and family members?).
8. Healthcare professionals can help their patients by helping them understand the risk of no treatment versus risk of treatment explaining these risks to their spouse, child or caregiver as appropriate, and with consent.

The burden of nonadherence and poor implementation or compliance to osteoporosis therapies is large both in terms of societal costs of the burden of fractures but equally important in terms of the effects of fracture on quality of life of the individual with fractures.

Conclusion

Adherence or persistence to osteoporosis medications and to healthy behaviours such as calcium, vitamin D, exercise and balance training begins with effective communication of the risk of fractures and falls by the health care practitioner.

Communication of risk is complex, potentially influenced by gender and cultural differences as well as unconscious biases. The ability to comprehend the information is also limited by differences in the way individual patients understand this information. To help patients understand this information, there is a need for tools to help communicate information about risk as patients have different levels of numeracy, literacy and different learning styles (verbal or visual).

References

1. Borgström F, Karlsson L, Ortsäter G, et al. Fragility fractures in Europe: burden, management and opportunities. Arch Osteoporos. 2020;15(1):59. https://doi.org/10.1007/s11657-020-0706-y.
2. Hiligsmann M, Cornelissen D, Vrijens B, et al. Determinants, consequences and potential solutions to poor adherence to anti-osteoporosis treatment: results of an expert group meeting organized by the European Society for Clinical and Economic Aspects of osteoporosis, osteoarthritis and musculoskeletal. Osteoporos Int. 2019;30:2155–65. https://doi.org/10.1007/s00198-019-05104-5.
3. Lam WY, Fresco P. Medication adherence measures: an overview. Biomed Res Int. 2015;2015:217047. https://doi.org/10.1155/2015/217047.
4. World Health Organisation. Adherence to long-term therapies: evidence for action. http://www.who.int/chp/knowledge/publications/adherence_report/en/.
5. Dobbels F, Van Damme-Lombaert R, Vanhaecke J, De Geest S. Growing pains: non-adherence with the immunosuppressive regimen in adolescent transplant recipients. Pediatr Transplant. 2005;9:381–90. https://doi.org/10.1111/j.1399-3046.2005.00356.x.
6. Vrijens B, De Geest S, Hughes DA, et al. A new taxonomy for describing and defining adherence to medications. Br J Clin Pharmacol. 2012;73:691–705. https://doi.org/10.1111/j.1365-2125.2012.04167.x.
7. Lekkerkerker F, Kanis JA, Alsayed N, et al. Adherence to treatment of osteoporosis: a need for study. Osteoporos Int. 2007;18:1311–7. https://doi.org/10.1007/s00198-007-0410-4.
8. Anghel LA, Farcas AM, Oprean RN. An overview of the common methods used to measure treatment adherence. Med Pharm Rep. 2019;92:117–22. https://doi.org/10.15386/mpr-1201.
9. Vrijens B, Heidbuchel H. Non-vitamin K antagonist oral anticoagulants: considerations on once- vs. twice-daily regimens and their potential impact on medication adherence. Europace. 2015;17:514–23. https://doi.org/10.1093/europace/euu311.
10. Bonafede M, Johnson BH, Tang DH, et al. Etanercept-methotrexate combination therapy initiators have greater adherence and persistence than triple therapy initiators with rheumatoid arthritis. Arthritis Care Res. 2015;67:1656–63. https://doi.org/10.1002/acr.22638.
11. Chu LH, Kawatkar AA, Gabriel SE. Medication adherence and attrition to biologic treatment in rheumatoid arthritis patients. Clin Ther. 2015;37:660–6. https://doi.org/10.1016/j.clinthera.2014.10.022.
12. Kanis JA, Cooper C, Rizzoli R, et al. European guidance for the diagnosis and management of osteoporosis in postmenopausal women. Osteoporos Int. 2019;30:235–8. https://doi.org/10.1007/s00223-018-00512-x.
13. Rabenda V, Reginster JY. Overcoming problems with adherence to osteoporosis medication. Expert Rev Pharmacoecon Outcomes Res. 2010;10:677–89. https://doi.org/10.1586/erp.10.76.
14. Fischer MA, Stedman MR, Lii J, et al. Primary medication non-adherence: analysis of 195,930 electronic prescriptions. J Gen Intern Med. 2010;25:284–90. https://doi.org/10.1007/s11606-010-1253-9.

15. Reynolds K, Muntner P, Cheetham TC, et al. Primary non-adherence to bisphosphonates in an integrated healthcare setting. Osteoporos Int. 2013;24:2509–17. https://doi.org/10.1007/s00198-013-2326-5.
16. Fatoye F, Smith P, Gebrye T, Yeowell G. Real-world persistence and adherence with oral bisphosphonates for osteoporosis: a systematic review. BMJ Open. 2019;9:1–18. https://doi.org/10.1136/bmjopen-2018-027049.
17. Rabenda V, Mertens R, Fabri V, et al. Adherence to bisphosphonates therapy and hip fracture risk in osteoporotic women. Osteoporos Int. 2008;19:811–8. https://doi.org/10.1007/s00198-007-0506-x.
18. Koller G, Goetz V, Vandermeer B, et al. Persistence and adherence to parenteral osteoporosis therapies: a systematic review. Osteoporos Int. 2020;31:2093–102. https://doi.org/10.1007/s00198-020-05507-9.
19. Sato M, Tsujimoto M, Kajimoto K, et al. Effect of a patient-support program on once-daily teriparatide adherence and persistence in the Japan fracture observational study (JFOS). Arch Osteoporos. 2018;13(1):74. https://doi.org/10.1007/s11657-018-0487-8.
20. Blaschke TF, Osterberg L, Vrijens B, Urquhart J. Adherence to medications: insights arising from studies on the unreliable link between prescribed and actual drug dosing histories. Annu Rev Pharmacol Toxicol. 2012;52:275–301. https://doi.org/10.1146/annurev-pharmtox-011711-113247.
21. Sabate E, editor. Adherence to long-term therapies: evidence for action. Geneva: World Health Organization; 2003.
22. Kardas P, Lewek P, Matyjaszczyk M. Determinants of patient adherence: a review of systematic reviews. Front Pharmacol. 2013;4:1–16. https://doi.org/10.3389/fphar.2013.00091.
23. Yeam CT, Chia S, Tan HCC, et al. A systematic review of factors affecting medication adherence among patients with osteoporosis. Osteoporos Int. 2018;29:2623–37. https://doi.org/10.1007/s00198-018-4759-3.
24. Adler R, El-Hajj Fuleihan G, Bauer DC, Camacho PM, Clarke BL, Clines GA, Compston JE, Drake MT, Edwards BJ, Favus MJ, Greespan SL, McKinney R Jr, DE Pignolo RJS. Managing osteoporosis patients after long-term bisphosphonate treatment. J Bone Min Res. 2016;31:16–35. https://doi.org/10.1002/jbmr.2708.Managing.
25. Kendler DL, Macarios D, Lillestol MJ, et al. Influence of patient perceptions and preferences for osteoporosis medication on adherence behavior in the Denosumab adherence preference satisfaction study. Menopause. 2014;21:25–32. https://doi.org/10.1097/GME.0b013e31828f5e5d.
26. Barrett-Connor E, Wade SW, Do TP, et al. Treatment satisfaction and persistence among postmenopausal women on osteoporosis medications: 12-month results from POSSIBLE US™. Osteoporos Int. 2012;23:733–41. https://doi.org/10.1007/s00198-011-1620-3.
27. Hiligsmann M, Bours SPG, Boonen A. A review of patient preferences for osteoporosis drug treatment. Curr Rheumatol Rep. 2015;17(9):61. https://doi.org/10.1007/S11926-015-0533-0.
28. Danila MI, Outman RC, Rahn EJ, et al. Evaluation of a multimodal, direct-to-patient educational intervention targeting barriers to osteoporosis care: a randomized clinical trial. J Bone Miner Res. 2018;33:763–72. https://doi.org/10.1002/jbmr.3395.
29. Siris ES, Selby PL, Saag KG, et al. Impact of osteoporosis treatment adherence on fracture rates in North America and Europe. Am J Med. 2009;122:S3. https://doi.org/10.1016/j.amjmed.2008.12.002.
30. Ross S, Samuels E, Gairy K, et al. A meta-analysis of osteoporotic fracture risk with medication nonadherence. Value Heal. 2011;14:571–81. https://doi.org/10.1016/j.jval.2010.11.010.
31. Imaz I, Zegarra P, González-Enríquez J, et al. Poor bisphosphonate adherence for treatment of osteoporosis increases fracture risk: systematic review and meta-analysis. Osteoporos Int. 2010;21:1943–51. https://doi.org/10.1007/s00198-009-1134-4.
32. Yu S, Burge RT, Foster SA, et al. The impact of teriparatide adherence and persistence on fracture outcomes. Osteoporos Int. 2012;23:1103–13. https://doi.org/10.1007/s00198-011-1843-3.

33. Ringe JD, Möller G. Differences in persistence, safety and efficacy of generic and original branded once weekly bisphosphonates in patients with postmenopausal osteoporosis: 1-year results of a retrospective patient chart review analysis. Rheumatol Int. 2009;30:213–21. https://doi.org/10.1007/s00296-009-0940-5.
34. Kanis JA, Reginster JY, Kaufman JM, et al. A reappraisal of generic bisphosphonates in osteoporosis. Osteoporos Int. 2012;23:213–21. https://doi.org/10.1007/s00198-011-1796-6.
35. Hiligsmann M, McGowan B, Bennett K, et al. The clinical and economic burden of poor adherence and persistence with osteoporosis medications in Ireland. Value Health. 2012;15:604–12. https://doi.org/10.1016/j.jval.2012.02.001.
36. Hiligsmann M, Rabenda V, Gathon HJ, et al. Potential clinical and economic impact of non-adherence with osteoporosis medications. Calcif Tissue Int. 2010;86:202–10. https://doi.org/10.1007/s00223-009-9329-4.
37. Hiligsmann M, Rabenda V, Bruyère O, Reginster JY. The clinical and economic burden of non-adherence with oral bisphosphonates in osteoporotic patients. Health Policy (New York). 2010;96:170–7. https://doi.org/10.1016/j.healthpol.2010.01.014.
38. Hiligsmann M, Boonen A, Rabenda V, Reginster JY. The importance of integrating medication adherence into pharmacoeconomic analyses: the example of osteoporosis. Expert Rev Pharmacoecon Outcomes Res. 2012;12:159–66. https://doi.org/10.1586/erp.12.8.
39. Hiligsmann M, Reginster JY, Tosteson ANA, et al. Recommendations for the conduct of economic evaluations in osteoporosis: outcomes of an experts' consensus meeting organized by the European Society for Clinical and Economic Aspects of osteoporosis, osteoarthritis and musculoskeletal diseases (ESCEO) and the US branch of the International Osteoporosis Foundation. Osteoporos Int. 2019;30:45–57. https://doi.org/10.1007/s00198-018-4744-x.
40. Hiligsmann M, Salas M, Hughes DA, et al. Interventions to improve osteoporosis medication adherence and persistence: a systematic review and literature appraisal by the ISPOR Medication Adherence & Persistence Special Interest Group. Osteoporos Int. 2013;24:2907–18. https://doi.org/10.1007/s00198-013-2364-z.
41. Cornelissen D, de Kunder S, Si L, et al. Interventions to improve adherence to anti-osteoporosis medications: an updated systematic review. Osteoporos Int. 2020;31:1645–69. https://doi.org/10.1007/s00198-020-05378-0.
42. Beaton DE, Mamdani M, Zheng H, et al. Improvements in osteoporosis testing and care are found following the wide scale implementation of the Ontario fracture clinic screening program. Medicine (United States). 2017;96:1–7. https://doi.org/10.1097/MD.0000000000009012.
43. Tüzün Ş, Akyüz G, Eskiyurt N, et al. Impact of the training on the compliance and persistence of weekly bisphosphonate treatment in postmenopausal osteoporosis: a randomized controlled study. Int J Med Sci. 2013;10:1880–7. https://doi.org/10.7150/ijms.5359.
44. Roux S, Beaulieu M, Beaulieu MC, et al. Priming primary care physicians to treat osteoporosis after a fragility fracture: an integrated multidisciplinary approach. J Rheumatol. 2013;40:703–11. https://doi.org/10.3899/jrheum.120908.
45. Seuffert P, Sagebien CA, McDonnell M, O'Hara DA. Evaluation of osteoporosis risk and initiation of a nurse practitioner intervention program in an orthopedic practice. Arch Osteoporos. 2016;11:1–6. https://doi.org/10.1007/s11657-016-0262-7.
46. Hiligsmann M, Reginster JY. Cost-effectiveness of gastro-resistant risedronate tablets for the treatment of postmenopausal women with osteoporosis in France. Osteoporos Int. 2019;30:649–58. https://doi.org/10.1007/s00198-018-04821-7.
47. Oral A, Lorenc R, Sindel D, et al. Compliance, persistence, and preference outcomes of postmenopausal osteoporotic women receiving a flexible or fixed regimen of daily risedronate: a multicenter, prospective, parallel group study. Acta Orthop Traumatol Turc. 2015;49:67–74. https://doi.org/10.3944/AOTT.2015.14.0082.
48. Ducoulombier V, Luraschi H, Forzy G, et al. Contribution of phone follow-up to improved adherence to oral osteoporosis treatment. Am J Pharm Benefits. 2015;7:e81–9.

49. Stuurman-Bieze AGG, Hiddink EG, Van Boven JFM, Vegter S. Proactive pharmaceutical care interventions decrease patients' nonadherence to osteoporosis medication. Osteoporos Int. 2014;25:1807–12. https://doi.org/10.1007/s00198-014-2659-8.
50. Wu CH, Te Tu S, Chang YF, et al. Fracture liaison services improve outcomes of patients with osteoporosis-related fractures: a systematic literature review and meta-analysis. Bone. 2018;111:92–100. https://doi.org/10.1016/j.bone.2018.03.018.
51. Bachour F, Rizkallah M, Sebaaly A, et al. Fracture liaison service: report on the first successful experience from the Middle East. Arch Osteoporos. 2017;12:4–9. https://doi.org/10.1007/s11657-017-0372-x.
52. Axelsson KF, Jacobsson R, Lund D, Lorentzon M. Effectiveness of a minimal resource fracture liaison service. Osteoporos Int. 2016;27:3165–75. https://doi.org/10.1007/s00198-016-3643-2.
53. Grad R, Légaré F, Bell NR, et al. Shared decision making in preventive health care: what it is; what it is not. Can Fam Physician. 2017;63:682–4.
54. Montori VM, Shah ND, Pencille LJ, et al. Use of a decision aid to improve treatment decisions in osteoporosis: the osteoporosis choice randomized trial. Am J Med. 2011;124:549–56. https://doi.org/10.1016/j.amjmed.2011.01.013.
55. Delmas PD, Vrijens B, Eastell R, et al. Effect of monitoring bone turnover markers on persistence with risedronate treatment of postmenopausal osteoporosis. J Clin Endocrinol Metab. 2007;92:1296–304. https://doi.org/10.1210/jc.2006-1526.
56. Diez-Perez A, Adachi JD, Agnusdei D, et al. Treatment failure in osteoporosis. Osteoporos Int. 2012;23:2769–74. https://doi.org/10.1007/s00198-012-2093-8.
57. Diez-Perez A, Naylor KE, Abrahamsen B, et al. International osteoporosis foundation and European calcified tissue society working group. Recommendations for the screening of adherence to oral bisphosphonates. Osteoporos Int. 2017;28:767–74. https://doi.org/10.1007/s00198-017-3906-6.
58. Lloyd AJ. The extent of patients' understanding of the risk of treatments. Qual Heal Care. 2001;10:i14–8. https://doi.org/10.1136/qhc.0100014.
59. Weinstein ND. Optimistic biases about personal risks. Science (80-). 1989;246:1232–3. https://doi.org/10.1126/science.2686031.
60. Siris ES, Gehlbach S, Adachi JD, et al. Failure to perceive increased risk of fracture in women 55 years and older: the global longitudinal study of osteoporosis in women (GLOW). Osteoporos Int. 2011;22:27–35. https://doi.org/10.1007/s00198-010-1211-8.
61. Science of Patient Input Communication Working Group Consortium of the Medical Device Innovation. Best practices for communicating benefit, risk, and uncertainty for medical devices. https://mdic.org/resource/best-practices-for-communicating-benefit-risk-and-uncertainty-for-medical-devices/. Accessed Sept 2020.
62. Schrager S. Five ways to communicate risks so that patients understand. Fam Pract Manag. 2018;25:28–31.
63. Fischhoff B, Brewer N, Downs JE. Communicating risks and benefits: an evidence-based user's guide [Internet]. Silver Spring: U.S. Dep. Heal. Hum. Serv. Food Drug Adm; 2011. [Cited 2013 Feb 27].
64. Fagerlin A, Zikmund-Fisher BJ, Ubel PA. Helping patients decide: ten steps to better risk communication. J Natl Cancer Inst. 2011;103:1436–43. https://doi.org/10.1093/jnci/djr318.
65. FDA. (2016). Patient preference information – voluntary submission R in PAA, humanitarian device exemption applications, and de novo requests and i in ds and, device labeling. https://www.fda.gov/media/92593/download. Accessed Sept 2020. No Title.
66. Kessels RPC. Patients' memory for medical information. J R Soc Med. 2003;96:219–22. https://doi.org/10.1258/jrsm.96.5.219.
67. Büchter RB, Fechtelpeter D, Knelangen M, et al. Words or numbers? Communicating risk of adverse effects in written consumer health information: a systematic review and meta-analysis. BMC Med Inform Decis Mak. 2014;14:1–11. https://doi.org/10.1186/1472-6947-14-76.

68. Wilson R, Crouch WA. Risk assessment and comparisons: an introduction. Sciences (New York). 1987;236:267–70.
69. Wiles MD, Duffy A, Neill K. The numerical translation of verbal probability expressions by patients and clinicians in the context of peri-operative risk communication. Anaesthesia. 2020;75:e39–45. https://doi.org/10.1111/anae.14871.
70. Fraenkel L, Stolar M, Swift S, et al. Subjective numeracy and the influence of order and amount of audible information on perceived medication value. Med Decis Mak. 2017;37:230–8. https://doi.org/10.1177/0272989X16650665.
71. Webster RK, Weinman J, Rubin GJ. Explaining all without causing unnecessary harm: is there scope for positively framing medical risk information? Patient Educ Couns. 2019;102:602–3. https://doi.org/10.1016/j.pec.2018.09.014.
72. Silverman S, Age Q, Curtis J. (2014). Understanding physicians' perceptions of patients' barriers to osteoporosis medication initiation. Present. ASBMR. https://www.asbmr.org/education/abstractdetail?aid=8F4Fc96a-8ef1-4f7b-8dda-fa7d2747da1c.
73. Park DC, Lautenschlager G, Hedden T, et al. Models of visuospatial and verbal memory across the adult life span. Psychol Aging. 2002;17:299–320. https://doi.org/10.1037/0882-7974.17.2.299.
74. Schwartz LM, Woloshin S, Black WC, Welch HG. The role of numeracy in understanding the benefit of screening mammography. Ann Intern Med. 1997;127:966–72. https://doi.org/10.7326/0003-4819-127-11-199712010-00003.
75. Lipkus et al. General performance.
76. Peters E, Västfjäll D, Slovic P, et al. Numeracy and decision making. Psychol Sci. 2006;17:407–13. https://doi.org/10.1111/j.1467-9280.2006.01720.x.
77. Yamagishi K. When a 12. 86% mortality is more dangerous than 24.14%: implications for risk communication. Appl Cognit Psycol. 1997;11:495–506.
78. Schapira MM, Nattinger AB, McHorney CA. Frequency or probability? A qualitative study of risk communication formats used in health care. Med Decis Mak. 2001;21:459–67. https://doi.org/10.1177/0272989X0102100604.
79. Zipkin DA, Umscheid CA, Keating NL, et al. Evidence-based risk communication: a systematic review. Ann Intern Med. 2014;161:270–80. https://doi.org/10.7326/M14-0295.
80. Akl EA, Oxman AD, Herrin J, et al. Using alternative statistical formats for presenting risks and risk reductions. Cochrane Database Syst Rev. 2011;2011(3):CD006776. https://doi.org/10.1002/14651858.cd006776.pub2.
81. Covey J. A meta-analysis of the effects of presenting treatment benefits in different formats. Med Decis Mak. 2007;27:638–54. https://doi.org/10.1177/0272989X07306783.
82. Bodemer N, Meder B, Gigerenzer G. Communicating relative risk changes with baseline risk: presentation format and numeracy matter. Med Decis Mak. 2014;34:615–26. https://doi.org/10.1177/0272989X14526305.
83. Cheung YB, Wee HL, Thumboo J, et al. Risk communication in clinical trials: a cognitive experiment and a survey. BMC Med Inform Decis Mak. 2010;10:55. https://doi.org/10.1186/1472-6947-10-55.
84. Pighin S, Savadori L, Barilli E, et al. The 1-in-X effect on the subjective assessment of medical probabilities. Med Decis Mak. 2011;31:721–9. https://doi.org/10.1177/0272989X11403490.
85. Sheridan SL, Pignone MP, Lewis CL. A randomized comparison of patients' understanding of number needed to treat and other common risk reduction formats. J Gen Intern Med. 2003;18:884–92. https://doi.org/10.1046/j.1525-1497.2003.21102.x.
86. Trevena LJ, Zikmund-Fisher BJ, Edwards A, et al. Presenting quantitative information about decision outcomes: a risk communication primer for patient decision aid developers. BMC Med Inform Decis Mak. 2013;13:S7. https://doi.org/10.1186/1472-6947-13-S2-S7.
87. Sprague D, Russo JE, Lavallie DL, Buchwald DS. Influence of framing and graphic format on comprehension of risk information among American Indian tribal college students. J Cancer Educ. 2012;27:752–8. https://doi.org/10.1007/s13187-012-0372-x.

88. Waters EA, Weinstein ND, Colditz GA, Emmons K. Formats for improving risk communication in medical tradeoff decisions. J Health Commun. 2006;11:167–82. https://doi.org/10.1080/10810730500526695.
89. Garcia-Retamero R, Cokely ET. Designing visual AIDS that promote risk literacy: a systematic review of Health Research and evidence-based design heuristics. Hum Factors. 2017;59:582–627. https://doi.org/10.1177/0018720817690634.
90. Oudhoff JP, Timmermans DRM. The effect of different graphical and numerical likelihood formats on perception of likelihood and choice. Med Decis Mak. 2015;35:487–500. https://doi.org/10.1177/0272989X15576487.
91. Ancker JS, Senathirajah Y, Kukafka R, Starren JB. Design features of graphs in health risk communication: a systematic review. J Am Med Inform Assoc. 2006;13:608–18. https://doi.org/10.1197/jamia.M2115.
92. Barnes AJ, Hanoch Y, Miron-Shatz T, Ozanne EM. Tailoring risk communication to improve comprehension: do patient preferences help or hurt? Health Psychol. 2016;35:1007–16. https://doi.org/10.1037/hea0000367.
93. Hawley ST, Zikmund-Fisher B, Ubel P, et al. The impact of the format of graphical presentation on health-related knowledge and treatment choices. Patient Educ Couns. 2008;73:448–55. https://doi.org/10.1016/j.pec.2008.07.023.
94. Feldman-Stewart D, Kocovski N, McConnell BA, et al. Perception of quantitative information for treatment decisions. Med Decis Mak. 2000;20:228–38. https://doi.org/10.1177/0272989X0002000208.
95. Staff RC, Zwanziger L, Wiley J, Group NP. Communicating risks and benefits. Pharm Pract. 2003;13:289.
96. Garcia-Retamero R, Galesic M. Communicating treatment risk reduction to people with low numeracy skills: a cross-cultural comparison. Am J Public Health. 2009;99:2196–202. https://doi.org/10.2105/AJPH.2009.160234.
97. McCaffery KJ, Dixon A, Hayen A, et al. The influence of graphic display format on the interpretations of quantitative risk information among adults with lower education and literacy: a 1y. Med Decis Mak. 2012;32:532–44. https://doi.org/10.1177/0272989X11424926.
98. Lühnen J, Steckelberg A, Buhse S. Pictures in health information and their pitfalls: focus group study and systematic review. Z Evid Fortbild Qual Gesundhwes. 2018;137–138:77–89. https://doi.org/10.1016/j.zefq.2018.08.002.
99. Dolan JG, Iadarola S. Risk communication formats for low probability events: an exploratory study of patient preferences. BMC Med Inform Decis Mak. 2008;8:14. https://doi.org/10.1186/1472-6947-8-14.
100. Carrigan N, Raynor DK, Knapp P. Adequacy of patient information on adverse effects: an assessment of patient information leaflets in the UK. Drug Saf. 2008;31:305–12. https://doi.org/10.2165/00002018-200831040-00004.
101. Trevena LJ, Davey HM, Barratt A, et al. A systematic review on communicating with patients about evidence. J Eval Clin Pract. 2006;12:13–23. https://doi.org/10.1111/j.1365-2753.2005.00596.x.
102. Zikmund-Fisher BJ, Fagerlin A, Ubel PA. A demonstration of "less can be more" in risk graphics. Med Decis Mak. 2010;30:661–71. https://doi.org/10.1177/0272989X10364244.
103. Lewiecki EM. The role of risk communication in the care of osteoporosis. Curr Osteoporos Rep. 2011;9:141–8. https://doi.org/10.1007/s11914-011-0056-1.
104. Sale JEM, Hawker G, Cameron C, et al. Perceived messages about bone health after a fracture are not consistent across healthcare providers. Rheumatol Int. 2015;35:97–103. https://doi.org/10.1007/s00296-014-3079-y.
105. Dewan N, MacDermid JC, MacIntyre NJ, Grewal R. Therapist's practice patterns for subsequent fall/osteoporotic fracture prevention for patients with a distal radius fracture. J Hand Ther. 2019;32:497–506. https://doi.org/10.1016/j.jht.2018.03.001.
106. Meyer G, Steckelberg A, Mühlhauser I. Analysis of consumer information brochures on osteoporosis prevention and treatment. Ger Med Sci. 2007;5:Doc01.

107. Litwic AE, Westbury LD, Carter S, et al. Self-perceived fracture risk in the global longitudinal study of osteoporosis in women: its correlates and relationship with bone microarchitecture. Calcif Tissue Int. 2020;106:625–36. https://doi.org/10.1007/s00223-020-00680-9.
108. Kanis JA, Harvey NC, McCloskey E, et al. Algorithm for the management of patients at low, high and very high risk of osteoporotic fractures. Osteoporos Int. 2020;31:1–12. https://doi.org/10.1007/s00198-019-05176-3.
109. Barrett-Connor E, Sajjan SG, Siris ES, et al. Wrist fracture as a predictor of future fractures in younger versus older postmenopausal women: results from the National Osteoporosis Risk Assessment (NORA). Osteoporos Int. 2008;19:607–13. https://doi.org/10.1007/s00198-007-0508-8.
110. O'Reilly C, Keogan F, Breen R, et al. Falls risk factors and healthcare use in patients with a low-trauma wrist fracture attending a physiotherapy clinic. Int J Ther Rehabil. 2013;20:480–6. https://doi.org/10.12968/ijtr.2013.20.10.480.
111. Hakestad KA, Nordsletten L, Torstveit MK, Risberg MA. Postmenopausal women with osteopenia and a healed wrist fracture have reduced physical function and quality of life compared to a matched, healthy control group with no fracture. BMC Womens Health. 2014;14:92. https://doi.org/10.1186/1472-6874-14-92.
112. Hvas L, Reventlow S, Malterud K. Women's needs and wants when seeing the GP in relation to menopausal issues. Scand J Prim Health Care. 2004;22:118–21. https://doi.org/10.1080/02813430410005964.
113. Kasper MJ, Peterson MG, Allegrante JP. The need for comprehensive educational osteoporosis prevention programs for young women: results from a second osteoporosis prevention survey. Arthritis Rheum. 2001;45:28–34. https://doi.org/10.1002/1529-0131(200102)45:1<28::AID-ANR80>3.0.CO;2-G.
114. Yen PH, Leasure AR. Use and effectiveness of the teach-Back method in patient education and health outcomes. Fed Pract. 2019;36:284–9.
115. Prochnow JA, Meiers SJ, Scheckel MM. Improving patient and caregiver new medication education using an innovative teach-back toolkit. J Nurs Care Qual. 2019;34:101–6. https://doi.org/10.1097/NCQ.0000000000000342.
116. Lewiecki EM. Risk communication and shared decision making in the care of patients with osteoporosis. J Clin Densitom. 2010;13:335–45. https://doi.org/10.1016/j.jocd.2010.06.005.
117. Ettinger B. A personal perspective on fracture risk assessment tools. Menopause. 2008;15:1023–6. https://doi.org/10.1097/gme.0b013e31817f3e4d.
118. Roblin DW, Cram P, Lou Y, et al. Diet and exercise changes following bone densitometry in the patient activation after DXA result notification (PAADRN) study. Arch Osteoporos. 2018;13(1):4. https://doi.org/10.1007/s11657-017-0402-8.
119. Roblin DW, Zelman D, Plummer S, et al. Evaluation of a "just-in-time" nurse consultation on bone health: a pilot randomized controlled trial. Perm J. 2017;21:1–12. https://doi.org/10.7812/TPP/16-112.
120. Wolinsky FD, Lou Y, Edmonds SW, et al. Activating patients with a tailored bone density test results letter and educational brochure: the PAADRN randomized controlled trial. J Clin Densitom. 2017;20:464–71. https://doi.org/10.1016/j.jocd.2016.08.012.
121. Wu F, Wills K, Laslett LL, et al. Individualized fracture risk feedback and long-term benefits after 10 years. Am J Prev Med. 2018;54:266–74. https://doi.org/10.1016/j.amepre.2017.10.018.
122. Nadler M, Alibhai S, Catton P, et al. The impact of bone mineral density testing, fracture assessment, and osteoporosis education in men treated by androgen deprivation for prostate cancer: a pilot study. Support Care Cancer. 2014;22:2409–15. https://doi.org/10.1007/s00520-014-2183-6.
123. Brask-Lindemann D, Cadarette SM, Eskildsen P, Abrahamsen B. Osteoporosis pharmacotherapy following bone densitometry: importance of patient beliefs and understanding of DXA results. Osteoporos Int. 2011;22:1493–501. https://doi.org/10.1007/s00198-010-1365-4.

124. Dunniway DL, Camune B, Baldwin K, Crane JK. FRAX® counseling for bone health behavior change in women 50 years of age and older. J Am Acad Nurse Pract. 2012;24:382–9. https://doi.org/10.1111/j.1745-7599.2012.00700.x.
125. Solomon DH, Finkelstein JS, Polinski JM, et al. A randomized controlled trial of mailed osteoporosis education to older adults. Osteoporos Int. 2006;17:760–7. https://doi.org/10.1007/s00198-005-0049-y.
126. Edmonds SW, Cram P, Lu X, et al. Improving bone mineral density reporting to patients with an illustration of personal fracture risk. BMC Med Inform Decis Mak. 2014;14:1–12. https://doi.org/10.1186/s12911-014-0101-y.
127. Kalluru R, Petrie KJ, Grey A, et al. Randomised trial assessing the impact of framing of fracture risk and osteoporosis treatment benefits in patients undergoing bone densitometry. BMJ Open. 2017;7:1–8. https://doi.org/10.1136/bmjopen-2016-013703.
128. Stephens MH, Grey A, Fernandez J, et al. 3-D bone models to improve treatment initiation among patients with osteoporosis: a randomised controlled pilot trial. Psychol Health. 2016;31:487–97. https://doi.org/10.1080/08870446.2015.1112389.
129. Feldstein A, Elmer PJ, Smith DH, et al. Electronic medical record reminder improves osteoporosis management after a fracture: a randomized, controlled trial. J Am Geriatr Soc. 2006;54:450–7. https://doi.org/10.1111/j.1532-5415.2005.00618.x.

Chapter 9
Fracture Liaison Services

Z. Mohsin and M. K. Javaid

Introduction

A fracture after a fall from standing height or less in an adult aged 50 years and over is an accepted critical signal to assess and treat osteoporosis, secondary fracture prevention. Despite consistent and robust evidence to support the clinical effectiveness of this approach from large scale randomised controlled trials [1–10], natural experiments [11] and real world data [12], a large proportion of patients presenting to healthcare professionals with a clear fragility fracture remain undiagnosed and untreated [13, 14] in the so-called 'Treatment Gap' [15]. It is estimated that only 20% of fractured patients are assessed and treated appropriately, varying by country and fracture site [16]. As a result, most patients with a fragility fracture continue to lose bone and have potentially avoidable fractures with significant mortality, loss of independence and cost to healthcare, social care and wider society. To address this treatment gap, national and international clinical guidelines [17–19] and systematic reviews from the academic community [20, 21] recommend the use of a Fracture Liaison Service (FLS) in order to effectively close this treatment gap.

Secondary Fracture Prevention: The Solutions

The core components for secondary fracture prevention are to ensure all adults aged 50 years and over presenting with a fragility fracture after a minimal trauma (a fall from standing height or less) are systematically assessed, recommended therapy and then monitored for at least 12 months [18, 22, 23] (Fig. 9.1). Fractures of the digits,

Z. Mohsin · M. K. Javaid (✉)
NDORMS, University of Oxford, Oxford, UK
e-mail: zaineb.mohsin@ndorms.ox.ac.uk; kassim.javaid@ndorms.ox.ac.uk

E. Dennison (ed.), *Osteoporosis Treatment*, https://doi.org/10.1007/978-3-030-78128-6_9

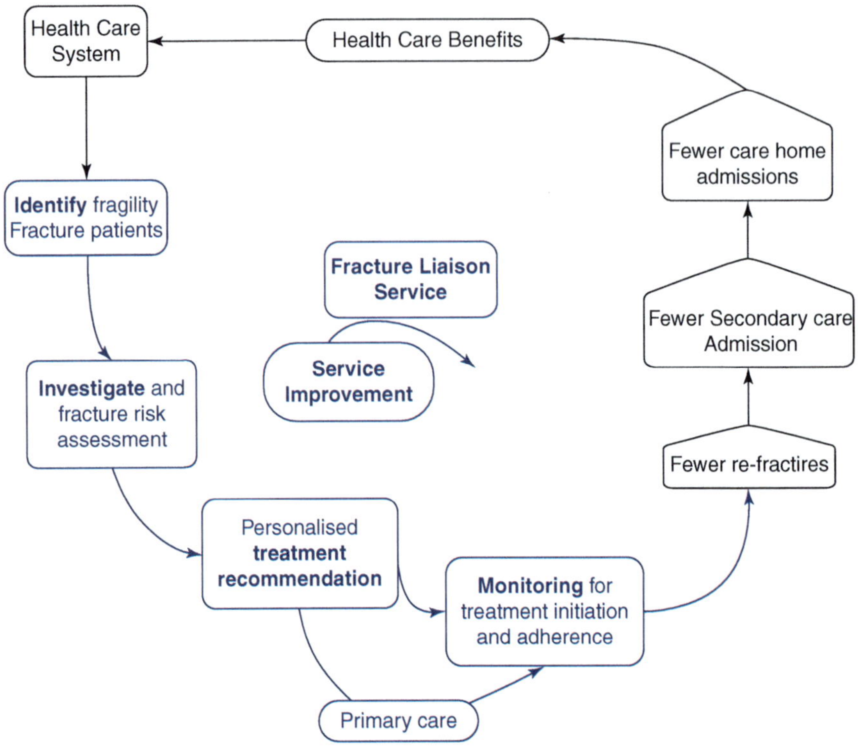

Fig. 9.1 Conceptual Model of a Fracture Liaison Service

scaphoid, face and skull are usually not considered as fragility fractures in this context. A number of health service models have been used to close the treatment gap, collectively labelled as Post Fracture Care systems. These can be grouped into services that exclusively deliver these components such as Fracture Liaison Services (FLSs) or models that include secondary fracture prevention. They also include other healthcare provider roles such as Osteoporosis Liaison Services, that also include primary prevention or Orthogeriatric Liaison Services, that also include other aspects of orthogeriatric care coordination an integrated orthopaedic solutions, rather than secondary fracture prevention which is embedded in the routine trauma care pathway [24]. While each of the above have their strengths and weaknesses, services that only deliver education or refer/ ask other healthcare providers to do additional work are not effective [25]. Any successful model serves two main purposes; one to ensure patients eligible for anti-osteoporosis therapy start treatment early and adhere; two: to constantly evaluate service performance to optimise effectiveness, efficiency and patient experience [26]. In this chapter we will use the acronym FLS to encompass the different secondary fracture prevention models of care.

The outline model for the key steps for secondary fracture prevention is depicted in Fig. 9.2.

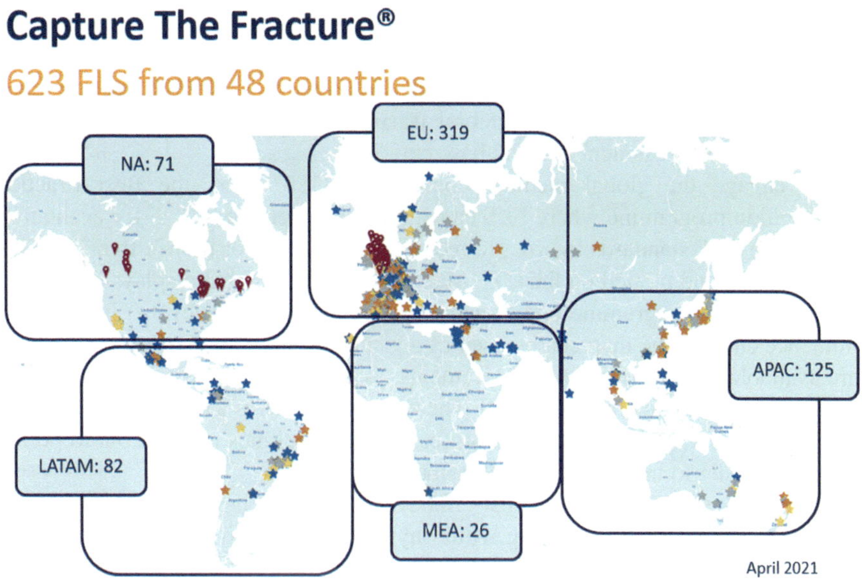

Fig. 9.2 The Map of Best Practice recognises over 400 FLS that identify over 345,000 patients every year across the globe. (© Capture the Fracture®/International Osteoporosis Foundation, Reprinted with permission from the IOF. All rights reserved)

Evidence for Effectiveness of FLS

The International Osteoporosis Foundation (IOF) Capture the Fracture® (CTF) initiative has allowed effective mapping of FLS across the globe (Fig. 9.2). In 2013, there were 57 FLS worldwide registered with the IOF Capture the Fracture programme. In the same year, FLS coverage was assessed in 19 of 27 European countries. It was estimated that there was an FLS in less than 10% of their healthcare institutions [16]. The story was even more concerning in the Asia-Pacific region with 9 out of 16 countries reporting that none of their hospitals had an FLS [27] and only Singapore reported an established FLS in over half of their hospitals [28]. By 2018 the total number of FLS had risen to 327 (identifying over 345,000 fracture patients/year) with 80 new FLS in that year alone, and three new countries registering their first FLS; The Philippines, Sri Lanka, and Saudi Arabia.

It was previously considered difficult to compare 'inter-service' efficacy and performance due to the wide range of service models in use [21], however, the CTF programme (launched in 2012) has drawn up standards against which services can be assessed. This 'Best Practice Framework' identifies 13 criteria and standards including patient identification, patient evaluation, post-assessment timing, vertebral fracture identification, assessment guidelines, assessment of secondary causes of osteoporosis, falls prevention services, multifaceted nature of assessment, medication initiation, medication review, communication strategy, long-term management and database curation. Each of these standards are graded as bronze, silver or gold depending on the quality of the particular facet of the service. The FLS is then scored according to 5 domains composed of 4 different fracture types (hip, inpatient, outpatient and vertebral fractures) and an organizational domain (including falls assessment and database curation).

To engage the global medical community, CTF offers the Best Practice Recognition programme where FLS can submit their service to IOF for evaluation against the BPF standards in order to receive a gold, silver or bronze star. The FLS is showcased and plotted on the CTF Map of Best Practice that displays participating FLS in the programme and their respective achievement level (Fig. 9.2). To influence change, the map can be used as a visual representation of services which are available worldwide, their achievements, as well as the areas for improvement in secondary fracture prevention [29]. The map also serves as a policy advocacy tool that can be leveraged by healthcare professionals and clinics to reach out to policy makers in order to influence changes at national levels.

Analyses of the clinical and cost-effectiveness of FLS have been performed in recent years, including modelling within hypothetical cohorts. McLellan and colleagues used a cost-effectiveness and budget-impact model (developed using 8 years of FLS data in a UK population) to show that, by implementing an FLS, 18 fractures could be prevented per year (for a hypothetical cohort of 1000 fragility fracture patients) providing an overall saving of £21,000 [30]. A similar study of a hypothetical cohort of 1000 patients in a Swedish population used a Markov microsimulation model to demonstrate that FLS implementation prevented 22 fractures with an incremental cost per QALY for FLS vs. usual care of €14,029 [31].

In 2016, Hawley and colleagues examined the impact of FLS introduction or expansion on hip fracture outcomes in the UK using the Hospital Episode Statistics database. Their natural experiment included patients across 11 acute hospital trusts in England who had sustained a hip fracture between 2003 and 2013 and were aged over 60 years. Using time-series analyses, 30 day and 1 year mortality and second hip fracture were examined before and after the change in fracture prevention services. Of the 33,152 primary hip fractures included in the study, 1288 (4.2%) went on to sustain a second hip fracture within 2 years, 3033 (9.5%) patients died within 30 days of their primary hip fracture and 9662 (29.8%) died within 1 year [32]. The introduction or expansion of a nurse-led fracture liaison service was protective for 30 day mortality (Hazard Ratio (HR) 0.80, 95% CI 0.71–0.91) and 1 year mortality (HR 0.84, 95% CI 0.77–0.93) [32]. However, there was no effect on the occurrence of second hip fracture and there was no account of whether patients were actually seen by the FLS. A parallel qualitative study was undertaken for the sites and identified ensuring good adherence as key for service effectiveness [33]. The findings of this study provide substantial evidence that delegating monitoring and adherence to existing primary care services blunts the effectiveness of FLSs and supports the need to include monitoring, at least in the short to medium term, within the FLS specification.

The cost-effectiveness of FLS was addressed in 2017 by Leal and colleagues who used Markov models to estimate the lifetime impact of an orthogeriatrician-led FLS, nurse-led FLS and usual care. They estimated that, for a female aged 83 years, an orthogeriatrician-led service was effective at £22,709 per QALY for all costs and £12,860 per QALY for healthcare costs. For males the cost-effectiveness of healthcare costs was £14,525 per QALY. These findings demonstrate that there is a significant economic rationale for the introduction of FLS. A more recent systematic review that included any study of FLSs irrespective of study design has also demonstrated the potential benefits from introduction of an FLS [34, 35].

The workforce impact and issues surrounding the running of an FLS were assessed in a qualitative analysis of interviews with 43 health professionals in the UK, all of whom had been involved in FLS [36]. Significant themes included communication, resourcing and adherence. It was felt that fracture prevention coordinators improved communication within the multidisciplinary team, however, communication between secondary and primary care was sometimes a challenge. It was noted that the writing of a business case (a fundamental step en route to establishing an FLS in a hospital trust in the UK) was challenging and that there was under-resourcing of FLS in some sectors. Patient adherence to treatment was observed to be a weakness of the current FLS model and led to calls to improved medication monitoring.

In conclusion, an increasingly substantial body of research data supports the use of FLS by demonstrating a 50% reduction in hip fracture mortality, a 20% reduction in secondary fracture and reduced drug therapy and cost in regions served by an FLS.

How to Implement an FLS (a Step-by-Step Guide)

The key stages to the development of an FLS are developing national prioritisation, the business case, implementation and sustainability. The first step is prioritization for FLS at the policy level nationally or regionally. This involves a national coalition of professional societies, patient groups, existing FLS champions and relevant policy makers at the regional and national level. Central to the process of prioritisation is the data pack that links current and projected burden of fragility fracture with the patient, family, health care and societal benefits from national implementation of secondary fracture prevention services, options for integration within existing and planned healthcare policy initiatives and a framework for evaluation.

At the local level, there are key steps to getting started. These include identifying the FLS champion, assembling a team including multiple disciplines and patient representatives; identifying key influencers; mapping the current and desired care pathway for secondary fracture prevention; collecting audit and other data to develop a business case (Fig. 9.3). A coherent multi-disciplinary team should be identified and recruited including a lead champion for osteoporosis, orthopaedic (likely hip) surgeon, physicians (likely to come from specialties including geriatrics, rheumatology or endocrinology), DXA-specialist radiologists, specialist nurses, physiotherapists and an FLS coordinator. The project team should also include representation from relevant stakeholders including pharmacy, primary care physicians, health system administration, patient champions, charity sector and the

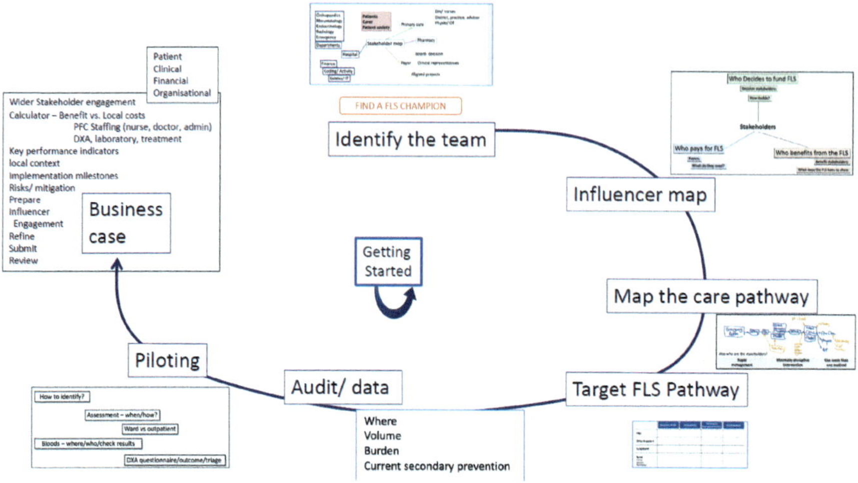

Fig. 9.3 Capture the Fracture Mentorship roadmap for getting FLSs started

health system management funders. This team will provide a holistic overview and ensure that the FLS is structured to perform the functions required by all stakeholders. An initial audit should be performed in order to provide a 'pre-FLS' baseline for future analyses of quality improvement. The data collected should include the number of individuals aged ≥50 years who attend with a hip fragility fracture, with a previous fragility fracture in the last 2 years, already receiving anti-osteoporosis medications and discharged on anti-osteoporosis medication. Additional information on length of stay, discharge destination, healthcare costs and extension to other fracture types will depend on the availability of contemporary national data.

Effective staged implementation of the FLS is often needed. This involves starting with a specific subgroup such as individuals with a hip fracture, women, those aged 60–75 or at specific clinic sites or weeks of the year and introducing the care pathway from identification to monitoring as a minimum scalable unit. Learning from this small-scale implementation then informs wider roll out till all eligible patients can be managed.

A FLS business case is then developed that reflects the local benefits of FLS implementation as well as the local FLS costs and inter-dependencies. This may need to be informed by pilot studies to ascertain the optimal minimally disruptive pathway for patients through the different stages of identification, investigation, treatment recommendation and monitoring [37]. Effective patient engagement is key to ensure the pathway is patient centred.

Benchmarking the Service: Delivering the Expected Benefit

Following implementation, service improvement is essential to ensure services are delivering on their expectations and should be supported by local, regional and national and peer-peer and peer-expert forums for discussion and sharing learning [23]. Tools to deliver these programmes of work are being developed by the Capture the Fracture working group and include different methods for mentoring FLSs through implementation and sustainability of their services.

Core to service improvement is the Best Practice Framework developed by the IOF to measure the organisational elements of the service to ensure the correct pathways and resources are in place [22]. A questionnaire based on the Framework is also available in multiple languages and is key to getting evaluated on the Capture the Fracture Map (https://www.capturethefracture.org/get-mapped) [38].

This is supported by the CTF Educational Programme, and includes webinars with the aim to engage with the FLS community of CTF and provide relevant knowledge on FLS and secondary fracture prevention. (https://capturethefracture.org/webinars).

The 13 benchmarking criteria are graded as Level 1, 2 or 3 (3 being the best example of practice), as seen in Table 9.1 and include the following:

Table 9.1 The Capture the Fracture® Best Practice Framework for the international benchmarking of fracture liaison services

BPF standard	Level 1	Level 2	Level 3
1. Patient Identification	Patents ID'd, **not** tracked	Patents ID'd, **are** tracked	Patients ID'd, tracked & **Independent review**
2. Patient Evaluation	**50%** assessed	**70%** assessed	**90%** assessed
3. Post Fracture Assessment Timing	Within **13–16 weeks**	Within **9–12 weeks**	Within **8 weeks**
4. Vertebral Fracture (VF) ID	Known VF assessed	Routinely assesses for VF	Radiologists identify VF
5. Assessment Guidelines	Local	Regional	National
6. Secondary Causes of Osteoporosis	**50%** of patients screened	**70%** of patients screened	**90%** of patients screened
7. Falls Prevention Services	**50%** of patients evaluated	**70%** of patients evaluated	**90%** of patients evaluated
8. Multifaceted Assessment	**50%** of patients screened	**70%** of patients screened	**90%** of patents screened
9. Medication Initiation	**50%** of patients initiated	**70%** of patients initiated	**90%** of patients initiated
10. Medication Review	**50%** assessed	**70%** assessed	**90%** assessed
11. Communication Strategy	Communicates to doctor	Communicates to doctor w/ %**50** criteria	Communicates to doctor w/%**90** criteria[a]
12. Long-term Management	**1 year** follow-up		**6 month** follow-up & **1 year** follow-up
13. Database	Local	Regional	National

[a]Criteria: FRAX, DXA, Vertebral DXAIx-ray. primary risk factors, secondary risk factors, falls risk, current medications, medication compliance, follow-up plan, lifestyle risk-factors, time since last fracture

1. Patient identification—patients with fragility fractures may be identified (level 1), tracked through the health system and may be independently reviewed by the FLS (level 2 and 3).
2. Patient evaluation—assesses the percentage of patients with a fragility fracture are evaluated for the risk of future fracture via a clinical prediction tool (FRAX®) or assessment of bone mineral density
3. Post-fracture assessment timing—assesses how quickly patients with fragility fractures are assessed with a formal fracture risk assessment by the FLS in weeks since the fracture
4. Vertebral fracture identification—despite being the most common fragility fracture many vertebral fractures are identified by chance (for example as incidental findings in radiological investigations) due to variation in clinical presentation. To achieve the highest level of practice in this criterion it is necessary to liaise with radiology to ensure that they identify and report vertebral fractures and provide a coherent pathway for these patients to access the FLS
5. Assessment guidelines—evaluates whether the practice of the FLS is aligned to local, national or international guidance for the assessment of fragility fractures
6. Secondary causes of osteoporosis—assesses the percentage of patients with fragility fractures who are screened for secondary causes of osteoporosis
7. Falls prevention services—concerns the percentage of patients evaluated for referral to a falls service
8. Multifaceted assessment—addresses the assessment (and management) of lifestyle factors which may underlie the fracture
9. Medication initiation—includes the percentage of patients who were eligible for treatment receiving anti-osteoporosis medication
10. Medication review—includes the percentage of patients who are on anti-osteoporosis medication who have their compliance assessed and in whom alternative medications are considered
11. Communication strategy—assesses the quality of communication between the FLS and doctors in primary and secondary care including whether the following items are communicated; FRAX® scores, DXA outcomes, vertebral imaging, primary and secondary risk factors for fracture, falls risk, current medication and compliance, follow-up plan, lifestyle risk-factors and time since last fracture
12. Long-term management—assesses whether medication compliance and tolerance are assessed at 6 months and 1 year after commencement
13. Database—refers to whether the FLS contributes to a database for fragility fractures at a local, regional or national level

These criteria are similar to the data collected as part of national registries, including the Australian and New Zealand Hip Fracture Registry [39].

Services can use the questionnaire based on the BPF to apply for recognition on the Capture the Fracture Map. A star is awarded depending on the type of service. A blue star is given for sites that have just started and do not have enough information for a full assessment. A blue star is important as it recognises the initiation of FLS activity in the local healthcare provider site. This may be important to motivate decision makers to support local initiatives as well as provide a focus for other sites to form local networks or bone clubs for support and advocacy. Stars (bronze to gold) are awarded based on the organisational performance following completion of the BPF questionnaire. Completing the detailed questionnaire provides a structured review of services and supports the local team to identify areas of good practice to maintain as well as areas to improve by service redesign / improvement or by requesting additional resources.

At the patient level, a set of key performance indicators have been developed to inform service improvement (Fig. 9.4) [40]. These indicators measure the actual delivery of patient care across 11 indicators compared with the BPF which uses reported performance.

The indicators can be used in the local context for quality improvement through data driven identification of care pathway components that require improvement as well as evaluating the impact of any service change in real time (Fig. 9.5).

At the regional level, they can support peer to peer mentoring as well as identification of beacon services delivering more effective care (Fig. 9.6).

Finally at the national level they can be used to prioritise structural priorities that require high level policy or commissioning action. The England and Wales Fracture Liaison Service Database annual reports exemplifies the use of patient level indicators [41] (Fig. 9.7).

Potential Barriers and How to Overcome Them

In some cases the instigation of an FLS is hampered by barriers, both perceived and real.

Inadequate financial resources to afford an FLS nurse specialist is one such example with a potential solution being the employment (or re-deployment) of a member of secretarial staff to take on the administrative duties which form part of the FLS nurse specialist role. Language is a potential barrier to engaging with global

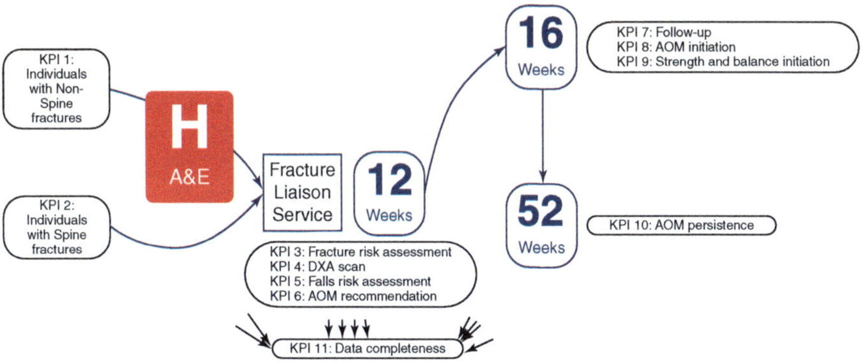

Fig. 9.4 Overview of key performance indicator set for FLSs. (Adapted from Javaid et al. [40]). *AOM* anti-osteoporosis medication

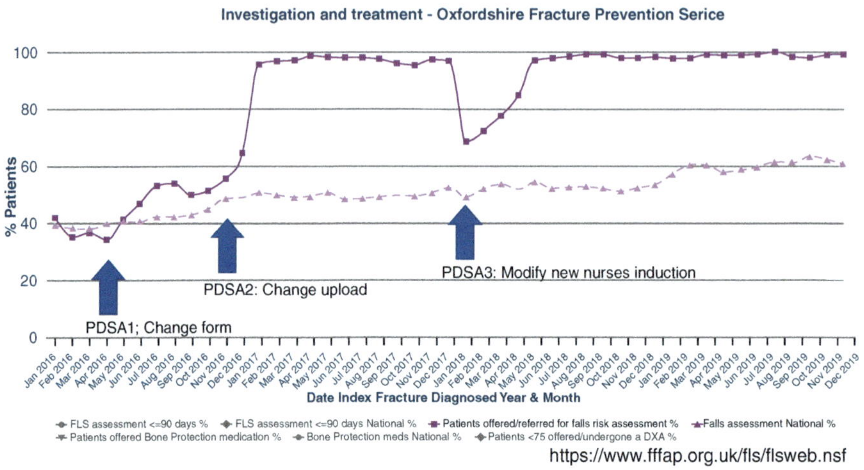

Fig. 9.5 Using the Key performance indicators to track delivery of falls assessment over time at the FLS level. (Data extracted from Public Run charts from Health and Quality Improvement Partnership Royal College of Physicians Fracture Liaison Service Database Audit for the Oxfordshire Fracture prevention service (https://www.fffap.org.uk/80257FC4002BDD96). Reprinted with permission. Copyright RCP and Crown Informatics Attribution)

Total records submitted	Cases identified	Spine fractures	Assessment within 90 days	DXA within 90 days	Falls risk assessment	Bone treatment	Strength & Balance by 16 weeks	16 week follow up	Treatment by 1st followup	1 year drug adhereance
3518	99	66.2	78.9	70.6	98.9	61.3	.4	52.9	46.4	43.7
1044	43.2	28	59.2	36.7	84	32.9	2.9	6	45.1	27.5
10	1.5	0	10	0	30	10	0	0	0	50
1062	52.4	10.9	66.4	57.9	66.4	30.2	.5	24	14.6	0
283	18.9	14	76.7	29.6	84.2	50.2	20.7	6.4	41.4	18.8
857	30.9	4	99.2	1.5	37.9	75.3	14.8	38.6	14.2	26.3
1983	78.7	76.8	70.8	70.5	98	46.1	17.4	56.6	42	33.5
2283	79.4	11	92.9	31.4	54.7	50.6	2.8	20.9	14.4	.1
1	.1	.3	100	0	100	100	0	0	0	0
1407	74.4	18.8	99.8	75.2	66.5	62.8	0	0	0	0
748	29.5	1.4	67.6	32.3	97.4	28.5	1.5	32.4	34.7	22.5
709	65	1.8	37	2.1	100	14.4	42.4	4.9	54.9	2.1
5	.5	0	80	0	40	100	0	80	60	0
3336	79.9	.7	99.4	.2	54.6	86.5	0	.3	.3	0
3518	99	66.2	78.9	70.6	98.9	61.3	.4	52.9	46.4	43.7
1122	58.6	61.9	41.3	60.6	67.6	24.6	18	39	44.3	38.6

Fig. 9.6 Using Key performance indicators to identify beacon sites with more effective delivery of secondary fracture prevention. Each row is a different FLS and for each indicator that actual performance for 2018 is shown together with a colour code of green >80%, orange 50–79% and red <50%. (Reprinted with permission. Copyright RCP and Crown Informatics Attribution)

resources (such as those available through CTF) however, the Best Practice Framework (BPF) document is currently available in 12 major languages: English; French; Spanish; German; Portuguese; Polish; Italian; Hebrew; Russian; Slovak; Chinese (both traditional and simplified forms); and Japanese and the BPF questionnaire (which is completed by all FLS joining the Capture the Fracture program) is now available in 8 languages: English; Polish; Spanish; Portuguese; Japanese;

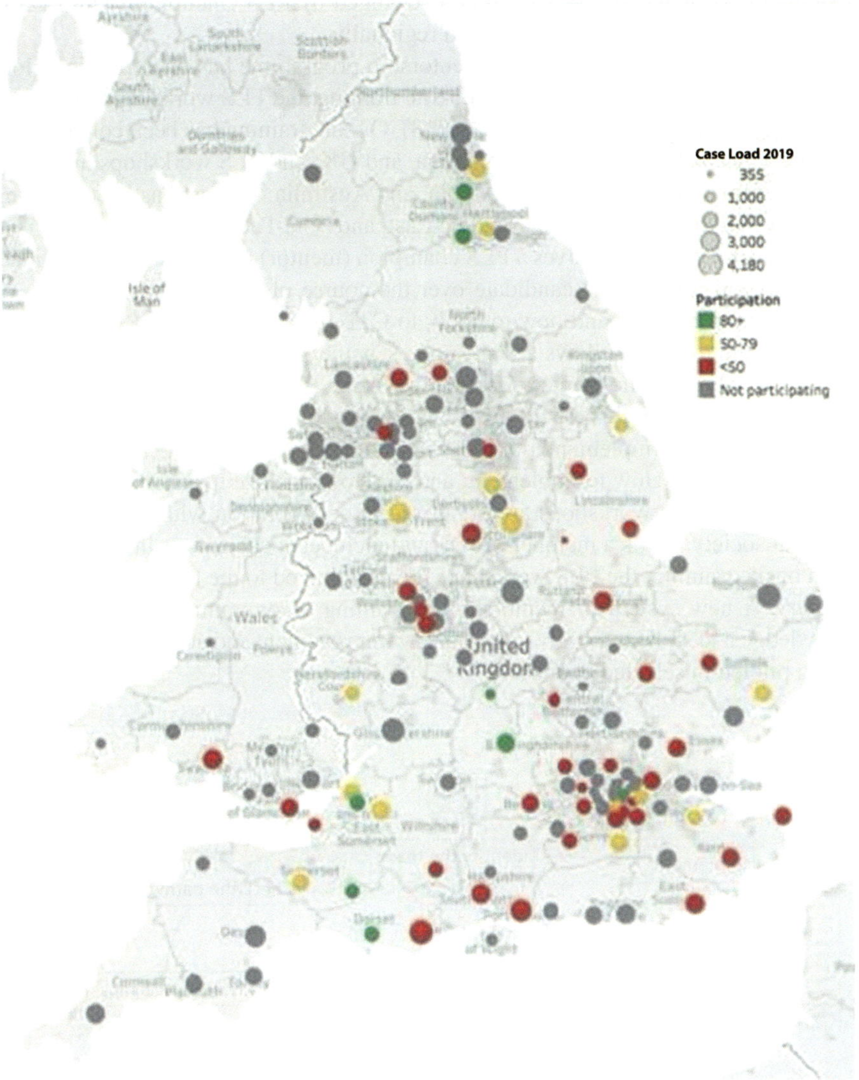

Fig. 9.7 Case identification in FLSs in England and Wales in 2019. Map of case identification for sites from modified from [41]

Russian; German; and Slovak. A Thai version is being developed in collaboration with local FLS experts and medical associations in 2019.

Lack of prior experience running an FLS can lead to a lack of confidence and halting of an FLS initiative. This can be addressed via educational tools and direct mentorship from experienced FLS providers.

The CTF mentorship programme, connects leading FLS experts with institutions willing to establish a new FLS. The programme creates the platform on which essential knowledge and skills can be exchanged by FLS champions with FLS in early stage of development, locally and regionally.

Since its inception in 2016, the mentorship programme has been running globally, offering a combination of both on-site training and FLS workshops to provide guidance on FLS implementation (Fig. 9.8). On-site training has been conducted in France, Canada, Russia, Brazil, Argentina, and UK; and FLS workshops in Russia, Mexico, Brazil, Argentina, Saudi Arabia, and Australia. Interest has been growing especially in the Latin America, Middle East, and Asia-Pacific regions.

The onsite training involves a FLS champion (mentor) hosting an FLS candidate (mentee) and training the candidate over the course of a day on the key steps of implementing an FLS, and how to apply to CTF by submitting the BPF questionnaire. As the training follows a one-to-one scheme, the content is tailored to meet the precise needs of the mentee. On the other hand, FLS workshops involve a larger audience, often more than 15–20 FLS candidates within the same country. The four key steps of FLS implementation: (1) Developing policy case; (2) Developing a business case; (3) How to implement; and (4) How to make it sustainable, are covered in 1 day. The workshops are organized in collaboration with local patient or medical society that is a member of IOF and includes local experts in the panel. As with onsite training, the FLS workshops are customized to the health system of the country. A new system of mentorship by training a community of mentors with knowledge and skills in FLS but also quality improvement and adult learning is now being piloted in selected countries.

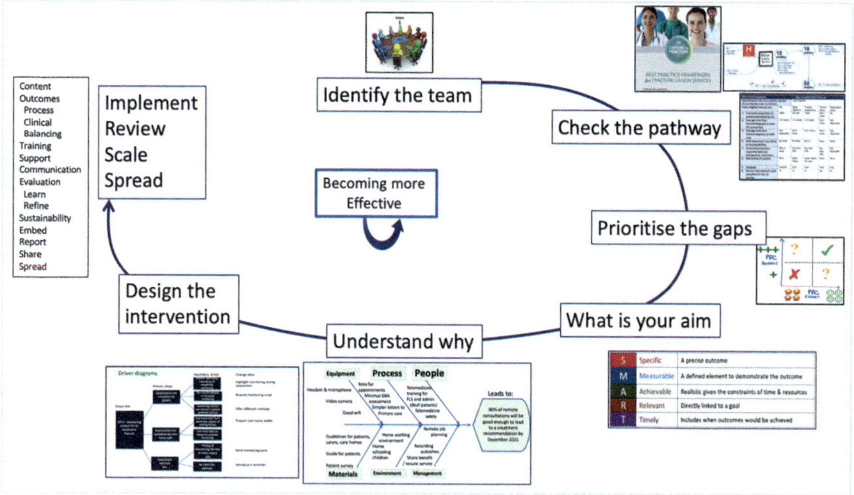

Fig. 9.8 Steps in making the FLS program more effective

Implementation in a Low Resource Setting

Fracture Liaison Services should seek to address the issue of fragility fractures within their given locality, and, of course, there will be variation in demographics of the patient group [42] and the healthcare resources available. However, the resources required to implement a fracture are actually fairly limited. The only technological components are a DXA scanner and a computer, and if neither of these are available then paper copies of the FRAX® tool are available for use in low-resource settings and treatment decisions made without bone mineral density data. In some areas, initiation of a single dose of zoledronate is triggered by the orthopaedic team in patients with hip fracture and normal laboratory results with calcium and vitamin D supplementation, reserving FLS for those patients with less severe fractures or abnormal laboratory findings [24]. The CTF mentorship scheme, described above provides expert support and advice to those setting up an FLS in a transitioning economy (though it should also be noted that a paucity of resources is not only a problem to transitioning economies).

Conclusions

In conclusion, there is substantial evidence to demonstrate the clinical efficacy and cost-effectiveness of setting up a Fracture Liaison Service. In this chapter we have outlined a step-by-step guide for how to set up an FLS and benchmark it against other services internationally.

References

1. Black DM, Cummings SR, Karpf DB, et al. Randomised trial of effect of alendronate on risk of fracture in women with existing vertebral fractures. Fracture Intervention Trial Research Group. Lancet. 1996;348(9041):1535–41.
2. Reginster J, Minne HW, Sorensen OH, et al. Randomized trial of the effects of risedronate on vertebral fractures in women with established postmenopausal osteoporosis. Vertebral Efficacy with Risedronate Therapy (VERT) Study Group. Osteoporos Int. 2000;11(1):83–91.
3. Meunier PJ, Roux C, Seeman E, et al. The effects of strontium ranelate on the risk of vertebral fracture in women with postmenopausal osteoporosis. N Engl J Med. 2004;350(5):459–68.
4. Chesnut CH 3rd, Skag A, Christiansen C, et al. Effects of oral ibandronate administered daily or intermittently on fracture risk in postmenopausal osteoporosis. J Bone Miner Res. 2004;19(8):1241–9.
5. Ettinger B, Black DM, Mitlak BH, et al. Reduction of vertebral fracture risk in postmenopausal women with osteoporosis treated with raloxifene: results from a 3-year randomized clinical trial. Multiple Outcomes of Raloxifene Evaluation (MORE) Investigators. JAMA. 1999;282(7):637–45.
6. Cummings SR, San Martin J, McClung MR, et al. Denosumab for prevention of fractures in postmenopausal women with osteoporosis. N Engl J Med. 2009;361(8):756–65.

7. Lyles KW, Colon-Emeric CS, Magaziner JS, et al. Zoledronic acid and clinical fractures and mortality after hip fracture. N Engl J Med. 2007;357(18):1799–809.
8. Kendler DL, Marin F, Zerbini CAF, et al. Effects of teriparatide and risedronate on new fractures in post-menopausal women with severe osteoporosis (VERO): a multicentre, double-blind, double-dummy, randomised controlled trial. Lancet. 2018;391(10117):230–40.
9. Miller PD, Hattersley G, Riis BJ, et al. Effect of Abaloparatide vs placebo on new vertebral fractures in postmenopausal women with osteoporosis: a randomized clinical trial. JAMA. 2016;316(7):722–33.
10. Saag KG, Petersen J, Brandi ML, et al. Romosozumab or alendronate for fracture prevention in women with osteoporosis. N Engl J Med. 2017;377(15):1417–27.
11. Axelsson KF, Johansson H, Lundh D, Möller M, Lorentzon M. Association between recurrent fracture risk and implementation of fracture liaison services in Four Swedish Hospitals: a cohort study. J Bone Miner Res. 2020;35(7):1216–23.
12. Hawley S, Leal J, Delmestri A, et al. Anti-osteoporosis medication prescriptions and incidence of subsequent fracture among primary hip fracture patients in England and Wales: an interrupted time-series analysis. J Bone Miner Res. 2016;
13. Hernlund E, Svedbom A, Ivergard M, et al. Osteoporosis in the European Union: medical management, epidemiology and economic burden. A report prepared in collaboration with the International Osteoporosis Foundation (IOF) and the European Federation of Pharmaceutical Industry Associations (EFPIA). Arch Osteoporos. 2013;8:136.
14. Solomon DH, Johnston SS, Boytsov NN, McMorrow D, Lane JM, Krohn KD. Osteoporosis medication use after hip fracture in U.S. patients between 2002 and 2011. J Bone Miner Res 2014; 29(9): 1929–1937.
15. Harvey NC, McCloskey EV, Mitchell PJ, et al. Mind the (treatment) gap: a global perspective on current and future strategies for prevention of fragility fractures. Osteoporos Int. 2017;28(5):1507–29.
16. Kanis JA, Borgstrom F, Compston J, et al. SCOPE: a scorecard for osteoporosis in Europe. Arch Osteoporos. 2013;8:144.
17. Kanis JA, Cooper C, Rizzoli R, Reginster JY. European guidance for the diagnosis and management of osteoporosis in postmenopausal women. Osteoporos Int. 2019;30(1):3–44.
18. Eisman JA, Bogoch ER, Dell R, et al. Making the first fracture the last fracture: ASBMR task force report on secondary fracture prevention. J Bone Miner Res. 2012;27(10):2039–46.
19. Marsh D, Akesson K, Beaton DE, et al. Coordinator-based systems for secondary prevention in fragility fracture patients. Osteoporos Int. 2011;22(7):2051–65.
20. Ganda K, Puech M, Chen JS, et al. Models of care for the secondary prevention of osteoporotic fractures: a systematic review and meta-analysis. Osteoporos Int. 2013;24(2):393–406.
21. Sale JE, Beaton D, Posen J, Elliot-Gibson V, Bogoch E. Systematic review on interventions to improve osteoporosis investigation and treatment in fragility fracture patients. Osteoporos Int. 2011;22(7):2067–82.
22. Akesson K, Marsh D, Mitchell PJ, et al. Capture the fracture: a best practice framework and global campaign to break the fragility fracture cycle. Osteoporos Int. 2013;24(8):2135–52.
23. Mitchell PJ, Cooper C, Fujita M, et al. Quality improvement initiatives in fragility fracture care and prevention. Curr Osteoporos Rep. 2019;17(6):510–20.
24. Senay A, Delisle J, Giroux M, et al. The impact of a standardized order set for the management of non-hip fragility fractures in a fracture liaison service. Osteoporos Int. 2016;27(12):3439–47.
25. Weil YA, Rivkin G, Safran O, Liebergall M, Foldes AJ. The outcome of surgically treated femur fractures associated with long-term bisphosphonate use. J Trauma. 2011;71(1):186–90.
26. Berwick DM. A primer on leading the improvement of systems. BMJ. 1996;312(7031):619–22.
27. Mithal A, Bansal B, Kyer CS, Ebeling P. The Asia-Pacific regional audit-epidemiology, costs, and burden of osteoporosis in India 2013: a report of International Osteoporosis Foundation. Indian J Endocrinol Metab. 2014;18(4):449–54.
28. Chandran M, Tan MZ, Cheen M, Tan SB, Leong M, Lau TC. Secondary prevention of osteoporotic fractures—an “OPTIMAL” model of care from Singapore. Osteoporos Int. 2013;24(11):2809–17.

29. Mitchell P, Åkesson K, Chandran M, Cooper C, Ganda K, Schneider M. Implementation of models of care for secondary osteoporotic fracture prevention and orthogeriatric models of care for osteoporotic hip fracture. Best Pract Res Clin Rheumatol. 2016:536–58.
30. McLellan AR, Wolowacz SE, Zimovetz EA, et al. Fracture liaison services for the evaluation and management of patients with osteoporotic fracture: a cost-effectiveness evaluation based on data collected over 8 years of service provision. Osteoporos Int. 2011;22(7):2083–98.
31. Jonsson EB, F.; Ström, C. Cost effectiveness evaluation of fracture liaison services for the management of osteoporosis in Sweden. Value Health. 2016;19:A347–766.
32. Hawley S, Javaid MK, Prieto-Alhambra D, et al. Clinical effectiveness of orthogeriatric and fracture liaison service models of care for hip fracture patients: population-based longitudinal study. Age Ageing. 2016;45(2):236–42.
33. Drew S, Judge A, Cooper C, Javaid MK, Farmer A, Gooberman-Hill R. Secondary prevention of fractures after hip fracture: a qualitative study of effective service delivery. Osteoporos Int. 2016;27(5):1719–27.
34. Wu CH, Kao IJ, Hung WC, et al. Economic impact and cost-effectiveness of fracture liaison services: a systematic review of the literature. Osteoporos Int. 2018;29(6):1227–42.
35. Wu CH, Tu ST, Chang YF, et al. Fracture liaison services improve outcomes of patients with osteoporosis-related fractures: a systematic literature review and meta-analysis. Bone. 2018;111:92–100.
36. Judge A, Javaid MK, Leal J, et al. Health Services and Delivery Research. Models of care for the delivery of secondary fracture prevention after hip fracture: a health service cost, clinical outcomes and cost-effectiveness study within a region of England. Southampton (UK): NIHR Journals Library Copyright (c) Queen's Printer and Controller of HMSO 2016. This work was produced by Judge et al. under the terms of a commissioning contract issued by the Secretary of State for Health. This issue may be freely reproduced for the purposes of private research and study and extracts (or indeed, the full report) may be included in professional journals provided that suitable acknowledgement is made and the reproduction is not associated with any form of advertising. Applications for commercial reproduction should be addressed to: NIHR Journals Library, National Institute for Health Research, Evaluation, Trials and Studies Coordinating Centre, Alpha House, University of Southampton Science Park, Southampton SO16 7NS, UK.; 2016
37. May C, Montori VM, Mair FS. We need minimally disruptive medicine. BMJ. 2009;339:b2803.
38. Javaid MK, Kyer C, Mitchell PJ, et al. Effective secondary fracture prevention: implementation of a global benchmarking of clinical quality using the IOF capture the fracture(R) best practice framework tool. Osteoporos Int. 2015;26(11):2573–8.
39. Australian and New Zealand Hip Fracture Registry, Annual Report, 2019.
40. Javaid MK, Sami A, Lems W, et al. A patient-level key performance indicator set to measure the effectiveness of fracture liaison services and guide quality improvement: a position paper of the IOF Capture the Fracture Working Group, National Osteoporosis Foundation and Fragility Fracture Network. Osteoporos Int. 2020;31(7):1193–204.
41. Javaid MK, Wiles B, Amusan L, Dickinson R, Sheshi N, Hawley S, Pinedo-Villanueva R. et al. Fracture Liaison Service database annual report benchmarking FLS improvement and performance in 2019: Pre-COVID. London: Royal College of Physicians; 2021.
42. Tsabasvi M, Davey S, Temu R. Hip fracture pattern at a major Tanzanian referral hospital: focus on fragility hip fractures. Arch Osteoporos. 2017;12(1):47.

Chapter 10
The Interplay of Muscle and Bone in Later Life

Faidra Laskou, Elaine Dennison, and Harnish Patel

Sarcopenia: An Introduction

Osteoporosis has been described in detail in this book, and represents the loss of bone with age. Sarcopenia, the age associated loss of skeletal muscle strength, function and mass, was first described much later, in 1988 [1]. Over the last few years, several international groups have developed definitions of sarcopenia, adding muscle function assessment to muscle mass although there is still no international consensus for the definition of sarcopenia. Most recently the European working group on sarcopenia in older people (EWGSOP) has developed a diagnostic and management pathway [2]. There have been several further international definitions of sarcopenia encompassing the measurement of muscle function and muscle mass including those from the International Working Group on Sarcopenia (IWGS), the Asian Working Group for Sarcopenia (AWGS) and an initiative from the Foundation for the National Institutes of Health (FNIH). However, despite excellent progress in defining and implementing diagnostic criteria, there is still no consensus for global diagnostic criteria based on cut-off values for muscle strength, muscle function and muscle mass accounting for gender and ethnicity.

Sarcopenia is associated with a range of adverse physical and metabolic outcomes in terms of disability, morbidity, impaired quality of life and mortality which are, and will be, highly relevant in the context of global population ageing [2]. In terms of cost, sarcopenia incurred an estimated $18.5billion in health care costs to the USA in 2000 [3].

F. Laskou (✉) · H. Patel
MRC Lifecourse Epidemiology Centre, Southampton, UK
e-mail: hp@mrc.soton.ac.uk

E. Dennison
MRC Lifecourse Epidemiology Centre, University of Southampton, Southampton, UK
e-mail: emd@mrc.soton.ac.uk

E. Dennison (ed.), *Osteoporosis Treatment*, https://doi.org/10.1007/978-3-030-78128-6_10

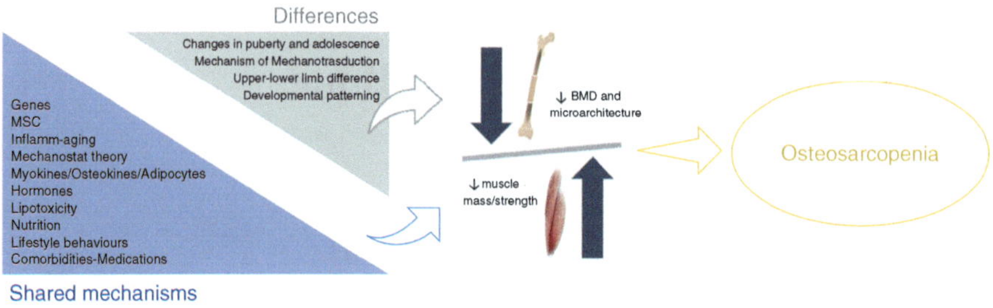

Fig. 10.1 Shared mechanisms and differences in 'muscle-bone unit' progressing to osteosarcopenia (Adapted from the book 'Osteosarcopenia: Bone, muscle and Fat interactions' by Gustavo Duque [78])

Osteosarcopenia

Growing interest has emerged in the coexistence of sarcopenia and osteoporosis in an individual, with several terms used in the past including sarco-porosis, sarco-osteopenia, sarco-osteoporosis and dysmotility syndrome [4]. The most common term describing coexisting poor bone and muscle health currently is osteosarcopenia (Fig. 10.1).

Definitional Approaches to Osteosarcopenia

Diagnosis of Contributing Conditions

The diagnostic approaches to osteoporosis are described elsewhere in Chaps. 1 and 2. The most widely used definition for sarcopenia was proposed by the European Working Group on sarcopenia in Older People (EWGSOP2) and represents an update of previous guidance, supported by the Asian Working Group on Sarcopenia in Older People definition which used different cut-off values for muscle strength, muscle mass indices and function that accounts for differences found in Asian populations [2]. The European Working Group on Sarcopenia in Older People (EWGSOP2) diagnostic algorithm recommends the use of the SARC-F questionnaire to identify possible symptomatic cases (Fig. 10.2). A score of >4 suggests individuals are symptomatic of sarcopenia. This is then followed by the use of normative grip strength reference values for young healthy adults where possible, with cut-off points usually set at −2 or −2.5 standard deviations compared to mean reference values [2]. Sarcopenia is probable when low muscle strength is present (grip <27 kg for men, <16 kg for women) or time taken to complete five chair rises is greater than 15 s [5]. A diagnosis of sarcopenia is confirmed by the presence of low muscle quantity where appendicular lean mass (ALM) measured by dual-energy Xray-absorptiometry (DXA) scanning expressed as a function of the square of body

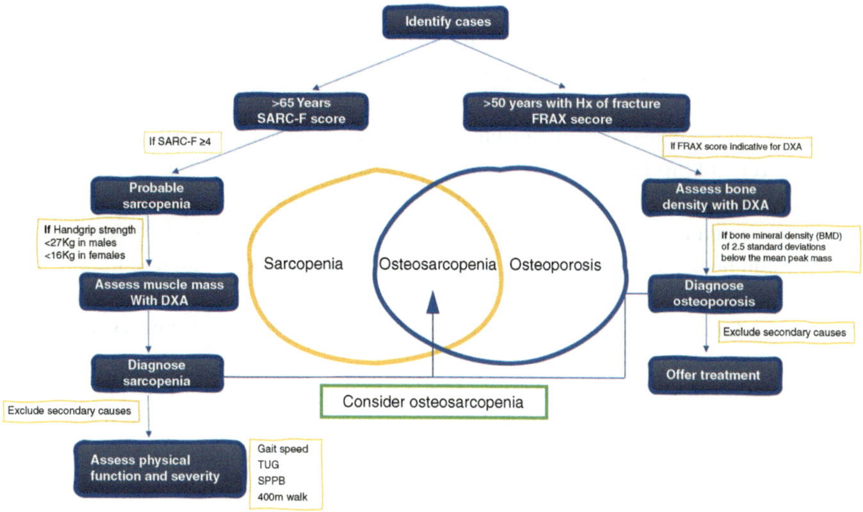

Fig. 10.2 Proposed pathway to identify and diagnose patients with osteosarcopenia based on recent EWGSOP2 criteria for sarcopenia and NICE criteria for osteoporosis. (Adapted from Kirk B et al., Osteosarcopenia: epidemiology, diagnosis, and treatment—facts and numbers [100])

height (ALM/ht^2) is <7.0 kg/m^2 for men and <6.0 kg/m^2 for women. If these parameters are accompanied by poorer objective physical performance measures e.g. gait speed ≤0.8 m/s, then sarcopenia is considered severe.

Prevalence of Coexistence of Low Bone and Muscle Mass

The idea that individuals with low bone mass might also have low muscle mass is not new. Several epidemiological studies have considered the association between total body bone mineral content (BMC) and lean body mass (LBM). In 1998, a study assessed the relationship between whole body BMC and lean mass in both genders between 2 and 87 years of age [6]. The Finnish Twin Cohort Study concluded that lean mass was a better predictor of whole body BMD than fat mass [7]. In other work in the Hertfordshire Cohort Study, muscle size and muscle strength were positively associated with bone size and strength [8] while the European Male Ageing Study reported that men with sarcopenia had lower BMD and were more likely to have osteoporosis compared to men without sarcopenia [9]. In the KHANES survey, low lean mass was an independent risk factor for osteoporosis in men [10]. Decreased relative skeletal muscle mass in men was associated with narrower bones and thinner cortices resulting in a lower bending strength, and a lower section modulus of distal radius and femoral neck in the MINOS study [11]. A difference was also observed in total body skeletal muscle mass and appendicular lean muscle mass between groups with osteoporosis and osteopenia in a study of Ecuadorian patients, the majority of whom were women [12]. The STRAMBO study, which recruited men >60 years of age, concluded that low upper limb appendicular lean mass (ALM) and low grip strength were independently associated with lower cortical bone area and thickness at the distal radius [13]. A positive longitudinal relationship between muscle and bone mass decline, an increase in the risk of fracture, and a clinically relevant decline in muscle strength was associated with a decrease in spine BMD and hip BMD was recognised over a period of 1 year in older individuals in the SarcoPhage cohort [14]. At all sites, BMD was lower among individuals with sarcopenia and a diagnosis of sarcopenia increased the risk of osteoporosis in the Copenhagen Sarcopenia study [15]. Finally, In a Japanese study, a significant association between sarcopenia and osteopenia/osteoporosis was shown in women; relative skeletal muscle index (RSMI) was positively correlated with BMD of the lumbar spine and total hip [16].

Sarcopenia has also been identified as a predictor of fracture risk [17]. In one study, individuals diagnosed with both sarcopenia and osteoporosis were more likely to be older and have a history of falling [18]. The idea that the decline in bone mass was more rapid in the presence of sarcopenia was proposed here, as the authors observed that the group which progressed from sarcopenia to osteosarcopenia did so faster compared to the group that progressed from osteoporosis to osteosarcopenia.

Despite these studies, few researchers have reported the prevalence of these conditions coexisting. In those studies that report this, the prevalence of osteosarcopenia among community dwelling populations has been observed to increase with age and is greater in women than men. Estimates range between 5 and 37% depending on the population and definition of sarcopenia used, with the highest rates observed in those subjects with fractures [15, 19]. The prevalence of osteosarcopenia will, however, almost inevitably increase as the population grows older [20].

Risk Factors for Bone and Muscle Loss in Older Adults

Sex Hormones

Sex hormones exert several effects on muscle and bone and constitute an important role in musculoskeletal health. With ageing, tissues become less sensitive to sex-steroids through altered serum levels and trophic activity. Broadly speaking, androgens exert anabolic effects on muscle and oestrogens have an anti-resorptive effect on bone. Menopause characterised by a sharp decline in circulating prostaglandin (PG) E2 in women, is an important contributor to decline in muscle and bone; the same abrupt decline does not apply to men. Sex steroid receptors have been identified in other cells such as mesenchymal, myeloid precursors [(myocytes and satellite cells in muscle, osteoblasts and osteoclasts in bone [21–23]]. Effects of oestrogens on muscle mass growth and maintenance seem weaker compared to their effects on the bone. Androgens seem to have more potent effects than oestrogens on muscle in both sexes. This raises the question as to whether testosterone may be the more significant sex hormone in the regulation of skeletal muscle homeostasis in both genders [24]. In patients who are receiving androgen deprivation and aromatase inhibitors therapies for prostate and breast cancer respectively, a catabolic effect on bone, muscle and fat has been noted [25–27].

Lifestyle Factors and Nutrition

Lifestyle factors affect the ‘muscle-bone unit’. Smoking decreases bone density through deleterious effects on bone quality mediated by direct and indirect effects of nicotine and other toxins [28]. Current smoking has associated with lower cortical and trabecular BMD in males [29] and active smoking has also been associated with sarcopenia in the MINOS study [30]; a meta-analysis reported that cigarette smoking may be a contributor factor for the development of sarcopenia [31].

Specific nutrients affect both bone and muscle – for example, vitamin D plays a major role in both muscle and bone health. Undernutrition is commonly observed in older people and being malnourished has been proposed as a major cause of musculoskeletal decline [32]. Low levels of Vitamin D are commonly found in osteosarcopenic patients [18] although the benefits of supplementation have not been thoroughly studied [33]. In one Korean study, Vitamin D deficiency was associated with low BMD and was more pronounced in those with sarcopenia [34] while low ALM was associated with low Vitamin D in the MINOS Study [30]. Low Vitamin D levels are likely to contribute to muscle weakness and increased risk of falls in addition to increased bone fragility [35, 36]. Previous studies have considered a role for raised PTH in the pathogenesis of osteosarcopenia [18, 37]. A recent cross sectional study showed that older individuals who reported more falls per year, lower grip strength, lower BMD and slower gait velocity had raised PTH levels which were not secondary to Vitamin D deficiency [38]. Finally vitamin K is essential for the effective function of proteins including those involved for bone remodelling and it has been shown that in vitro vitamin K improves the proliferation and migration of bovine skeletal muscle [18]. Vitamin K serves as a connection agent in muscle-bone interactions through several mechanisms facilitating muscle-bone cross talk [39]. However, it appears to have no effect on postural sway or physical function in older people [40].

Osteosarcopenic Obesity

Bone, muscle and fat share the same type of mesenchymal stem cells (MSCs) precursors and the capacity of MSC to differentiate into chrondrocytes, osteoblasts and others is reduced with aging. An increase in their differentiation into adipocytes has been noted. Adipokines and fatty acids, factors that are secreted by adipocytes, have a major effect on bones and muscles. Lipotoxic lipids have also an impact on cell function and survival as a mechanism that is described as lipoapoptosis [41]. The bone marrow microenvironment becomes toxic with ageing secondary to adipocyte infiltration [41]. Studies have suggested that elevated lipotoxic lipids such as palmitic acid are a causative mediator for sarcopenia and osteoporosis [42–44].

Accumulation of fat in skeletal muscle is linked to reduced muscle quality and muscle dysfunction. A separate entity, osteosarcopenic obesity, was first described in 2014 [42]. In a definition that was initially proposed by Ilich et al., researchers included the presence of hip or lumbar spine T-score ≤ -1.0, ALM normalized to height ≤ 5.45 (women) or ≤ 7.26 kg/m^2 (men), and total body fat >40% (women) or >30% (men) [42]. Grip strength and Short Physical Performance Battery (SBBP) was then added as the proposed definition of sarcopenia also was modified [45].

Some studies have suggested that osteosarcopenic obesity is associated with poorer outcomes compared to osteoporosis and sarcopenia alone. Similar to the pathophysiology of osteosarcopenia, cellular and endocrine changes as well as bone, muscle and fat cross talk via osteokines, myokines and adipokines may lead to the development of osteosarcopenic obesity [46]. Osteosarcopenic obesity has been associated with poor function in postmenopausal women [47], poor physical performance and frailty in an older Mexican population [48], and dyslipidaemia and hypertension in an older Chinese population [49, 50]. It has also been suggested that OSO increases the risk of fracture, falls and long term frailty [51].

Higher body fat for BMI has been associated with lower BMD in women, suggesting that increased fat mass without an accompanying increase in lean mass may be deleterious to bone [51]. In contrast, other studies have suggested that obesity can be a protective factor against bone loss with a positive correlation between BMD and BMI and a lower incidence of hip and vertebral fractures in obese subjects [52, 53]. Insulin resistance (IR) has been associated with low muscle mass and sarcopenia. The KHANES study found that osteosarcopenic obesity may not have a stronger association with insulin resistance compared to obesity only, and obesity co-existent with other conditions [54].

The relationship between diet and OSO remains unclear. However, in other work a pro-inflammatory diet, based on the dietary inflammatory index (DII) [51], was associated with an increased odds of osteopenic and osteosarcopenic obesity in a cross-sectional study in postmenopausal Korean women [55]. It has also been suggested that the microbiome plays a role in osteosarcopenic obesity [56].

Recognizing the coexistence and possibly the co-development of osteoporosis, sarcopenia and obesity as osteosarcopenic obesity may assist in the development of targeted and improved treatment plans [57].

Management of Osteosarcopenia

Multicomponent intervention is required to manage osteosarcopenia. Exercise and nutritional support remain the core. Commonalities in pathophysiology advocate potential targets for treatment such as IGF1, selective androgen receptor modulators

(SARMs), Vitamin D and targets involved in the muscle-bone cross talk such as activin signalling inhibitors, myostatin antibodies, recombinant follistatin derivatives and myokines [58, 59]. Currently there are few randomised controlled trials that have investigated a common pharmacological target in osteosarcopenia. Randomised controlled trials have demonstrated the efficacy of progressive resistance exercise to stimulate osteoblastogenesis and muscle protein synthesis [60, 61]. Multi-modal programs which incorporate traditional and high velocity progressive resistance training, weight bearing exercises and balance/mobility activities have been suggested as the best approach [19].

Nonpharmacological Interventions and Treatment

Nutritional Approaches

The nutrition approach focuses on Vitamin D, calcium and protein intake, and has been discussed in detail with regard to bone health in Chap. 3. It has been suggested that adequate protein intake should be ensured; the recommended dietary allowance of protein of 0.8 g protein/kg/day although this might not be adequate for older people to meet their metabolic and physiological needs and might need to be increased [62]. An international study group suggested that in healthy older individuals both endurance and resistance type exercises are recommended in combination with higher protein intakes of at least 1/2 g/kg body weight/day in those who remain active [63]—adequate protein intake has benefited patients with osteosarcopenia [64]. A recent systematic review and meta regression analysis of randomised trials showed that lean mass gain was associated with protein supplementation and muscle strengthening exercise in elderly patients with a high risk of sarcopenia [65]. Meta-analyses have reported an increase in lean mass accompanied by significant strength gain or improvement in physical activity when protein intake is combined with muscle strengthening exercises, but conflicting results have also been reported [66–69].

The role of protein intake in bone health has also been described showing that protein is essential nutrient for bone health as it contributes to the regulation of IGF1, has a role in the moderation of calcium absorption and impacts on sex hormone binding globulin concentration [70]. Dairy foods which provide nutrients such as calcium, phosphate and protein promote the maintenance of good bone health. An interaction of dietary protein and mechanical loading on skeletal muscle mass and function has been reported [32].

Leucine is described as the most marked anabolic amino acid which triggers initiation of protein synthesis [71]. Studies have evaluated the role of a leucine enriched diet on muscle and bone health. In a study where leucine-enriched protein supplement was given alongside exercise in community dwelling older patients, physical exercise was found to improve myoelectrical muscle fatigue but a leucine enriched diet did not enhance this response [61, 72]. In contrast, the PROVIDE study concluded that 13 weeks of nutritional supplementation with Vitamin D and leucine-enriched whey protein may attenuate low grade inflammation, a significant factor which contributes to frailty and sarcopenia, when there are mobility restrictions and exercise intervention is limited [73]. Creatine has also been reported to increase muscle mass and strength as well as bone density although further studies are required to establish the benefit of creatine in osteosarcopenic patients [63].

Higher baseline Vitamin D concentrations and dietary protein intake have been associated with greater gain in appendicular muscle mass, skeletal muscle index and relative appendicular muscle mass in response to nutritional interventions [74]. Administration alfacalcidol, an activated form of Vitamin D has also been associated with increased muscle mass [75]. By contrast, annual oral administration of high-dose cholecalciferol resulted in an increased risk of falls and fractures [76], highlighting the uncertainties in this area [33].

Vitamin E has been found to inhibit Connexin 43, a protein component of gap junctions, which allow for gap junction intercellular communication between cells to regulate cell death, proliferation, and differentiation. Vitamin E may reduce muscle atrophy especially when caused by long term corticosteroids use and it may be a potential treatment for steroid induced osteosarcopenia [77].

Exercise

Finally, several training methods have been proposed to improve muscle and bone health such as endurance, resistance and combined training. Long term resistance or combined training is proposed to have beneficial effects in preserving bone mass [60, 78]. Resistance exercise is proven to have a positive impact on muscle quantity and quality [79] but endurance exercise could improve functional capabilities [78]. To date there is no strong evidence to support a specific model of training superior to others for osteosarcopenia, but combined training can potentially benefit muscle and bone health.

Pharmacologic Treatments

There are no approved pharmacological agents for osteosarcopenia so the focus on pharmacological treatment relies on osteoporosis treatment. Denosumab, a RANKL ligand inhibitor, has shown promising effects on muscle and bone health [80]. In the FREEDOM trial, denosumab was associated with reduced falls but no causative mechanism was described [81]. Handgrip strength and LBM was increased significantly with denosumab therapy when compared to IV zoledronic acid [80]. In a non-randomised study of community dwelling older adults, denosumab has shown improvement on balance, fear of falling and physical action when compared to IV zoledronic acid [82].

Testosterone levels drop with age and they are considered an important cause of age-related musculoskeletal disorders. It has been shown that replacement of testosterone improves muscle mass and function in older adults [83]. Community dwelling frail older [84, 85] and healthy individuals [86] benefited from testosterone administration with regard to muscle strength and gait but those effects did not last post discontinuation of testosterone. In a review of testosterone trials, increase in the distance walked, and in volumetric BMD was reported in older individuals but it was also noted the increased coronary plaque volume which have been associated with more cardiovascular events.More trial data are required to determine the significance of these findings [87].

Fear regarding side effects of testosterone promoted the study of Selective Androgen Receptor Modulators (SARMs)as they achieve tissue selectivity [86]; Andarine and Ostarine were shown to increase lean mass and physical function in older males and post-menopausal females [88, 89]. However, no clear advantage of SARMs has been proven in bone health in humans.

Myostatin inhibitors have also been suggested as a possible treatment for osteosarcopenia. In a phase II trial in older adults with a history of falls, antimyostatin antibodies increased LBM and improved functional measures associated with muscle strength [90] but the benefit in bone health has not been established in clinical trials.

Bimagrumab, a human monoclonal antibody which binds to type II activin receptors and prevents the binding of myostatin and activin A, has demonstrated significant increases in muscle mass and strength in older adults with sarcopenia (defined by ASMI as per EWGSOP 2010 criteria but gait speed between 0.4–1.0 m/s) [91], and also reduced fat mass in overweight and obese adults with insulin resistance in early trials, which might have a role in osteosarcopenic obesity [92]. Further trials are required to confirm these findings and identify effective treatment for osteosarcopenia and osteosarcopenic obesity.

Oral GH has not been shown to have any clear benefit in muscle mass, function or strength and as it has been associated with soft tissue oedema, arthralgia, carpal tunnel syndrome, and gynecomastia as well as increased mortality and morbidity in patients in intensive care units, so it is not recommended as a treatment [93, 94]. In animal work, administration of exogenous IGF-1 attenuated effects of advanced glycation end products (AGEs) in mouse myoblastic cells, representing a potential treatment which required validation [95]. Irisin has also been suggested as a target to treat older osteosarcopenic subjects as it retrieves disuse-induced bone loss and muscle atrophy in mice. Finally melatonin has also been suggested as a potential treatment; It affects mitochondrial function, reduces oxidative stress and autophagic alterations in bone and muscle cells [96].

Finally an interesting novel therapeutic target could be the prevention of fat infiltration. Use of cerulenin, an inhibitor of fatty acid synthase, led to recovery in bone mass associated with higher levels of bone formation and an increase in subcutaneous muscle volumes also noted in the cerulenin treated group [97]. Further studies targeting fatty acid synthase are essential [98]. Exosomes have the role of messengers on intercellular communications and they have been considered as a potential target for treatment in osteosarcopenia. Release of exosomes with physical exercise and evidence that they can increase muscle regeneration after skeletal muscle injury would support this theory but the underlying mechanism is not fully understood [99].

Conclusion

Osteoporosis and sarcopenia are related diseases associated with morbidity and mortality in older people. Their prevalence is expected to increase in coming years, leading to devastating consequences for individuals and healthcare systems globally. These two conditions share common pathophysiological mechanisms and hence an interest and attempt to treat and manage these pathologies as one is growing. Clinicians should now become increasingly alert of the interrelationship of muscle and bone which will facilitate the early identification, diagnosis and management of individuals suffering from osteosarcopenia similar to osteoporosis alone.

References

1. Rosenberg IH. Sarcopenia: origins and clinical relevance. Clin Geriatr Med. 2011;27(3):337–9.
2. Cruz-Jentoft AJ, Bahat G, Bauer J, Boirie Y, Bruyère O, Cederholm T, et al. Sarcopenia: revised European consensus on definition and diagnosis European Working Group on sarcopenia in older people 2 (EWGSOP2), and the extended group for EWGSOP2. Age Ageing [Internet]. 2019;48:16–31. [cited 2020 Jun 16]. https://academic.oup.com/ageing/article-abstract/48/1/16/5126243.
3. Janssen I, Shepard DS, Katzmarzyk PT, Roubenoff R. The healthcare costs of sarcopenia in the United States. J Am Geriatr Soc. 2004;52(1):80–5.
4. Binkley N, Krueger D, Buehring B. What's in a name revisited: should osteoporosis and sarcopenia be considered components of "dysmobility syndrome?". Osteoporos Int. 2013;24(12):2955–9.
5. Cruz-Jentoft AJ, Sayer AA. Sarcopenia. Lancet [Internet]. 2019 [cited 2020 Jun 18]. https://doi.org/10.1016/S0140-6736.
6. Ferretti JL, Capozza RF, Cointry GR, García SL, Plotkin H, Filgueira MLA, et al. Gender-related differences in the relationship between densitometric values of whole-body bone mineral content and lean body mass in humans between 2 and 87 years of age. Bone. 1998;22(6):683–90.
7. Bogl LH, Latvala A, Kaprio J, Sovijärvi O, Rissanen A, Pietiläinen KH. An investigation into the relationship between soft tissue body composition and bone mineral density in a young adult twin sample. J Bone Miner Res [Internet]. 2011 Jan [cited 2020 Jul 17];26(1):79–87. https://pubmed.ncbi.nlm.nih.gov/20658559/.
8. Edwards MH, Gregson CL, Patel HP, Jameson KA, Harvey NC, Sayer AA, et al. Muscle size, strength, and physical performance and their associations with bone structure in the Hertfordshire Cohort Study. J Bone Miner Res [Internet]. 2013 Nov [cited 2020 Jul 23];28(11):2295–304. https://pubmed.ncbi.nlm.nih.gov/23633238/.
9. Verschueren S, Gielen E, O'Neill TW, Pye SR, Adams JE, Ward KA, et al. Sarcopenia and its relationship with bone mineral density in middle-aged and elderly European men. Osteoporos Int. 2013;24(1):87–98.

10. Kim S, Won CW, Kim BS, Choi HR, Moon MY. The association between the low muscle mass and osteoporosis in elderly Korean people. J Korean Med Sci. 2014;29(7):995–1000.
11. Szulc P, Beck TJ, Marchand F, Delmas PD. Low skeletal muscle mass is associated with poor structural parameters of bone and impaired balance in elderly men—the MINOS study. J Bone Miner Res. 2005;20(5):721–9.
12. Intriago M, Maldonado G, Guerrero R, Messina OD, Rios C. Bone mass loss and sarcopenia in Ecuadorian patients. J Aging Res. 2020;2020:1072675.
13. Szulc P, Blaizot S, Boutroy S, Vilayphiou N, Boonen S, Chapurlat R. Impaired bone microarchitecture at the distal radius in older men with low muscle mass and grip strength: the STRAMBO study. J Bone Miner Res. 2013;28(1):169–78.
14. Locquet M, Beaudart C, Reginster JY, Bruyère O. Association between the decline in muscle health and the decline in bone health in older individuals from the SarcoPhAge cohort. Calcif Tissue Int. 2019;104(3):273–84.
15. Nielsen BR, Andersen HE, Haddock B, Hovind P, Schwarz P, Suetta C. Prevalence of muscle dysfunction concomitant with osteoporosis in a home-dwelling Danish population aged 65–93 years - the Copenhagen sarcopenia study. Exp Gerontol. 2020;138:110974.
16. Miyakoshi N, Hongo M, Mizutani Y, Shimada Y. Prevalence of sarcopenia in Japanese women with osteopenia and osteoporosis. J Bone Miner Metab. 2013;31(5):556–61.
17. Oliveira A, Vaz C. The role of sarcopenia in the risk of osteoporotic hip fracture. Clin Rheumatol. 2015;34(10):1673–80.
18. Huo YR, Suriyaarachchi P, Gomez F, Curcio CL, Boersma D, Muir SW, et al. Phenotype of Osteosarcopenia in older individuals with a history of falling. J Am Med Dir Assoc [Internet] 2015;16(4):290–5. https://doi.org/10.1016/j.jamda.2014.10.018.
19. Fahimfar N, Zahedi Tajrishi F, Gharibzadeh S, Shafiee G, Tanha K, Heshmat R, et al. Prevalence of Osteosarcopenia and its association with cardiovascular risk factors in Iranian older people: Bushehr elderly health (BEH) program. Calcif Tissue Int. 2020;106(4):364–70.
20. Nielsen BR, Abdulla J, Andersen HE, Schwarz P, Suetta C. Sarcopenia and osteoporosis in older people: a systematic review and meta-analysis. Vol. 9, European Geriatric Medicine. Springer International Publishing; 2018. p. 419–34.
21. Almeida M, Laurent MR, Dubois V, Claessens F, O'Brien CA, Bouillon R, et al. Estrogens and androgens in skeletal physiology and pathophysiology. Physiol Rev [Internet]. 2017 [cited 2020 Jul 27];97(1):135–87. https://www.physiology.org/, https://doi.org/10.1152/physrev.00033.2015.
22. Kim YJ, Tamadon A, Park HT, Kim H, Ku S-Y. The role of sex steroid hormones in the pathophysiology and treatment of sarcopenia. Osteoporos Sarcopenia [Internet]. 2016 [cited 2020 Jul 27];2(3):140–55. https://doi.org/10.1016/j.afos.2016.06.002.
23. Kawano H, Sato T, Yamada T, Matsumoto T, Sekine K, Watanabe T, et al. Suppressive function of androgen receptor in bone resorption. Proc Natl Acad Sci U S A [Internet]. 2003 [cited 2020 Jul 27];100(16):9416–21. www.pnas.orgcgi, https://doi.org/10.1073pnas.1533500100.
24. Carson JA, Manolagas SC. Effects of sex steroids on bones and muscles: similarities, parallels, and putative interactions in health and disease. Bone. 2015;80:67–78.
25. Sestak I, Singh S, Cuzick J, Blake GM, Patel R, Gossiel F, et al. Changes in bone mineral density at 3 years in postmenopausal women receiving anastrozole and risedronate in the IBIS-II bone substudy: an international, double-blind, randomised, placebo-controlled trial. Lancet Oncol [Internet]. 2014;15:1460–8. [cited 2020 Jul 27]. www.thelancet.com/oncology.
26. Cheung AS, Gray H, Schache AG, Hoermann R, Lim Joon D, Zajac JD, et al. Androgen deprivation causes selective deficits in the biomechanical leg muscle function of men during walking: a prospective case-control study. 2016;
27. Lam T, Birzniece V, McLean M, Gurney H, Hayden A, Cheema BS. The adverse effects of androgen deprivation therapy in prostate cancer and the benefits and potential anti-oncogenic mechanisms of progressive resistance training [Internet]. Sports Med Open. Springer. 2020;6:1–14. https://link.springer.com/articles/10.1186/s40798-020-0242-8.

28. Cusano NE. Skeletal Effects of Smoking. Curr Osteoporos Rep [Internet]. 2015;13(5):302–9. [cited 2020 Jun 17]. http://www.ncbi.nlm.nih.gov/pubmed/26205852.
29. Oliver H, Jameson KA, Sayer AA, Cooper C, Dennison EM. Growth in early life predicts bone strength in late adulthood: the Hertfordshire Cohort Study. Bone [Internet]. 2007;41(3):400–5. [cited 2020 Jul 24]. https://doi.org/10.1016/j.bone.2007.05.007.
30. Szulc P, Duboeuf F, Marchand F, Delmas PD. Hormonal and lifestyle determinants of appendicular skeletal muscle mass in men: the MINOS study [Internet]. Am J Clin Nutr. 2004;80:1–3 [cited 2020 Jul 26]. https://academic.oup.com/ajcn/article-abstract/80/2/496/4690338.
31. Steffl M, Bohannon RW, Petr M, Kohlikova E, Holmerova I, Kohlíková E. Relation between cigarette smoking and sarcopenia: meta-analysis. Physiol Res [Internet]. 2015;64:419–26. [cited 2020 Jul 26]. www.biomed.cas.cz/physiolres.
32. Bonjour J-P, Kraenzlin M, Levasseur R, Warren M, Whiting S. Dairy in adulthood: from foods to nutrient interactions on bone and skeletal muscle health. J Am Coll Nutr [Internet]. 2013;32(4):251–63. [cited 2020 Jun 12]. http://www.tandfonline.com/doi/abs/10.1080/07315724.2013.816604.
33. Bruyère O, Cavalier E, Reginster JY. Vitamin D and osteosarcopenia: An update from epidemiological studies. Curr Opin Clin Nutr Metab Care. 2017;20(6):498–503.
34. Lee SG, Lee YH, Kim KJ, Lee W, Kwon OH, Kim JH. Additive association of vitamin D insufficiency and sarcopenia with low femoral bone mineral density in noninstitutionalized elderly population: the Korea National Health and Nutrition Examination Surveys 2009–2010. Osteop Int. Springer; 2013;24:2789–99.
35. Gunton JE, Girgis CM. Vitamin D and muscle. Bone Rep. 2018;8:163–7.
36. Reid IR, Bolland MJ. Skeletal and nonskeletal effects of vitamin D: is vitamin D a tonic for bone and other tissues? [Internet]. Osteop Int. Springer-Verlag London Ltd. 2014;25:2347–57. [cited 2020 Jul 27]. https://link.springer.com/article/10.1007/s00198-014-2749-7.
37. Visser M, Deeg DJH, Lips P. Low vitamin d and high parathyroid hormone levels as determinants of loss of muscle strength and muscle mass (Sarcopenia): the Longitudinal Aging Study Amsterdam. 2003 [cited 2020 Jul 27]. https://academic.oup.com/jcem/article-abstract/88/12/5766/2661478.
38. Suriyaarachchi P, Gomez F, Curcio CL, Boersma D, Murthy L, Grill V, et al. High parathyroid hormone levels are associated with osteosarcopenia in older individuals with a history of falling. Maturitas [internet]. 2018;113(December 2017):21–5. https://doi.org/10.1016/j.maturitas.2018.04.006.
39. Gordeladze JO, Haugen HJ, Johnsen GF, Møller M. Vitamin K2 facilitating inter-organ cross-talk. In: Vitamin K2 - vital for health and wellbeing [Internet]. InTech; 2017 [cited 2020 Jul 27]. https://doi.org/10.5772/67153.
40. Witham MD, Price RJG, Band MM, Hannah MS, Fulton RL, Clarke CL, et al. Effect of vitamin K2 on postural sway in older people who fall: a randomized controlled trial. J Am Geriatr Soc [Internet]. 2019;67(10):2102–7. [cited 2020 Jun 18]. https://onlinelibrary.wiley.com/doi/abs/10.1111/jgs.16024.
41. Guerra DAP, Paiva AE, Sena IFG, Azevedo PO, Luiz Batista M, Mintz A, et al. Adipocytes role in the bone marrow niche. Cytometry A. 2018;93(2):167–71.
42. Ilich JZ, Kelly OJ, Inglis JE, Panton LB, Duque G, Ormsbee MJ. Interrelationship among muscle, fat, and bone: connecting the dots on cellular, hormonal, and whole body levels. Ageing Res Rev [Internet] 2014;15(1):51–60. https://doi.org/10.1016/j.arr.2014.02.007.
43. Budui SL, Rossi AP, Zamboni M. The pathogenetic bases of sarcopenia. Clin Cases Min Bone Metab. 2015;12:22–6.
44. Gunaratnam K, Vidal C, Boadle R, Thekkedam C, Duque G. Mechanisms of palmitate-induced cell death in human osteoblasts. Biol Open. 2013;2(12):1382–9.
45. Ilich JZ, Kelly OJ, Inglis JE. Osteosarcopenic obesity syndrome: what is it and how can it be identified and diagnosed? Curr Gerontol Geriatr Res [Internet]. 2016;2016. [cited 2020 Jul 29]. https://doi.org/10.1155/2016/7325973.

46. Kelly OJ, Gilman JC, Boschiero D, Ilich JZ. Osteosarcopenic obesity: current knowledge, revised identification criteria and treatment principles. Nutrients. 2019;11(4):747.
47. Ilich JZ, Inglis JE, Kelly OJ, McGee DL. Osteosarcopenic obesity is associated with reduced handgrip strength, walking abilities, and balance in postmenopausal women. Osteoporos Int [Internet]. 2015;26(11):2587–95. [cited 2020 Jul 31]. https://link.springer.com/article/10.1007/s00198-015-3186-y.
48. Szlejf C, Parra-Rodríguez L, Rosas-Carrasco O. Osteosarcopenic obesity: prevalence and relation with frailty and physical performance in middle-aged and older women. J Am Med Dir Assoc [Internet]. 2017;18(8):733.e1–733.e5. [cited 2020 Jul 31]. https://doi.org/10.1016/j.jamda.2017.02.023.
49. Mo D, Hsieh P, Yu H, Zhou L, Gong J, Xu L, et al. Osteosarcopenic obesity and its relationship with dyslipidemia in women from different ethnic groups of China. Arch Osteoporos [Internet]. 2018;13(1):1–9. [cited 2020 Jul 31]. https://doi.org/10.1007/s11657-018-0481-1.
50. Chen X, Kong C, Yu H, Gong J, Lan L, Zhou L, et al. Association between osteosarcopenic obesity and hypertension among four minority populations in China: A cross-sectional study. BMJ Open [Internet]. 2019;9(7). [cited 2020 Jul 31]. https://doi.org/10.1136/bmjopen-2018-026818.
51. Shivappa N, Steck SE, Hurley TG, Hussey JR, Hébert JR. Designing and developing a literature-derived, population-based dietary inflammatory index. Public Heal Nutr. 2014;17(8):1689–96.
52. Compston J. Obesity and fractures in postmenopausal women. Curr Opin Rheumatol. 2015;27(4):414–9.
53. De Laet C, Kanis JA, Odén A, Johanson H, Johnell O, Delmas P, et al. Body mass index as a predictor of fracture risk: a meta-analysis. Osteoporos Int [Internet]. 2005;16(11):1330–8. [cited 2020 Jul 29]. https://link.springer.com/article/10.1007/s00198-005-1863-y.
54. Lee K. Association of osteosarcopenic obesity and its components: osteoporosis, sarcopenia and obesity with insulin resistance. J Bone Miner Metab. 2020 Apr;25:1–7.
55. Park S, Na W, Sohn C. Relationship between osteosarcopenic obesity and dietary inflammatory index in postmenopausal Korean women: 2009 to 2011 Korea National Health and Nutrition Examination Surveys. J Clin Biochem Nutr [Internet]. 2018;63(3):211–6. [cited 2020 Jun 16]. https://www.jstage.jst.go.jp/article/jcbn/63/3/63_18-10/_article.
56. Inglis JE, Ilich JZ. The microbiome and osteosarcopenic obesity in older individuals in long-term care facilities [Internet]. Curr Osteop Rep. Current Medicine Group LLC 1. 2015;13:358–62. [cited 2020 Jul 26]. https://link.springer.com/article/10.1007/s11914-015-0287-7.
57. Bauer JM, Cruz-Jentoft AJ, Fielding RA, Kanis JA, Reginster JY, Bruyère O, et al. Is There enough evidence for osteosarcopenic obesity as a distinct entity? A critical literature review. Calcified Tissue International. Springer New York LLC. 2019;105:109–24.
58. Fatima M, Brennan-Olsen SL, Duque G. Therapeutic approaches to osteosarcopenia: insights for the clinician. Ther Adv Musculoskelet Dis. 2019;11:1759720X1986700.
59. Girgis CM, Mokbel N, DiGirolamo DJ. Therapies for musculoskeletal disease: Can we treat two birds with one stone?. Curr Osteop Rep. Current Medicine Group LLC 1. 2014;12:142–53.
60. Daly RM, Gianoudis J, Kersh ME, Bailey CA, Ebeling PR, Krug R, et al. Effects of a 12-month supervised, community-based, multimodal exercise program followed by a 6-month research-to-practice transition on bone mineral density, trabecular microarchitecture, and physical function in older adults: a randomized controlled trial. J Bone Miner Res [Internet]. 2020;35(3):419–29. [cited 2020 Aug 5]. https://onlinelibrary.wiley.com/doi/abs/10.1002/jbmr.3865.
61. Kirk B, Mooney K, Cousins R, Angell P, Jackson M, Pugh JN, et al. Effects of exercise and whey protein on muscle mass, fat mass, myoelectrical muscle fatigue and health-related quality of life in older adults: a secondary analysis of the Liverpool Hope University—Sarcopenia Ageing Trial (LHU-SAT). Eur J Appl Physiol [Internet]. 2020;120(2):493–503. [cited 2020 Aug 5]. https://doi.org/10.1007/s00421-019-04293-5.

62. Campbell WW, Trappe TA, Wolfe RR, Evans WJ. The recommended dietary allowance for protein may not be adequate for older people to maintain skeletal muscle [internet]. J Gerontol. 2001;56. [cited 2020 Jun 17]. https://academic.oup.com/biomedgerontology/article-abstract/56/6/M373/526427.
63. Bauer J, Biolo G, Cederholm T, Cesari M, Cruz-Jentoft AJ, Morley JE, et al. Evidence-based recommendations for optimal dietary protein intake in older people: a position paper from the PROT-AGE study group. 2013 [cited 2020 Aug 5]. https://doi.org/10.1016/j.jamda.2013.05.021.
64. De Rui M, Inelmen EM, Pigozzo S, Trevisan C, Manzato E, Sergi G. Dietary strategies for mitigating osteosarcopenia in older adults: a narrative review. Aging Clin Exp Res. Springer International Publishing. 2019;31:897–903.
65. Liao C-D, Chen H-C, Huang S-W, Liou T-H. The role of muscle mass gain following protein supplementation plus exercise therapy in older adults with sarcopenia and frailty risks: a systematic review and meta-regression analysis of randomized trials. Nutrients [Internet]. 2019. 11(8). [cited 2020 Jun 18]. http://www.ncbi.nlm.nih.gov/pubmed/31349606.
66. Morton RW, Murphy KT, Mckellar SR, Schoenfeld BJ, Henselmans M, Helms E, et al. A systematic review, meta-analysis and meta-regression of the effect of protein supplementation on resistance training-induced gains in muscle mass and strength in healthy adults. Br J Sport Med [Internet]. 2018;52:376–84. [cited 2020 Aug 4]. https://doi.org/10.1136/bjsports-2017-097608.
67. Luo D, Lin Z, Li S. Liu S-J. Effect of nutritional supplement combined with exercise intervention on sarcopenia in the elderly: a meta-analysis. Int J Nurs Sci [Internet]. 2017;4:389–401. [cited 2020 Aug 4]. https://doi.org/10.1016/j.ijnss.2017.09.004.
68. Finger D, Goltz FR, Umpierre D, Meyer E, Rosa LHT, Schneider CD. Effects of protein supplementation in older adults undergoing resistance training: a systematic review and meta-analysis [Internet]. Sports Med. Springer International Publishing; 2015;45:245–55. [cited 2020 Aug 4]. https://link.springer.com/article/10.1007/s40279-014-0269-4.
69. Liao C-D, Lee P-H, Hsiao D-J, Huang S-W, Tsauo J-Y, Chen H-C, et al. Effects of protein supplementation combined with exercise intervention on frailty indices, body composition, and physical function in frail older adults. [cited 2020 Aug 4]. www.mdpi.com/journal/nutrients.
70. Dolan E, Sale C. Conference on "nutrient-nutrient interaction" symposium 2: nutrient interactions and their role in protection from chronic diseases Protein and bone health across the lifespan. 2018 [cited 2020 Aug 5]; https://doi.org/10.1017/S0029665118001180.
71. Wilkinson DJ, Hossain T, Hill DS, Phillips BE, Crossland H, Williams J, et al. Effects of leucine and its metabolite β-hydroxy-β-methylbutyrate on human skeletal muscle protein metabolism. J Physiol [Internet]. 2013;591(11):2911–23. [cited 2020 Aug 5]. https://doi.org/10.1113/jphysiol.2013.253203.
72. Burtscher M, Brooks S V, Casagrande Figueiredo V, Kirk B, Mooney K, Amirabdollahian F, et al. Exercise and dietary-protein as a countermeasure to skeletal muscle weakness: liverpool hope university—sarcopenia aging trial (LHU-SAT). 2019 [cited 2020 Aug 5]. www.frontiersin.org.
73. Liberman K, Njemini R, Luiking Y, Forti LN, Sjors V, Bauer JM, et al. Thirteen weeks of supplementation of vitamin D and leucine-enriched whey protein nutritional supplement attenuates chronic low-grade inflammation in sarcopenic older adults: the PROVIDE study. Aging Clin Exp Res. 2019;31:845–54. [cited 2020 Aug 5]. https://doi.org/10.1007/s40520-019-01208-4.
74. Verlaan S, Maier AB, Bauer JM, Bautmans I, Brandt K, Donini LM, et al. Sufficient levels of 25-hydroxyvitamin D and protein intake required to increase muscle mass in sarcopenic older adults e The PROVIDE study. Clin Nutr [Internet]. 2018;37:551–7. [cited 2020 Aug 5]. https://doi.org/10.1016/j.clnu.2017.01.0050261-5614/.

75. Ito S, Harada A, Kasai T, Sakai Y, Takemura M, Matsui Y, et al. Use of alfacalcidol in osteoporotic patients with low muscle mass might increase muscle mass: an investigation using a patient database. Geriatr Gerontol Int. 2014;14(Suppl. 1):122–8.
76. Sanders KM, Stuart AL, Williamson EJ, Simpson JA, Kotowicz MA, Young D, et al. Annual high-dose oral vitamin D and falls and fractures in older women: a randomized controlled trial. J Am Med Assoc. 2010 May 12;303(18):1815–22.
77. Ishikawa M, Iwamoto T, Nakamura T, Doyle A, Fukumoto S, Yamada Y. Pannexin 3 functions as an ER Ca 2+ channel, hemichannel, and gap junction to promote osteoblast differentiation. J Cell Biol [Internet]. 2011;193(7):1257–74. [cited 2020 Jul 28]. https://doi.org/10.1083/jcb.201101050.
78. Osteosarcopenia: bone, muscle and fat interactions. Springer International Publishing; 2019.
79. Suetta C, Andersen JL, Dalgas U, Berget J, Koskinen S, Aagaard P, et al. Resistance training induces qualitative changes in muscle morphology, muscle architecture, and muscle function in elderly postoperative patients. J Appl Physiol [Internet]. 2008;105(1):180–6. [cited 2020 Oct 1]. https://doi.org/10.1152/japplphysiol.01354.2007.
80. Bonnet N, Bourgoin L, Biver E, Douni E, Ferrari S. RANKL inhibition improves muscle strength and insulin sensitivity and restores bone mass. J Clin Invest. 2019;129(8):3214–23.
81. Cummings SR, Martin JS, McClung MR, Siris ES, Eastell R, Reid IR, et al. Denosumab for prevention of fractures in postmenopausal women with osteoporosis. N Engl J Med [Internet]. 2009;361(8):756–65. [cited 2020 Aug 5]. http://www.nejm.org/doi/abs/10.1056/NEJMoa0809493.
82. Phu S, Bani Hassan E, Vogrin S, Kirk B, Duque G. Effect of denosumab on falls, muscle strength, and function in community-dwelling older adults. J Am Geriatr Soc. Blackwell Publishing Inc. 2019;67:2660–1.
83. Bhasin S, Woodhouse L, Casaburi R, Singh AB, Mac RP, Lee M, et al. Older men are as responsive as young men to the anabolic effects of graded doses of testosterone on the skeletal muscle. J Clin Endocrinol Metab [Internet]. 2005;90(2):678–88. [cited 2020 Aug 5]. https://academic.oup.com/jcem/article-lookup/doi/10.1210/jc.2004-1184.
84. O'Connell MDL, Roberts SA, Srinivas-Shankar U, Tajar A, Connolly MJ, Adams JE, et al. Do the effects of testosterone on muscle strength, physical function, body composition, and quality of life persist six months after treatment in intermediate-frail and frail elderly men? J Clin Endocrinol Metab [Internet]. 2011;96(2):454–8. [cited 2020 Aug 5]. https://academic.oup.com/jcem/article/96/2/454/2709511.
85. Travison TG, Basaria S, Storer TW, Jette AM, Miciek R, Farwell WR, et al. Clinical meaningfulness of the changes in muscle performance and physical function associated with testosterone administration in older men with mobility limitation. J Gerontol Ser A Biol Sci Med Sci. 2011;66A(10):1090–9.
86. Wittert GA, Chapman IM, Haren MT, Mackintosh S, Coates P, Morley JE. Oral testosterone supplementation increases muscle and decreases fat mass in healthy elderly males with low-normal gonadal status [Internet]. [cited 2020 Aug 5]. https://academic.oup.com/biomedgerontology/article-abstract/58/7/M618/544182.
87. Snyder PJ, Bhasin S, Cunningham GR, Matsumoto AM, Stephens-Shields AJ, Cauley JA, et al. Lessons from the testosterone trials. Endocr Rev [Internet]. 2018;39(3):369–86. [cited 2020 Aug 5]. https://academic.oup.com/edrv/article/39/3/369/4924422.
88. Dalton JT, Barnette KG, Bohl CE, Hancock ML, Rodriguez D, Dodson ST, et al. The selective androgen receptor modulator GTx-024 (enobosarm) improves lean body mass and physical function in healthy elderly men and postmenopausal women: results of a double-blind, placebo-controlled phase II trial. J Cachexia Sarcopenia Muscle. 2011;2(3):153–61.
89. Mohler ML, Bohl CE, Jones A, Coss CC, Narayanan R, He Y, et al. Nonsteroidal Selective Androgen Receptor Modulators (SARMs): dissociating the anabolic and androgenic activities of the androgen receptor for therapeutic benefit [Internet]. J Med Chem. American Chemical Society. 2009;52:3597–617. [cited 2020 Aug 5]. https://pubs.acs.org/sharingguidelines.

90. Becker C, Lord SR, Studenski SA, Warden SJ, Fielding RA, Recknor CP, et al. Myostatin antibody (LY2495655) in older weak fallers: a proof-of-concept, randomised, phase 2 trial. Lancet Diabetes Endocrinol [Internet]. 2015;3(12):948–57. https://doi.org/10.1016/S2213-8587(15)00298-3.
91. Rooks D, Praestgaard J, Hariry S, Laurent D, Petricoul O, Perry RG, et al. Treatment of sarcopenia with Bimagrumab: results from a phase II, randomized, controlled, proof-of-concept study. J Am Geriatr Soc. 2017;65(9):1988–95.
92. Garito T, Roubenoff R, Hompesch M, Morrow L, Gomez K, Rooks D, et al. Bimagrumab improves body composition and insulin sensitivity in insulin-resistant individuals. Diabetes Obes Metab. 2018;20(1):94–102.
93. Takala J, Ruokonen E, Webster NR, Nielsen MS, Zandstra DF, Vundelinckx G, et al. Increased mortality associated with growth hormone treatment in critically Ill adults. N Engl J Med [Internet]. 1999;341(11):785–92. [cited 2020 Aug 5]. http://www.nejm.org/doi/abs/10.1056/NEJM199909093411102.
94. Liu H, Bravata DM, Olkin I, Nayak S, Roberts B, Garber AM, et al. Systematic review: The safety and efficacy of growth hormone in the healthy elderly. Ann Internal Med. American College of Physicians. 2007;146:104–15.
95. Adachi N, Kanazawa I, Tanaka K-I, Takeno A, Notsu M, Tanaka S, et al. Insulin-like growth factor-I protects against the detrimental effects of advanced glycation end products and high glucose in myoblastic C2C12 cells. Calcif Tissue Int [Internet]. 2019;105(1):89–96. [cited 2020 Jul 26]. https://doi.org/10.1007/s00223-019-00537-w.
96. Coto-Montes A, Boga J, Tan D, Reiter R. Melatonin as a potential agent in the treatment of sarcopenia. Int J Mol Sci [Internet]. 2016;17(10):1771. [cited 2020 Jun 12]. http://www.mdpi.com/1422-0067/17/10/1771.
97. Bermeo S, Al Saedi A, Vidal C, Khalil M, Pang M, Troen BR, et al. Treatment with an inhibitor of fatty acid synthase attenuates bone loss in ovariectomized mice. Bone. 2019;122:114–22.
98. Kirk B, Al Saedi A, Duque G. Osteosarcopenia: a case of geroscience. AGING Med. 2019;2(3):147–56.
99. Rong S, Wang L, Peng Z, Liao Y, Li D, Yang X, et al. The mechanisms and treatments for sarcopenia: could exosomes be a perspective research strategy in the future? J Cachexia, Sarcopenia Muscle. Wiley Blackwell. 2020;11:348–65.
100. Kirk B, Zanker J, Duque G. Osteosarcopenia: epidemiology, diagnosis, and treatment—facts and numbers. J Cachexia Sarcopenia Muscle [Internet]. 2020;11(3):609–18. [cited 2020 Jun 16]. https://onlinelibrary.wiley.com/doi/abs/10.1002/jcsm.12567.

Chapter 11
Secondary Osteoporosis

A. E. Litwic, A. Dębska-Ślizień, and Elaine Dennison

Introduction

Osteoporosis is described as secondary when low bone mineral density or an increased risk of fragility fracture is caused by factors other than aging or postmenopausal status. A large number of factors cause secondary osteoporosis; the spectrum of diseases and medications associated with secondary osteoporosis are reported in Table 11.1. Osteoporosis is usually attributed to age-related bone loss in postmenopausal women, whereas idiopathic osteoporosis is more commonly diagnosed in younger adults [1]. While the prevalence of secondary causes of osteoporosis varies according to the population studied, as many as 50–55% of men and 40–50% of premenopausal women presenting with established osteoporosis have been found to have other conditions that may have contributed to their bone loss [2].

A. E. Litwic (✉)
MRC Lifecourse Epidemiology Centre, University of Southampton, Southampton, UK

Department of Nephrology, Transplantology and Internal Medicine,
Medical University of Gdańsk, Gdańsk, Poland

A. Dębska-Ślizień
Department of Nephrology, Transplantology and Internal Medicine,
Medical University of Gdańsk, Gdańsk, Poland
e-mail: adeb@gumed.edu.pl

E. Dennison
MRC Lifecourse Epidemiology Centre, University of Southampton, Southampton, UK
e-mail: emd@mrc.soton.ac.uk

E. Dennison (ed.), *Osteoporosis Treatment*, https://doi.org/10.1007/978-3-030-78128-6_11

Table 11.1 Causes of secondary osteoporosis

Causes of secondary osteoporosis
Endocrine diseases Acromegaly, adrenal insufficiency; Cushing syndrome (hypercortisolism); diabetes mellitus (types I and II); growth hormone deficiency; hyperparathyroidism and hyperthyroidism; pregnancy
Gastrointestinal conditions Inflammatory bowel disease Generalized malnutrition or inadequate intake including alcoholism-related malnutrition, deficiency of calcium, magnesium, protein and/or vitamin D; parenteral nutrition; anorexia nervosa and bulimia nervosa Malabsorption including bariatric surgery; gastric bypass surgery; coeliac disease; chronic pancreatitis; liver cirrhosis; chronic biliary tract obstruction; cystic fibrosis Alcoholic liver disease
Heamatologic disorders Multiple myeloma; leukaemia; lymphoma; systemic mastocytosis; myelofibrosis; monoclonal gammopathy of unknown significance
Rheumatological diseases Rheumatoid arthritis Spondylarthritis including ankylosing spondylitis Systemic lupus erythematosus Vasculitides
Renal diseases Chronic kidney disease-mineral and Bone disorder
Neurological disorders Multiple sclerosis; Parkinson's disease, states of prolonged immobilization and skeletal unloading including spinal cord injury
Infectious Human immunodeficiency virus (HIV)
Transplantation
Congenital and genetic conditions Structural collagen or connective tissue defects including osteogenesis imperfecta, Ehlers–Danlos syndrome, Marfan syndrome, pseudoxanthoma elasticum Disrupted calcium and/or phosphate homeostasis including hypophosphatasia, Idiopathic hypercalciuria Metabolic and storage disorders including cystic fibrosis, glycogen storage diseases, Gaucher disease, haemochromatosis, porphyria Haematologic disorders including haemophilia, sickle cell anaemia, thalassaemia Primary hypogonadal states including Turner syndrome; Klinefelter syndrome
Drugs

In addition secondary causes are found in approximately 30% of postmenopausal women with osteoporosis [2, 3].

Given the diversity of diseases, deficiencies and drugs that cause secondary osteoporosis (Table 11.1), a detailed discussion of each potential mechanism is not possible here, but rather we review the more common causes of secondary osteoporosis, with a focus on pathogenesis and treatment strategies.

Endocrine Diseases

Glucocorticoid Excess

Endogenous glucocorticoids have an important role in bone homeostasis [4]. An endogenous excess of glucocorticoids in the form of Cushing disease produces profound skeletal effects [5]. Similarly, glucocorticoids, when administered systemically, have a well-documented effect on bone health and increase the risk of fracture - the most common serious and preventable adverse event associated with these agents [6–8]. This is very important as approximately 1% of adults receive long-term oral glucocorticoids, mainly for the treatment of allergies, arthropathies, digestive system disorders or cancer [9, 10]. Systemic administration of glucocorticoids is the most common secondary cause of osteoporosis, glucocorticoid-induced osteoporosis (GIO), and the most common iatrogenic cause of the disease [11, 12].

There are two phases of bone loss caused by GIO: an initial phase, during the first year of treatment, with more rapid rate of bone mineral density (BMD) deterioration of around 6–12%, followed by a continued annual loss with ongoing therapy with a slower rate of BMD loss of around 3% per year [13]. However, the amount of bone loss varies greatly and depends on several factors that influence individual susceptibility to skeletal adverse effects including advanced age, low BMI, dose and duration of glucocorticoid, as well as other traditional factors [14–16]. There are five main methods by which fracture risk has been attributed to glucocorticoid exposure ("current use", "ever use", "daily dose", "cumulative dose" and "time-variant"), none of which consider the dose, duration and timing of treatment [17]. However, in a recent study Robinson et al. found that different aspects of oral glucocorticoids exposure affect the risk of fracture with increased risk for more recent doses, higher doses and a longer duration spent on oral glucocorticoids. Those complex individual patterns of steroid treatment should be considered by clinicians, as they are not incorporated into fracture risk calculators [18].

Glucocorticoids have direct and indirect effects on bone through their effect on bone cells (osteoblasts, osteocytes and osteoclasts), indirect effects on bone metabolism and muscle loss leading to an increased fall risk. The pathophysiology of GIO manifests as impaired or decreased bone formation through restricting differentiation and replication of osteoblasts and inducing apoptosis; and increased bone resorption that results from increases in expression of receptor activator of nuclear factor-κB ligand (RANKL), which lead to increases in the number of bone-resorbing osteoclasts [16]. Glucocorticoids also increase osteocyte apoptosis, that occurs early after treatment initiation, and decrease vascular endothelial growth factor expression, skeletal angiogenesis and cause disruption of fluid flow in the osteocyte–canalicular network leading to altered material properties of the surrounding bone [19–21]. In addition, glucocorticoids induce production of sclerostin and dickkopf-related protein 1 (DKK-1) by osteocytes, inhibiting Wnt signalling pathway, and reducing bone formation [22]. Glucocorticoids also indirectly affect bone metabolism through decreased production of oestrogen and testosterone, reduction in growth hormone (GH) secretion, alter renal and gastrointestinal calcium absorption and reduce muscle mass and strength, increasing falls risk [23]. There are many factors that influence fracture risk, either through bone mineral density (BMD) or through independent mechanisms. GIO risk is higher in women and among Caucasians, and is also higher in older patients and in those with low BMI, and/or underlying conditions such as rheumatoid arthritis, polymyalgia rheumatica, inflammatory bowel disease, chronic pulmonary disease, and transplantation [8, 24].

The increased risk of fracture is also related to oral glucocorticoids (GC) dose. van Staa and colleagues using data from >240,000 glucocorticoid-exposed cases and >240,000 controls from the UK General Practice Research database (GPRD) demonstrated that fracture risk increased in relation to daily GC dose with the risk of both hip and vertebral fractures [6]. Daily dose of prednisolone of 2.5 mg or less was associated with hip fracture risk of 0.99 (0.82–1.20) relative to control, and increased to 1.77 (1.55–2.02) at daily doses of 2.5–7.5 mg, and 2.27 (1.94–2.66) at doses of 7.5 mg or greater. The relative rates for vertebral fracture were higher at 1.55 (1.20–2.01), 2.59 (2.16–3.10), and 5.18 (4.25–6.31), respectively. All fracture risks declined after cessation of oral GC treatment toward baseline [6]. The risk of fractures is more strongly related to daily dose than to cumulative doses in GC users. Moreover, there is an increased fracture incidence among patients initiating oral GC therapy, of vertebral fracture, compared to chronic GC users [25]. For non-vertebral fracture, the annual rate is reported to be similar among GC initiators and among chronic GC users. This suggests that bone loss affects both axial and appendicular sites, but oral GCs have a predominant effect at the spine leading to vertebral fragility.

In contrast, users of inhaled glucocorticoids had excess fracture risk at non-vertebral, hip and vertebral sites, compared with users of non-glucocorticoid dilators, but fracture rates between those taking and not taking inhaled glucocorticoids are similar, suggesting that inhaled glucocorticoids do not convey additional fracture risk, but they are used by individuals with increased fracture risk [26].Therefore, a prescribing physician should use the lowest dose for the shortest period, and via the most appropriate route (preferably topical rather than systemic) for GC treatment. Bone mineral density measurement to assess the risk of fracture using a fracture risk assessment tool (FRAX) at the onset of therapy should also be performed [24]. For those clinicians managing the condition, an updated treatment guideline was recently published, and both anabolic and antiresorptive therapies may be used in addition to calcium and vitamin D supplementation [24].

Primary Hyperparathyroidism

Parathyroid hormone (PTH) helps to regulate calcium and phosphorus homeostasis. Primary hyperparathyroidism (PHPT) is observed three times more frequently in women than in men, with an incidence as high as 1 in 500 in postmenopausal females [20]. In PHPT persistently elevated levels of PTH are catabolic to the skeleton, and preferentially affect cortical rather than cancellous bone [27]. Thus, bone loss is most prominent at skeletal sites that consist of cortical bone (e.g. middle third of the forearm and femoral neck), while the spine, mainly composed of cancellous bone, is less severely affected [28]. Therefore, patients with PHPT should be evaluated for bone loss at the distal forearm, femoral neck and lumbar spine BMD by DXA if available [28].

The precise mechanism of bone loss in PHPT is not completely understood. Chronic PTH excess leads to a high bone turnover state and is associated with a low BMD and also with alterations in the mineralization density distribution and collagen crosslinks affecting material properties of the bone [29, 30]. PHPT has also been shown to increase bone resorption through an observed low OPG/RANKL ratio, at the cellular level [31]. As a consequence of these bone turnover alterations PHPT has been shown to increase both hip fracture risk [32] and vertebral fracture prevalence [33]. The primary treatment for primary hyperparathyroidism is surgical resection of the adenoma or hyperplastic glands and several studies have demonstrated the beneficial effects of surgery on indices of bone turnover, bone density and fracture risk in postoperative patients [34, 35].

Hyperthyroidism

Thyroid hormones have important effects on skeletal development and maintenance of bone mass [36]. TSH receptors are located on osteoblasts and osteoclasts [36]; and a direct action on bone tissue cells from this hormone leads to enhanced bone remodelling and hence osteoporosis. Hyperthyroidism causes acceleration of bone turnover and loss of mineral density, mainly in cortical bone, suggesting the need to screen distal forearm BMD as a preferred site of measurement [37, 38]. In this condition the cycle of bone remodelling is shortened and the balance of bone formation and bone resorption is disturbed. The phase of bone formation is significantly reduced and it causes overall net loss of bone at an estimated rate of 10% of mineralized bone per remodelling cycle [2]. Untreated thyrotoxicosis is associated with significantly reduced BMD at the spine and hip and is an independent risk factor for osteoporotic fracture [39, 40]. Wejda et al. reported that hyperthyroidism was found 2.5-fold more often in hip fracture patients than in controls [41]while Bauer et al. noted that postmenopausal women with decreased TSH concentrations (<0.1 mU/L), even in subclinical thyroid disease, had a threefold increased risk of hip and a fourfold increased risk of vertebral fracture compared with women with normal TSH levels [39]. Hyperthyroidism should be detected and controlled with medical and/or surgical therapies as required as there is evidence that use of anti-thyroid drugs was associated with a significantly reduced fracture risk independently of the dose used [42].

Diabetes Mellitus

Although the relationship between diabetes and osteoporosis has been widely investigated, it remains controversial. Diabetes could impact bone through several mechanisms, some of which may have contradictory effects. There is evidence that patients with both type 1 (T1DM) and 2 diabetes mellitus (T2DM) are predisposed to osteoporosis and are at increased fracture risk [43, 44].

Studies in patients with T1DM indicate an associated 12-fold increased risk of osteoporotic fracture [45]. This increase is associated with reduced BMD and a failure to achieve peak bone mass [46], as a result of absolute deficiency of insulin and insulin-like growth factor-1 (IGF-1). There is also a reported increased risk of fracture in patients with T2DM with a 1.7-fold higher risk of self-reported hip fracture than women without the disease [45]. In T2DM, however, the increased risk of fracture occurs with normal or increased BMD, implicating a decline in the quality of the bone as a contributor to fracture risk [47]. Other studies suggest structural changes in T2DM that may explain the higher fracture risk despite normal or elevated BMD including increased intracortical porosity and decreased material strength [48, 49]. The accumulation of end-products of advanced glycosylation and lower enzymatic collagen crosslinks contribute to altered bone quality in diabetes; it has been shown to be reduced by medications used for T2DM treatment [50]. The reduced bone quality in patients with T2DM could also be a result of hyperinsulinemia, hypercalciuria, renal failure, microangiopathy, and/or reduced serum levels of insulin-like growth factor 1.

Interestingly, T1DM and T2DM are not different regarding the effect on bone markers, although sclerostin levels are higher in T2DM, suggesting that bones are affected through an antagonizing effect on the WnT pathway in T2DM, but not in T1DM [51]. A reasonable assumption is that good diabetic control will reduce the risk of fractures in patients with T1DM or T2DM. However, addressing other factors that could contribute to an increased risk for falls and fractures in this population such as retinopathy-induced visual impairment, balance problems caused by neuropathy, renal osteodystrophy from dialysis, renal transplantation or sarcopenia is also important. In diabetic patients with established osteoporosis, standard osteoporosis therapies may be used.

Male Hypogonadism

Hypogonadism, whether from aging, surgery, or a medication, is a major cause of osteoporosis in men, as androgens are important for developing and maintaining skeletal health [52]. Testosterone signalling stimulates osteoblasts to form trabecular bone and helps osteocytes prevent trabecular bone loss. Decreased BMD and increased fracture risk are seen in men with both primary and secondary hypogonadism [53]. Testosterone also has an indirect effect on bone through its aromatization to estrogen via aromatase. Estrogens play a role in both bone resorption and bone formation in men. A relationship between low serum estradiol levels and low BMD and increased fracture risk has been demonstrated in men [54]. While there is evidence that testosterone replacement therapy can improve bone density at the spine and the hip, as well as trabecular architecture, and mechanical properties, whether it reduces fracture risk in hypogonadal bone disease is less clear [53] and further work is required to determine whether testosterone treatment of older men with low testosterone reduces fracture risk.

A major cause of androgen deficiency is iatrogenic therapy i.e.androgen deprivation therapy (ADT), for prostate cancer. Androgen deficiency is accompanied by a decline in BMD within the first 6–9 months of ADT and then continues at a rate of approximately 2–3% loss per annum; it results in an increase in fracture risk of nearly 20% after 5 years of therapy [55]. ADT increases the rate of bone turnover, which after 6 months after starting treatment stabilises [2]. Consequences of ADT related to bone health include loss of muscle mass and increased risk of falls and fractures. As hormone therapies are contraindicated in prostate cancer, bisphosphonates and denosumab have been used to suppress osteoclast function.

Gastrointestinal Conditions

Inflammatory Bowel Disease

Crohn's disease and ulcerative colitis are two forms of chronic inflammatory bowel disease (IBD) and are associated with bone loss, with patients with inflammatory bowel disease at higher risk of developing osteoporosis and osteopenia and increased fracture risk. The prevalence of osteoporosis and osteopenia in patients with inflammatory bowel disease varies in different epidemiological studies and ranges from 22%–77% and 17%–41%, respectively [56]. In a meta-analysis of 16 studies of BMD in IBD compared with controls, the mean Z-scores at all sites were lower in patients with IBD (mean difference ranging from −0.5 to −1) [57]. Although low BMD is a well-recognised risk for fracture, many individuals with IBD have normal BMD at the time of fracture diagnosis [58]. Risk of fracture in IBD is also elevated; with a recent, large study involving 83,435 patients with incident IBD, reporting a 42% increase in risk of hip fracture in IBD; risk of any fracture was also increased (HR 1.18, 95% CI 1.15–1.20) [59]. In a meta-analysis of studies that evaluated specific types of fractures in patients with IBD, there was an increase in risk of vertebral fracture (1.34 versus 0.56% in healthy controls, odds ratio [OR] 2.26, 95% CI 1.04–4.90) [57]. Elevated risk of fracture in patients with IBD is related to both disease severity and use of medication [60].

The pathophysiology is multifactorial and includes the use of oral corticosteroids, vitamin D deficiency, malabsorption, malnutrition, low BMI, hypogonadism, and systemic inflammation [60]. Inflammation is one of the factors that contribute to osteoporosis in IBD patients, and the main system that is involved in bone loss is likely RANK/RANKL/osteoprotegerin [61]. Chronic inflammatory states mediated by T cell-produced cytokines affect osteoblasts and osteoclasts. Activated T cells produce RANKL and its soluble form, which directly triggers bone loss *via* the induction and activation of osteoclasts by RANK [62]. The elevated OPG levels are felt to be a response to osteopenia and RANKL driven osteoclastogenesis [54].

A high prevalence of vitamin D deficiency has been demonstrated in IBD patients, with as many as 50% of patients with IBD reported as vitamin D deficient [63]. The cause for deficiency is likely to be multifactorial, but include low sun exposure, inadequate intake as well as factors related to inflammatory disease, such as terminal ileum resection and low absorption due to the inflammatory process [64]. In Crohn's disease (CD), the primary tissue involved is at the terminal ileum, where the majority of absorption of fat-soluble vitamins occurs; and in CD resection of the terminal ileum, the most common surgery, has been described as one of the most important determinants of developing osteoporosis [64]. Routine BMD testing, dietary questioning on calcium intake, and measuring of 25-OH vitamin D levels are therefore recommended for all patients at the onset of disease.

Celiac Disease

Celiac disease is characterized by inflammatory changes in the duodenum with villous atrophy affecting dietary absorption. While classically thought to begin in childhood, it is now recognized that along with this classic form of the disease there are other clinical and subclinical forms that may manifest later and in which there may be no intestinal symptoms; indeed bone metabolism disorders and a decrease in BMD may be the only signs of otherwise asymptomatic celiac disease [65]. The poor absorption induced by celiac disease leads to deficiencies of nutrients including vitamin D and calcium, essential for the maintenance of bone structure. The prevalence of celiac disease among osteoporotic patients (3.4%) is much higher than that among non-osteoporotic individuals (0.2%), suggesting the need for more intensive screening in this population [66]. Decreased BMD and increased fracture risk has been reported in celiac patients compared with controls [67].

The pathophysiology of bone loss in celiac disease is multifactorial, centred around inflammation, malabsorption, and decreased intestinal absorption. Chronic release of proinflammatory cytokines by immunologically competent cells of the gastrointestinal mucosa might induce bone remodelling, stimulating bone resorption by osteoclasts [65].

Intestinal mucosal lesions can lead to calcium malabsorption and decreased levels of serum calcium along with hypovitaminosis D [68]; these changes contribute to elevation in PTH [69] and can result in skeletal consequences of secondary hyperparathyroidism including increased bone turnover and decreased BMD [70]. Chronic release of proinflammatory cytokines by the cells of gastrointestinal mucosa might induce bone remodelling, stimulating bone resorption by osteoclasts

[65]. Another mechanism involved in bone loss in celiac disease is the perturbation of the RANK/RANKL/osteoprotegerin axis [71]. However addressing other factors that could contribute to the bone loss associated with celiac disease such as low BMI, hypogonadism, decreased physical activity is also important. Treatment of coeliac disease with a gluten free diet probably protects against further bone loss, and in the early stages is associated with a gain in bone mineral density [72].

Other Nutritional Deficiencies

There are other nutritional deficiencies that could result from general malnutrition or inadequate intake such as alcoholism-related malnutrition, deficiency of calcium, magnesium, protein and/or vitamin D; parenteral nutrition; anorexia nervosa and bulimia nervosa or related to malabsorption such as bariatric surgery; gastric bypass surgery; chronic pancreatitis; liver cirrhosis; chronic biliary tract obstruction; cystic fibrosis. Details of each condition and potential mechanisms are beyond the scope of this chapter.

Rheumatological Conditions

Rheumatoid Arthritis

Rheumatoid arthritis (RA) is the most common form of inflammatory arthritis in adults and is characterized by chronic, progressive, systemic inflammation. In RA, localized (marginal joint erosions, periarticular osteopenia) and generalized bone disease occur. In active RA pannus (inflammatory synovial tissue proliferation), attaches to the bone surface where osteoclast-like cells invade and focal bone resorption takes place, in the almost complete absence of bone repair. With regard to generalised bone loss, underlying disease activity and ongoing use of glucocorticoids can contribute to bone loss and risk for fractures. Patients with RA have a two- to three-fold increased risk of hip and vertebral fractures [73, 74].

Several cytokines involved in RA-associated inflammation such as IL-1, IL-6, TNF-α can promote osteoclastic activity; similarly RANKL is released by infiltrating T cells and synoviocytes in RA, promoting osteoclast activation [75]. In RA increased RANKL:OPG ratio, as well as elevated bone turnover markers levels were found to be predictors of rapid and persistent bone damage [76]. In addition to an increased RANKL:OPG ratio, increased levels of Dkk-1 (a potent inhibitor of Wnt signalling pathways) and sclerostin, inhibitors of bone formation, have been found in the serum of RA patients [77]. Treatment used for RA has been shown to prevent those changes, with evidence that anti-TNF antibodies can decrease systemic bone loss (207) and use of inhibitors of IL-6 lead to a decrease in the

RANKL:OPG ratio as well as a drop in the Dkk-1 and sclerostin levels, and less bone loss [77]. Therefore, early, aggressive treatment of RA is essential for stopping disease progression and its skeletal consequences. In RA with established osteoporosis, standard osteoporosis therapies may be used [2].

Ankylosing Spondylitis

Ankylosing spondylitis (AS) is a chronic arthritis characterized by inflammation in synovial joints as well as the entheses. In contrast to RA, the inflammation can be accompanied by localized bone formation rather than erosions, particularly at areas of entheseal inflammation. However, osteoporosis is a known complication of AS. Chronic systemic inflammation and progressive immobility contribute to the bone loss. Patients with AS are at high risk of osteoporosis and both vertebral and nonvertebral fractures [78]. Osteoporosis is seen in up to 25%, and osteopenia in up to 50%, of patients with AS. Patients with AS have worse bone mineral density, microarchitecture and strength when compared to non-AS subjects [79]. The etiology of bone loss in patients with AS is multifactorial with systemic inflammation mediated by TNF-α being the most important etiologic factor; it activates osteoclasts to cause bone resorption and also increases the osteoblast apoptosis and decreases osteoblast proliferation, inhibiting bone formation [80]. Therapy with TNF-specific antagonists has been shown to increase vertebral and hip BMD in this condition [80]. Similar to other forms of inflammatory arthritis, in AS with established osteoporosis, standard osteoporosis therapies may be used.

Systemic Lupus Erythematosus

Patients with systemic lupus erythematosus (SLE) are exposed to factors that can induce bone loss including glucocorticosteroids and lower age of menopause due to the disease itself, or its treatment with cytotoxic substances. Low dietary intake of calcium and vitamin D combined with avoidance of sun light can contribute to deficiency of vitamin D and result in reduced bone mass. Interactions between proinflammatory cytokines and bone cells play an important role in diseases with systemic inflammation like SLE and are thought to be similar to those described above in RA [2]. Studies have shown a lower bone mineral density and increased risk of fractures in SLE patients and higher fracture rates than in the healthy population [81, 82]. General measures to improve bone health should be considered in all patients with SLE and other inflammatory conditions, with a low threshold for measuring BMD with DXA. Control of inflammatory activity is desirable for improved disease outcomes. In patients with established osteoporosis, standard osteoporosis therapies should be used with optimization of intake of calcium and vitamin D. However, as

SLE commonly affects premenopausal females, bisphosphonates need to be used with caution in women of child bearing age.

Neurological Disorders

Spinal Cord Injury and the Role of Immobility

Spinal cord injury (SCI), or any situation that results in prolonged immobilization leads to bone loss that affects mainly the paralyzed extremities, and is associated with increased risk of fracture [83, 84]. Mechanical unloading after paralysis results in increased osteocyte expression of sclerostin, leading to reduced Wnt/β-catenin signaling in osteoblasts, suppressed bone formation, and indirect stimulation of bone resorption [85]. Sclerostin causes the up-regulation of RANKL and down-regulation of osteoprotegerin (OPG), increasing osteoclast differentiation and activity, and leading to bone resorption [85].

The rate of bone loss is greatest during the first year after SCI, with a reduction in proximal femoral bone mineral density (BMD) of 2.5–3.1% per month [86]. The rapid decrease in BMD by 50–70% in the lower extremities (femoral neck and diaphysis, proximal tibia) in the first few years after SCI seems to stabilize at later stages [84]. Long-term follow-up data suggest that as many as 50% of people with SCI will sustain a low-impact or an osteoporotic fracture at some point following their injury [87]. Zehnder et al. reported fracture incidence after SCI approximately 1% per year with increase to 3.4–4.6% 10 years post injury with a mean duration of 8.9 years until the first fracture [83].

There is currently no well-accepted clinical guidance on interventions to prevent SCI-induced osteoporosis and tools to inform clinicians of the risk for fragility fractures in SCI subjects [88]. Interventions used in this patient group include mechanical loading of the lower extremity using functional electrical stimulation, and mechanical stimulation via vibration therapy. While bisphosphonates have all demonstrated reduced fragility fracture rates in the general osteoporosis population, the clinical benefits have not been demonstrated in the SCI-induced osteoporosis population [89, 90]. Teriparatide and denosumab have been studied in the SCI population with promising results compared to control [91, 92], but further research analyzing the long-term efficacy of these drugs is needed.

Multiple Sclerosis

Multiple sclerosis is a chronic demyelinating neurologic condition frequently associated with significant disability and limitation of physical function. Bone mineral density is reduced at the lumbar spine, hip and total body in MS, with the degree of reduction being greatest at the hip [93]. Factors contributing to reduced BMD in this population include vitamin D deficiency, glucocorticoid therapy, female gender and the role of the inflammatory processes of the disease Degree of functional impairment and duration of disease also contribute significantly to the low BMD found in these patients [94]. Patients with multiple sclerosis may be at an increased risk of fracture due to a greater risk of falling and decreased bone mineral density, when compared with the general population [95]. In a large multinational longitudinal cohort of women (GLOW), that MS was one of the comorbidities that contributed significantly to fracture risk [96]; in this cohort high fracture rate was observed in women with MS, with an almost three-fold increased fracture risk [97]. General measures to improve bone health should be considered in all patients with MS, similar to other inflammatory conditions, with a low threshold for measuring BMD with DXA. In patients with established osteoporosis, standard osteoporosis therapies should be used with optimization of intake of calcium and vitamin D.

Haematological Disorders

Multiple Myeloma

Multiple myeloma (MM) is a clonal malignancy of terminally differentiated plasma cells and is the type most likely to involve bone. A classic presentation of MM is bone pain, which occurs in 60–70% of patients and is associated with osteolytic bone lesions; up to 60% of patients will develop a pathologic fracture during their course of MM [98].The clonal proliferation results in classic lytic lesions and reduced bone mass due to increased bone resorption and decreased bone formation. It results from the excess production of osteoclastogenic factors by myeloma cells such as RANKL, macrophage-colony stimulating factor, macrophage inflammatory protein-1α, IL-11, IL-3 and IL-6 [2]. The RANKL:OPG axis is altered in MM, with an increase in the ratio observed favoring production and survival of osteoclasts [99]. Suppression of osteoblast activity also occurs in multiple myeloma, which might reflect activity of DKK-1 on Wnt pathway signalling [100]. The effect of these changes is decreased bone formation and increased bone resorption, leading to osteoporosis. Bisphosphonates and targeted therapies for myeloma help reduce osteolysis, the risk of fractures and when given at induction of chemotherapy have shown to reduce mortality [101, 102]. Denosumab is a potential alternative for the prevention of skeletal-related complications in patients with MM with impaired renal function since the drug is not metabolized or excreted by the kidneys [103].

Thalassesmia Major

Thalassemias comprise a group of inherited disorders of hemoglobin synthesis, and mutations in the *BGLOBIN* gene lead to defective Beta globin production and anemia. The reported frequency of osteoporosis, even in well treated thalassemia major (TM) patients is as high as 50% [104]. Different acquired and genetic factors are involved in its pathogenesis. Contributing factors include delay in sexual maturation, hypogonadism, decreased growth hormone and IGF-1 levels, diabetes, hypothyroidism, and vitamin D deficiency [104]. The pathogenesis of bone changes in TM patients is not completely understood. In TM there is an unbalance in bone mineral turnover resulting with increased resorptive rates and suppression of osteoblast activity, resulting in diminished bone mineral density (BMD) more evident in the lumbar spine and increased risk of fractures has been described [105].

The management of patients presenting with thalassemia-associated osteoporosis should consist of the implementation of general measures, including control of anemia, adequate chelation therapy, healthy nutrition and lifestyle, regular exercise, adequate management of comorbid conditions, hormone replacement therapy in patients with hypogonadism, and vitamin D supplementation/therapy, and the prescription of a specific anti-osteoporotic medication (AOM) [106]. Bisphosphonates decrease bone remodeling and increase BMD in TM patients, although it is not known whether fracture risk is decreased with bisphosphonate therapy [106].

Renal Disease

Chronic Kidney Disease-Mineral and Bone Disorder (CKD-MBD)

CKD-MBD is a systemic disorder of mineral and bone metabolism due to chronic kidney disease (CKD). It manifests by either one or a combination of the following: (1) abnormalities of calcium, phosphorus, PTH, vitamin D metabolism, (2) abnormalities in bone turnover, mineralization, volume, linear growth, or strength and (3) vascular or other soft-tissue calcification. Renal osteodystrophy is defined as abnormal bone histology and is one component of the bone abnormalities of CKD-MBD that is quantifiable by histomorphometry of bone biopsy.

CKD-MBD associated skeletal changes are associated with bone loss and fractures; with fracture incidence rates over fourfold higher than in the general population [107] Prevalence of osteoporosis in CKD is reported to be twice as common among individuals with an eGFR < 60 mL/min compared with those with an eGFR > 60 mL/min [108]. The pathogenesis of CKD-associated osteoporosis and propensity to fracture is complex and remains to be fully elucidated and is beyond the scope of this chapter. Diagnosis of CKD-associated osteoporosis can be made on the basis of the 2017 Kidney Disease Improving Global Outcome (KDIGO) guidelines [109]. The guidelines recommend measurement of BMD to assess fracture risk in patients with CKD-MBD and/or clinical risk factors for osteoporosis [109]. Treatment in patients with CKD G1–G2 and with CKD G3a–G3b with PTH in the normal range and osteoporosis or high risk of fracture is recommended as for the general population. In patients with CKD G3a–G5D with evidence of CKD-MBD or risk factors for osteoporosis, BMD assessment by DXA should be considered as there is evidence that lower DXA BMD predicts incident fractures in this patient group [109]. However in patients with CKD G3a–G5D with biochemical abnormalities of CKD-MBD and low BMD and/or fragility fractures the reversibility of the biochemical abnormalities and the progression of CKD should be taken into account prior to decision regarding treatment. In this group bone biopsy should be considered if it altered management, but the inability to perform a bone biopsy should not lead to withholding antiresorptive therapy from patients at high risk of fracture [109]. Patients with CKD require a personalized approach to determine the underlying renal osteodystrophy type and appropriateness of administering one of the current antiosteoporotic agents. The KDIGO 2017 Update no longer suggests performing a bone biopsy prior to initiation of antiresorptive therapy, as there is growing body of evidence that these medications are effective in patients with CKD G3a to G3b and G4, and no robust evidence that these medications induce adynamic bone disease [109].

Transplantation Osteoporosis

Transplantation is the lifesaving treatment for patients with end-stage kidney, heart, lung, and liver diseases, as well as for several hematologic disorders. Improved survival of transplant recipients has increased awareness and recognition of post-transplant complications, such as osteoporosis. Osteoporosis and fracture frequently occur after solid organ or hematopoietic transplantation [110]. Historically, post-transplant fracture rates were high, from 10 to 65%. However, more recent studies report lower fracture rates [111, 112], which might be due to increased recognition of and earlier treatment for osteoporosis, changes in treatment regimens (eg, reduction in dose and duration of glucocorticoids), and improvement in nutrition.

Post-transplant bone loss is multifactorial. The primary contributors are the immunosuppressive medications, namely glucocorticoids and calcineurin inhibitors (CIs), though factors such as decreased mobility, poor nutrition and hypogonadism all play a role [113]. Strong consideration should also be given to any underlying pre transplant bone disease, which will differ according to the condition leading to the need for transplantation. Excess glucocorticoids effect on bone is discussed above under endocrine causes of osteoporosis. Cyclosporine and tacrolimus have been shown to cause bone loss by inducing high-turnover state of bone remodelling

[54]. There is limited information regarding the effects of other immunosuppressive drugs on BMD bone metabolism and fracture but, azathioprine, sirolimus, mycophenelate mofetil, and daclizumab may also protect the skeleton by reducing glucocorticoids use [114]. Studies have shown increased bone resorption and decreased bone formation suggestive of uncoupled bone turnover early after transplantation [115, 116], leading to rapid bone loss and a high incidence of fragility fractures, particularly during the first post-transplant year. In the later posttransplant period, after 6 months, with weaning of glucocorticoid doses, bone formation begins to increase and the biochemical pattern is more typical of a high-turnover osteoporosis. Therefore, preventive therapy should be considered in the immediate post-transplantation period in patients with osteopenia or osteoporosis, since further bone loss will occur immediately after transplantation. There is evidence that treatment with a bisphosphonate or active vitamin D metabolite during the first year after solid organ transplantation reduced by 50% the number of subjects with fractures, and number of vertebral fractures [117]. Long-term organ transplant recipients should also have bone mass measurement and treatment of osteoporosis if indicated.

Drug-Induced Osteoporosis

Drug-induced osteoporosis is common and can be caused by a variety of pharmacological agents, including those used for the treatment of endocrine, central nervous system, autoimmune, cardiovascular and gastrointestinal disorders (Table 11.2). The effects of glucocorticoids, calcineurin inhibitors and ADT are described in previous sections of this chapter. This section will focus on four drug groups associated with secondary osteoporosis and widely used in clinical practice: acid-suppression therapies, aromatase inhibitors, selective serotonin reuptake inhibitors and thiazolinediones for diabetes.

Aromatase Inhibitors

In oestrogen receptor-positive breast cancer, aromatase inhibitors [AI] have become first-line adjuvant therapy to prevent breast cancer recurrence. These drugs work on the peripheral aromatization of androgens, reducing endogenous production of oestrogens by 80–90%. AI largely replaced Tamoxifen, because of better efficacy and fewer serious side effects. Tamoxifen was reported to be bone protective in postmenopausal (but not premenopausal) women [118], and use of tamoxifen in general was not associated with any significant change in the risk of any fracture [119]. In contrast AI, by preventing peripheral estrogen production, leads to increase of bone resorption, with a two- to four-fold increased bone loss compared to physiologic

Table 11.2 Drugs associated with osteoporosis

Drugs associated with osteoporosis
Androgen deprivation therapy
Anticoagulants: warfarin, heparin, unfractionated heparins
Anticonvulsants: sodium valproate; phenytoin; carbamazepine
Aromatase inhibitors,
Anti-psychotic therapies
Anti-retroviral therapies
Cytotoxic drugs: ciclosporins and tacrolimus
Diuretics: furosemide
Glucocorticoids
Gonadotrophin-releasing hormone analogues: buserelin; goserelin; cyproterone acetate
Lipase inhibitors: orlistat
Medroxyprogesterone acetate
Proton pump inhibitors
Selective serotonin reuptake inhibitors
Thiazolidinediones: rosiglitazone; pioglitazone
Thyroid hormone: L-thyroxine

postmenopausal BMD, resulting in increased risk for fractures and consequent increased morbidity and mortality [120].

It has been reported that breast cancer patients have fracture incidence rate ratios of 1.25 (95% CI: 1.23–1.28) compared to the general population [121]. In that study women taking AI were at an increased risk of fracture as compared with women taking tamoxifen (HR 1.48; 95% CI: 0.98–2.22). Furthermore, breast cancer patients hospitalized for a bone fracture had a higher risk of death (HR 1.83; 95% CI: 1.50–2.22) compared with those without bone fracture [121]. After cessation of AI treatment, bone turnover normalizes, and hence BMD and fracture risk can partially recover.

Therefore timely osteoporosis prevention strategies for women receiving AI are recommended. Guidance published in 2017 by several interdisciplinary cancer and bone societies involved in the management of AI-associated bone loss (AIBL) [120] recommended that all women treated with aromatase inhibitors should be evaluated for fracture risk and advice with regard to exercise and calcium/vitamin D supplementation should be given. Bone-directed therapy should be given to all patients with a T-score <-2.0 or with a T-score of <-1.5 SD with one additional RF, or with ≥ 2 risk factors (without BMD) for the duration of AI treatment. Patients with T-score >-1.5 SD and no risk factors should be managed based on BMD loss during the first year and the local guidelines for postmenopausal osteoporosis. Although the evidence for fracture prevention is strongest for denosumab, available data support additional anticancer benefits from adjuvant bisphosphonate treatment in postmenopausal women, because of a 34% relative risk reduction in bone metastasis and 17% breast cancer specific mortality achieved with this therapy [120].

Acid-Suppressive Medications

In recent years concerns have been raised about potential adverse drug events associated with the use of chronic acid-suppressive medications, proton-pump inhibitors (PPIs) and H2 receptor antagonists (H2RAs), including fractures. Initial reports related to histamine H2 receptor (H2R) blocker cimetidine; it was found to be an independent risk factor for hip fracture in a male cohort [122] Further evaluation in a case–control study showed a reduced risk of fractures in individuals exposed to H2R antagonists, but a significantly increased risk of fracture in those exposed to proton pump inhibitors (PPIs) [123]. Yang et al. also reported that PPI use was associated with an increased risk of fractures at the proximal femur, specifically among long-term (>12 months) users of PPI, especially at high doses (OR 1.44, 95% CI 1.31.59) [124]. These findings were supported by a more recent meta-analysis, that suggested that there is an increased risk of fractures at the hip, spine and overall fractures with PPI use [125].

Observational data on the risk of fracture with acid suppression therapy is consistent for PPIs but less so for H2R antagonists. Acid suppression therapies impact intestinal calcium absorption due to altered stomach pH, effect seems small and unlikely to explain the increased risk of fracture [126]. Studies evaluating PPI use and BMD have found no clear association, suggesting that other properties of bone metabolism or bone strength are altered with PPI exposure [127]. The mechanism of adverse skeletal events in the setting of acid suppression in not fully understood, but the use of long-term high-dose PPIs should be regarded as a risk factor for fracture. Furthermore, it has been suggested that patients on bisphosphonates who also take PPIs have a further increased risk of fracture [128, 129]. Lee and colleagues reported in a population based study OR for hip fracture related to PPI use was 1.34 [95% confidence interval (CI) 1.24–144] but was increased to 1.7 (95% CI 1.31–2.23) in patients taking bisphosphonates and PPIs [129]. Similar results were reported from Spanish cohort; they found that PPI use was associated with fractures in bisphosphonate users with an OR of 1.22 (95% CI 1.02–1.46) [130]. Based on these data, H2 blockers should be considered when possible in patients already taking a bisphosphonate.

Thiazolidinediones

Thiazolidinediones (TZDs) are agonists of the peroxisome proliferator activated receptor-γ (PPAR-γ) protein that promote insulin sensitisation and improve glycaemic control in patients with T2DM.TZDs have been associated with an increased risk of fracture [131]. Findings from observational studies suggest an increased risk of fracture in the axial skeleton with TZD use in both women and men [132]. Similar results been found in post-hoc analyses of randomised controlled trials (RCTs) which have also shown a consistently increased risk of fractures in women receiving TZDs [2].

The mechanism by which TZDs increase fracture risk remains unclear. TZDs target peroxisome proliferator-activated receptor-γ (PPAR-γ) protein, a key regulator of energy metabolism in fat tissue. PPAR-γ regulates lipogenesis and lipolysis. In bone, PPARγ influences maturation of mesenchymal stem cells towards osteoblasts and adipocytes and haematopoietic progenitors towards osteoclasts. In addition, PPAR-γ controls production of a variety of cytokines, which support hematopoiesis, including RANKL, which supports osteoclastogenesis. Findings from the meta-analysis suggest that TZDs decrease BMD at the lumbar spine, total hip and forearm; and those changes may not be reversed 1 year after cessation of treatment [133]. Therefore, evaluation of bone health should be undertaken before prescribing TZDs for DM, and if fracture risk is elevated, other hypoglycemic medications should be considered.

Selective Serotonin Reuptake Inhibitors

Selective serotonin reuptake inhibitors (SSRIs) are antidepressants used widely. They act by blocking the serotonin transporters (5-HTT) which are located in the CNS as well as in the periphery [134]. In this more peripheral role, serotonin may exert effects on the skeleton [135]. SSRIs are associated with bone loss and an increase in the risk of fractures in individuals ≥50 years of age [136]. The exact mechanism of bone loss among users of SSRI is unknown, but the focus has been on the effect of serotonin on osteoblasts, as circulating serotonin of gut origin was shown to reduce osteoblast proliferation [54]. There are currently no specific guidelines for the prevention of the bone loss associated with SSRIs. Patients considering treatment with SSRIs who have other risk factors for osteoporosis or fracture might benefit from DXA or FRAX analysis.

Conclusions

As outlined in this chapter, there are many disease states and medications that can affect the metabolic activity of bone, its density and risk of fracture. Understanding of mechanisms of osteoporosis is gradually increasing as new pathways and cell signalling systems are identified. Patients presenting with a new diagnosis of osteoporosis should be screened for the most common secondary causes. This approach can help to limit the added morbidity and mortality of an osteoporotic fracture to their other comorbid conditions.

References

1. Rubin MR, et al. Idiopathic osteoporosis in premenopausal women. Osteoporos Int. 2005;16:526–33.
2. Walker-Bone K. Recognizing and treating secondary osteoporosis. Nat Rev Rheumatol. 2012;8:480–92.
3. Harper KD, Weber TJ. Secondary osteoporosis: diagnostic considerations. Endocrinol Metab Clin N Am. 1998;27:325–48.
4. Caplan A, Fett N, Rosenbach M, Werth VP, Micheletti RG. Prevention and management of glucocorticoid-induced side effects: a comprehensive review: a review of glucocorticoid pharmacology and bone health. J Am Acad Dermatol. 2017;76:1–9.
5. Kaltsas G, Makras P. Skeletal diseases in Cushing's syndrome: osteoporosis versus arthropathy. Neuroendocrinology. 2010;92:60–4.
6. Van Staa TP, Leufkens HGM, Abenhaim L, Zhang B, Cooper C. Use of oral corticosteroids and risk of fractures. J Bone Miner Res. 2000;15:993–1000.
7. Hoes JN, Jacobs JWG, Verstappen SMM, Bijlsma JWJ, Van Der Heijden GJMG. Adverse events of low- to medium-dose oral glucocorticoids in inflammatory diseases: a meta-analysis. Ann Rheum Dis. 2009;68:1833–8.
8. Weinstein RS. Glucocorticoid-induced bone disease. N Engl J Med. 2011;365:62–70.
9. Overman RA, Yeh JY, Deal CL. Prevalence of oral glucocorticoid usage in the United States: a general population perspective. Arthritis Care Res. 2013;65:294–8.
10. Walsh LJ, Wong CA, Pringle M, Tattersfield AE. Use of oral corticosteroids in the community and the prevention of secondary osteoporosis: a cross sectional study. Br Med J. 1996;313:344–6.
11. Briot K, Roux C. Glucocorticoid-induced osteoporosis. RMD Open. 2015;1:e000014.
12. Compston J. Glucocorticoid-induced osteoporosis: an update. Endocrine. 2018;61:7–16.
13. LoCascio V, et al. Bone loss in response to long-term glucocorticoid therapy. Bone Miner. 1990;8:39–51.
14. Van Staa TP, Leufkens HGM, Abenhaim L, Zhang B, Cooper C. Oral corticosteroids and fracture risk: relationship to daily and cumulative doses. Rheumatology. 2000;39:1383–9.
15. Oshagbemi OA, et al. Use of high-dose intermittent systemic glucocorticoids and the risk of fracture in patients with chronic obstructive pulmonary disease. Bone. 2018;110:238–43.
16. Weinstein RS. Glucocorticoid-induced osteoporosis and osteonecrosis. Endocrinol Metab Clin N Am. 2012;41:595–611.
17. Robinson DE, Dennison EM, Cooper C, van Staa TP, Dixon WG. A review of the methods used to define glucocorticoid exposure and risk attribution when investigating the risk of fracture in a rheumatoid arthritis population. Bone. 2016;90:107–15.
18. Robinson DE, van Staa TP, Dennison EM, Cooper C, Dixon WG. The limitations of using simple definitions of glucocorticoid exposure to predict fracture risk: a cohort study. Bone. 2018;117:83–90.
19. O'Brien CA, et al. Glucocorticoids act directly on osteoblasts and osteocytes to induce their apoptosis and reduce bone formation and strength. Endocrinology. 2004;145:1835–41.
20. Hofbauer LC, Hamann C, Ebeling PR. Approach to the patient with secondary osteoporosis. Eur J Endocrinol. 2010;162:1009–20.
21. Weinstein RS, Jilka RL, Michael Parfitt A, Manolagas SC. Inhibition of osteoblastogenesis and promotion of apoptosis of osteoblasts end osteocytes by glucocorticoids potential mechanisms of their deleterious effects on bone. J Clin Invest. 1998;102(2):274–82. https://doi.org/10.1172/JCI2799.
22. Weinstein RS. Glucocorticoids, osteocytes, and skeletal fragility: the role of bone vascularity. Bone. 2010;46:564–70.
23. Chotiyarnwong P, McCloskey EV. Pathogenesis of glucocorticoid-induced osteoporosis and options for treatment. Nat Rev Endocrinol. 2020;16:437–47.

24. Buckley L, Humphrey MB. Glucocorticoid-induced osteoporosis. N Engl J Med. 2018;379:2547–56.
25. Amiche MA, et al. Fracture risk in oral glucocorticoid users: a Bayesian meta-regression leveraging control arms of osteoporosis clinical trials. Osteoporos Int. 2016;27:1709–18.
26. Van Staa TP, Leufkens HGM, Cooper C. Use of inhaled corticosteroids and risk of fractures. J Bone Miner Res. 2001;16:581–8.
27. Bandeira F, et al. Doença óssea no hiperparatiroidismo primário. Arq Bras Endocrinol Metabol. 2014;58:553–61.
28. Bilezikian JP, et al. Guidelines for the management of asymptomatic primary hyperparathyroidism: summary statement from the fourth international workshop. J Clin Endocrinol Metab. 2014;99:3561–9.
29. Roschger P, et al. New observations on bone quality in mild primary hyperparathyroidism as determined by quantitative backscattered electron imaging. J Bone Miner Res. 2007;22:717–23.
30. Zoehrer R, et al. Bone quality determined by Fourier transform infrared imaging analysis in mild primary hyperparathyroidism. J Clin Endocrinol Metab. 2008;93:3484–9.
31. Szymczak J, Bohdanowicz-Pawlak A. Osteoprotegerin, RANKL, and bone turnover in primary hyperparathyroidism: the effect of parathyroidectomy and treatment with alendronate. Horm Metab Res. 2013;45:759–64.
32. Di Monaco M, Vallero F, Di Monaco R, Mautino F, Cavanna A. Primary hyperparathyroidism in elderly patients with hip fracture. J Bone Miner Metab. 2004;22:491–5.
33. Cipriani C, et al. Prevalence of kidney stones and vertebral fractures in primary hyperparathyroidism using imaging technology. J Clin Endocrinol Metab. 2015;100:1309–15.
34. Rubin MR, et al. The natural history of primary hyperparathyroidism with or without parathyroid surgery after 15 years. J Clin Endocrinol Metab. 2008;93:3462–70.
35. Vestergaard P, Mosekilde L. Cohort study on effects of parathyroid surgery on multiple outcomes in primary hyperparathyroidism. Br Med J. 2003;327:530–3.
36. Bassett JHD, et al. Thyroid status during skeletal development determines adult bone structure and mineralization. Mol Endocrinol. 2007;21:1893–904.
37. Greenspan SL, Greenspan FS. The effect of thyroid hormone on skeletal integrity. Ann Intern Med. 1999;130:750–8.
38. Svare A, et al. Hyperthyroid levels of TSH correlate with low bone mineral density: the HUNT 2 study. Eur J Endocrinol. 2009;161:779–86.
39. Bauer DC, Ettinger B, Nevitt MC, Stone KL. Risk for fracture in women with low serum levels of thyroid-stimulating hormone. Ann Intern Med. 2001;134:561–8.
40. Vestergaard P, Mosekilde L. Hyperthyroidism, bone mineral, fracture risk—a meta-analysis. Thyroid. 2003;13:585–93.
41. Wejda B, Hintze G, Katschinski B, Olbricht T, Benker G. Hip fractures and the thyroid: a case-control study. J Intern Med. 1995;237:241–7.
42. Vestergaard P, Rejnmark L, Mosekilde L. Influence of hyper- and hypothyroidism, and the effects of treatment with antithyroid drugs and levothyroxine on fracture risk. Calcif Tissue Int. 2005;77:139–44.
43. Inzerillo AM, Epstein S. Osteoporosis and diabetes mellitus. Rev Endocr Metab Disord. 2004;5:261–8.
44. Epstein S, LeRoith D. Diabetes and fragility fractures—a burgeoning epidemic? Bone. 2008;43:3–6.
45. Nicodemus KK, Folsom AR. Type 1 and type 2 diabetes and incident hip fractures in postmenopausal women. Diabetes Care. 2001;24:1192–7.
46. Pan H, Wu N, Yang T, He W. Association between bone mineral density and type 1 diabetes mellitus: a meta-analysis of cross-sectional studies. Diabetes Metab Res Rev. 2014;30:531–42.
47. Ma L, et al. Association between bone mineral density and type 2 diabetes mellitus: a meta-analysis of observational studies. Eur J Epidemiol. 2012;27:319–32.

48. Burghardt AJ, et al. High-resolution peripheral quantitative computed tomographic imaging of cortical and trabecular bone microarchitecture in patients with type 2 diabetes mellitus. J Clin Endocrinol Metab. 2010;95:5045–55.
49. Farr JN, et al. In vivo assessment of bone quality in postmenopausal women with type 2 diabetes. J Bone Miner Res. 2014;29:787–95.
50. Hofbauer LC, Brueck CC, Singh SK, Dobnig H. Osteoporosis in patients with diabetes mellitus. J Bone Miner Res. 2007;22:1317–28.
51. Gennari L, et al. Circulating Sclerostin levels and bone turnover in type 1 and type 2 diabetes. J Clin Endocrinol Metab. 2012;97:1737–44.
52. Clarke BL, Khosla S. Androgens and bone. Steroids. 2009;74:296–305.
53. Snyder PJ, et al. Effect of testosterone treatment on volumetric bone density and strength in older men with low testosterone a controlled clinical trial. JAMA Intern Med. 2017;177:471–9.
54. Emkey GR. Secondary osteoporosis. In: Encyclopedia of endocrine diseases. 2018. p 253–269. https://doi.org/10.1016/B978-0-12-801238-3.65820-8.
55. Shahinian VB, Kuo YF, Freeman JL, Goodwin JS. Risk of fracture after androgen deprivation for prostate cancer. N Engl J Med. 2005;352:154–64.
56. Ali T, Lam D, Bronze MS, Humphrey MB. Osteoporosis in inflammatory bowel disease. Am J Med. 2009;122:599–604.
57. Szafors P, et al. Risk of fracture and low bone mineral density in adults with inflammatory bowel diseases. A systematic literature review with meta-analysis. Osteoporos Int. 2018;29:2389–97.
58. Stockbrügger RW, et al. Discordance between the degree of osteopenia and the prevalence of spontaneous vertebral fractures in Crohn's disease. Aliment Pharmacol Ther. 2002;16:1519–27.
59. Ludvigsson JF, et al. Fracture risk in patients with inflammatory bowel disease: a nationwide population-based cohort study from 1964 to 2014. Am J Gastroenterol. 2019;114:291–304.
60. Van Staa TP, et al. Inflammatory bowel disease and the risk of fracture. Gastroenterology. 2003;125:1591–7.
61. Reinshagen M. Osteoporosis in inflammatory bowel disease. J Crohns Colitis. 2008;2:202–7.
62. Clowes JA, Riggs BL, Khosla S. The role of the immune system in the pathophysiology of osteoporosis. Immunol Rev. 2005;208:207–27.
63. Ulitsky A, et al. Vitamin D deficiency in patients with inflammatory bowel disease: association with disease activity and quality of life. J Parenter Enter Nutr. 2011;35:308–16.
64. Lima CA. Risk factors for osteoporosis in inflammatory bowel disease patients. World J Gastrointest Pathophysiol. 2015;6:210.
65. Bianchi ML, Bardella MT. Bone in celiac disease. Osteoporos Int. 2008;19:1705–16.
66. Stenson WF, Newberry R, Lorenz R, Baldus C, Civitelli R. Increased prevalence of celiac disease and need for routine screening among patients with osteoporosis. Arch Intern Med. 2005;165:393–9.
67. Heikkilä K, Pearce J, Mäki M, Kaukinen K. Celiac disease and bone fractures: a systematic review and meta analysis. J Clin Endocrinol Metab. 2015;100:25–34.
68. Zanchi C, et al. Bone metabolism in celiac disease. J Pediatr. 2008;153:262–5.
69. Keaveny AP, Freaney R, McKenna MJ, Masterson J, O'Donoghue DP. Bone remodeling indices and secondary hyperparathyroidism in celiac disease. Am J Gastroenterol. 1996;91:1226–31.
70. Valdimarsson T, Toss G, Löfman O, Ström M. Three years' follow-up of bone density in adult coeliac disease: significance of secondary hyperparathyroidism. Scand J Gastroenterol. 2000;35:274–80.
71. Fiore CE, et al. Altered osteoprotegerin/RANKL ratio and low bone mineral density in celiac patients on long-term treatment with gluten-free diet. Horm Metab Res. 2006;38:417–22.
72. Kemppainen T, et al. Bone recovery after a gluten-free diet: a 5-year follow-up study. Bone. 1999;25:355–60.

73. Huusko TM, et al. Threefold increased risk of hip fractures with rheumatoid arthritis in Central Finland. Ann Rheum Dis. 2001;60:521–2.
74. Brennan SL, et al. Rheumatoid arthritis and incident fracture in women: a case-control study. BMC Musculoskelet Disord. 2014;15
75. Ferrari-Lacraz S, Ferrari S. Do RANKL inhibitors (denosumab) affect inflammation and immunity? Osteoporos Int. 2011;22:435–46.
76. Geusens PP, et al. The ratio of circulating osteoprotegerin to RANKL in early rheumatoid arthritis predicts later joint destruction. Arthritis Rheum. 2006;54:1772–7.
77. Terpos E, et al. Early effects of IL-6 receptor inhibition on bone homeostasis: a pilot study in women with rheumatoid arthritis. Clin Exp Rheumatol. 2011;29:921–5.
78. Prieto-Alhambra D, et al. Ankylosing spondylitis confers substantially increased risk of clinical spine fractures: a nationwide case-control study. Osteoporos Int. 2014;26:85–91.
79. Nigil Haroon N, et al. Alterations of bone mineral density, bone microarchitecture and strength in patients with ankylosing spondylitis: a cross-sectional study using high-resolution peripheral quantitative computerized tomography and finite element analysis. Arthritis Res Ther. 2015;17:377.
80. Nigil Haroon N, Sriganthan J, Al Ghanim N, Inman RD, Cheung AM. Effect of TNF-alpha inhibitor treatment on bone mineral density in patients with ankylosing spondylitis: a systematic review and meta-analysis. Semin Arthritis Rheum. 2014;44:155–61.
81. Coimbra IB, Costallat LTL. Bone mineral density in systemic lupus erythematosus and its relation to age at disease onset, plasmatic estradiol and immunosuppressive therapy. Joint Bone Spine. 2003;70:40–5.
82. Yee CS, et al. Prevalence and predictors of fragility fractures in systemic lupus erythematosus. Ann Rheum Dis. 2005;64:111–3.
83. Zehnder Y, et al. Long-term changes in bone metabolism, bone mineral density, quantitative ultrasound parameters, and fracture incidence after spinal cord injury: a cross-sectional observational study in 100 paraplegic men. Osteoporos Int. 2004;15:180–9.
84. Frotzler A, et al. Osteoporosis in the lower extremities in chronic spinal cord injury. Spinal Cord. 2020;58:441–8.
85. Battaglino RA, Lazzari AA, Garshick E, Morse LR. Spinal cord injury-induced osteoporosis: pathogenesis and emerging therapies. Curr Osteoporos Rep. 2012;10:278–85.
86. Edwards WB, Schnitzer TJ, Troy KL. Bone mineral loss at the proximal femur in acute spinal cord injury. Osteoporos Int. 2013;24:2461–9.
87. Szollar M, Martin EME, Sartoris DJ, Parthemore JG, Deftos LJ. Bone mineral density and indexes of bone metabolism in spinal cord injury. Am J Phys Med Rehabil. 1998;77:28–35.
88. Anderson D, Park AJ. Prophylactic treatment of osteoporosis after SCI: promising research, but not yet indicated. Spinal Cord Series Cases. 2019;5:25.
89. Bryson JE, Gourlay ML. Bisphosphonate use in acute and chronic spinal cord injury: a systematic review. J Spinal Cord Med. 2009;32:215–25.
90. Bauman WA, et al. Zoledronic acid administration failed to prevent bone loss at the knee in persons with acute spinal cord injury: an observational cohort study. J Bone Miner Metab. 2015;33:410–21.
91. Gordon KE, Wald MJ, Schnitzer TJ. Effect of parathyroid hormone combined with gait training on bone density and bone architecture in people with chronic spinal cord injury. PM R. 2013;5:663–71.
92. Gifre L, et al. Denosumab increases sublesional bone mass in osteoporotic individuals with recent spinal cord injury. Osteoporos Int. 2016;27:405–10.
93. Gibson JC, Summers GD. Bone health in multiple sclerosis. Osteoporos Int. 2011;22:2935–49.
94. Bazelier MT, et al. Risk of fractures in patients with multiple sclerosis: a population-based cohort study. Neurology. 2012;78:1967–73.
95. Bazelier MT, et al. The risk of fracture in patients with multiple sclerosis: the UK general practice research database. J Bone Miner Res. 2011;26:2271–9.

96. Dennison EM, et al. Effect of co-morbidities on fracture risk: findings from the Global Longitudinal Study of Osteoporosis in Women (GLOW). Bone. 2012;50:1288–93.
97. Gregson CL, et al. Disease-specific perception of fracture risk and incident fracture rates: GLOW cohort study. Osteoporos Int. 2014;25:85–95.
98. Kyle RA, et al. Review of 1027 patients with newly diagnosed multiple myeloma. Mayo Clin Proc. 2003;78:21–33.
99. Giuliani N, Bataille R, Mancini C, Lazzaretti M, Barillé S. Myeloma cells induce imbalance in the osteoprotegerin/osteoprotegerin ligand system in the human bone marrow environment. Blood. 2001;98:3527–33.
100. Tian E, et al. The role of the Wnt-signaling antagonist DKK1 in the development of osteolytic lesions in multiple myeloma. N Engl J Med. 2003;349:2483–94.
101. Mhaskar R, et al. Bisphosphonates in multiple myeloma: a network meta-analysis. Cochrane Database Syst Rev. 2012:CD003188. https://doi.org/10.1002/14651858.cd003188.pub3
102. Morgan GJ, et al. First-line treatment with zoledronic acid as compared with clodronic acid in multiple myeloma (MRC myeloma IX): a randomised controlled trial. Lancet. 2010;376:1989–99.
103. Hageman K, Patel KC, Mace K, El Papel de Cooper MR. Denosumab para la Prevención de Complicaciones Músculo-Esqueletales Debido a Mieloma Múltiple. Ann Pharmacother. 2013;47:1069–74.
104. De Sanctis V, et al. Osteoporosis in thalassemia major: an update and the I-CET 2013 recommendations for surveillance and treatment. Pediatr Endocrinol Rev. 2013;11:167–80.
105. Voskaridou E, Terpos E. New insights into the pathophysiology and management of osteoporosis in patients with beta thalassaemia. Br J Haematol. 2004;127:127–39.
106. Giusti A, Pinto V, Forni GL, Pilotto A. Management of beta-thalassemia-associated osteoporosis. Ann N Y Acad Sci. 2016;1368:73–81.
107. Alem AM, et al. Increased risk of hip fracture among patients with end-stage renal disease. Kidney Int. 2000;58:396–9.
108. Nickolas TL, McMahon DJ, Shane E. Relationship between moderate to severe kidney disease and hip fracture in the United States. J Am Soc Nephrol. 2006;17:3223–32.
109. Ketteler M, et al. Executive summary of the 2017 KDIGO chronic kidney disease–mineral and bone disorder (CKD-MBD) guideline update: what's changed and why it matters. Kidney Int. 2017;92:26–36.
110. Yu TM, et al. Osteoporosis and fractures after solid organ transplantation: a nationwide population-based cohort study. Mayo Clin Proc. 2014;89:888–95.
111. Premaor MO, et al. Fracture incidence after liver transplantation: results of a 10-year audit. QJM. 2011;104:599–606.
112. Hariman A, Alex C, Heroux A, Camacho P. Incidence of fractures after cardiac and lung transplantation: a single center experience. J Osteoporos. 2014;2014:573041.
113. Epstein S, Inzerillo AM, Caminis J, Zaidi M. Disorders associated with acute rapid and severe bone loss. J Bone Miner Res. 2003;18:2083–94.
114. Ebeling PR. Transplantation osteoporosis. Curr Osteoporos Rep. 2007;5:29–37.
115. Goodman GR, et al. Immunosuppressant use without bone loss—implications for bone loss after transplantation. J Bone Miner Res. 2001;16:72–8.
116. Cohen A, Sambrook P, Shane E. Management of bone loss after organ transplantation. J Bone Miner Res. 2004;19:1919–32.
117. Stein EM, Ortiz D, Jin Z, McMahon DJ, Shane E. Prevention of fractures after solid organ transplantation: a meta-analysis. J Clin Endocrinol Metab. 2011;96:3457–65.
118. Bjarnason NH, Hitz M, Jorgensen NR, Vestergaard P. Adverse bone effects during pharmacological breast cancer therapy. Acta Oncol. 2008;47:747–54.
119. Vestergaard P, Rejnmark L, Mosekilde L. Effect of tamoxifen and aromatase inhibitors on the risk of fractures in women with breast cancer. Calcif Tissue Int. 2008;82:334–40.

120. Hadji P, et al. Management of aromatase inhibitor-associated bone loss (AIBL) in postmenopausal women with hormone sensitive breast cancer: joint position statement of the IOF, CABS, ECTS, IEG, ESCEO IMS, and SIOG. J Bone Oncol. 2017;7:1–12.
121. Colzani E, et al. Risk of hospitalisation and death due to bone fractures after breast cancer: a registry-based cohort study. Br J Cancer. 2016;115:1400–7.
122. Grisso JA, et al. Risk factors for hip fracture in men. Am J Epidemiol. 1997;145:786–93.
123. Vestergaard P, Rejnmark L, Mosekilde L. Proton pump inhibitors, histamine H2 receptor antagonists, and other antacid medications and the risk of fracture. Calcif Tissue Int. 2006;79:76–83.
124. Yang YX, Lewis JD, Epstein S, Metz DC. Long-term proton pump inhibitor therapy and risk of hip fracture. J Am Med Assoc. 2006;296:2947–53.
125. Zhou B, Huang Y, Li H, Sun W, Liu J. Proton-pump inhibitors and risk of fractures: an update meta-analysis. Osteoporos Int. 2016;27:339–47.
126. O'Connell MB, Madden DM, Murray AM, Heaney RP, Kerzner LJ. Effects of proton pump inhibitors on calcium carbonate absorption in women: a randomized crossover trial. Am J Med. 2005;118:778–81.
127. Targownik LE, Lix LM, Leung S, Leslie WD. Proton-pump inhibitor use is not associated with osteoporosis or accelerated Bone mineral density loss. Gastroenterology. 2010;138:896–904.
128. De Vries F, Cooper AL, Cockle SM, Van Staa TP, Cooper C. Fracture risk in patients receiving acid-suppressant medication alone and in combination with bisphosphonates. Osteoporos Int. 2009;20:1989–98.
129. Lee J, et al. A population-based case-control study: proton pump inhibition and risk of hip fracture by use of bisphosphonate. J Gastroenterol. 2013;48:1016–22.
130. Prieto-Alhambra D, et al. Predictors of fracture while on treatment with oral bisphosphonates: a population-based cohort study. J Bone Miner Res. 2014;29:268–74.
131. Loke YK, Singh S, Furberg CD. Long-term use of thiazolidinediones and fractures in type 2 diabetes: a meta-analysis. Can Med Assoc J. 2009;180:32–9.
132. Solomon DH, et al. A cohort study of thiazolidinediones and fractures in older adults with diabetes. J Clin Endocrinol Metab. 2009;94:2792–8.
133. Billington EO, Grey A, Bolland MJ. The effect of thiazolidinediones on bone mineral density and bone turnover: systematic review and meta-analysis. Diabetologia. 2015;58:2238–46.
134. Bliziotes MM, Eshleman AJ, Zhang XW, Wiren KM. Neurotransmitter action in osteoblasts: expression of a functional system for serotonin receptor activation and reuptake. Bone. 2001;29:477–86.
135. Warden SJ, Robling AG, Haney EM, Turner CH, Bliziotes MM. The emerging role of serotonin (5-hydroxytryptamine) in the skeleton and its mediation of the skeletal effects of low-density lipoprotein receptor-related protein 5 (LRP5). Bone. 2010;46:4–12.
136. Eom CS, Lee HK, Ye S, Park SM, Cho KH. Use of selective serotonin reuptake inhibitors and risk of fracture: a systematic review and meta-analysis. J Bone Miner Res. 2012;27:1186–95.

Chapter 12
Bone Health in Children

Rebecca J. Moon and Justin H. Davies

Introduction

Fractures in childhood are common. Approximately one third of boys and a fifth of girls will sustain at least one fracture before their 18th birthday [1]. The majority of fractures in children occur in those with normal bone strength due to trauma. However, reduced bone strength due to impaired bone mineralization and alterations in bone microarchitecture, as observed in osteoporotic bone, increases the propensity to fracture. Whilst osteoporosis is usually considered a disease of older age and is most typically seen in post-menopausal women, childhood osteoporosis does occur, albeit far less commonly than in later life. Importantly, the principles of diagnosis and management of osteoporosis in adults cannot be extrapolated to the immature growing skeleton.

Definition of Osteoporosis in Children

As discussed in Chap. 2, in adults the diagnosis of osteoporosis is based on a measure of bone mineral density (BMD) by dual energy X-ray absorptiometry (DXA). Independent of age and sex, an individual's measured BMD is compared to data

R. J. Moon (✉)
Paediatric Endocrinology, University Hospitals Southampton NHS Foundation Trust, Southampton, UK

MRC Lifecourse Epidemiology Centre, University of Southampton, Southampton, UK
e-mail: Rm3w07@soton.ac.uk

J. H. Davies
Paediatric Endocrinology, University Hospitals Southampton NHS Foundation Trust, Southampton, UK
e-mail: justin.davies@uhs.nhs.uk

E. Dennison (ed.), *Osteoporosis Treatment*, https://doi.org/10.1007/978-3-030-78128-6_12

from a reference population comprised of healthy young adult females to generate a standard deviate "T-score [2]. In contrast, the definition of childhood osteoporosis, as proposed by the International Society of Clinical Densitometry (ISCD) in 2013 (and updated in 2019) includes a clinical component [3, 4]. One or more vertebral compression fractures in the absence of local disease or high energy trauma is considered indicative of osteoporosis. A measurement of BMD is not needed to define osteoporosis when a vertebral fracture is present as these have been observed to occur in children with a BMD Z-score > −2 [5], although a DXA measurement may be undertaken subsequently as part of the investigative process. In the absence of a vertebral fracture, osteoporosis is defined by both the presence of a clinically significant fracture history and a BMD Z-score ≤ −2.0. A clinically significant fracture history is considered as two or more low/moderate energy long bone fractures by age 10 years or three or more long bone fractures at any age up to age 19 years [3]. This definition was proposed, largely based on expert opinion, to prevent over-diagnosis of skeletal fragility in children, but recently it has been argued that such a strict criteria is likely to result in both under-diagnosis and delays in diagnosis whilst waiting for second and subsequent fractures to occur [6].

Aetiology of Childhood Osteoporosis

The causes of childhood osteoporosis can broadly be divided into primary and secondary. Primary osteoporosis is typically due to a genetic abnormality. Secondary osteoporosis occurs as a consequence of another underlying medical condition and/or its treatments.

Genetic Abnormalities Leading to Low Bone Density

Osteogenesis Imperfecta (OI)

The most common genetic cause of recurrent fracture in childhood is osteogenesis imperfecta (OI), a collection of genetically and clinically diverse disorders of connective tissue, which are associated with abnormal bone microarchitecture, low bone mass and propensity to fracture. OI affects approximately 1 in 10,000 live-births [7] and varies markedly in severity from perinatal lethality to increased fracture frequency with minimal trauma without chronic bony deformity. OI was originally classified into four types by Sillence et al. in 1979 based on clinical and radiological characteristics [8], with the later addition of more subtypes based on genetic abnormalities rather than clinical phenotypes [9]. However, with the increased availability of molecular genetic testing, an ever-expanding number of genes associated with bone fragility have been identified. As such, in 2010 (revised 2015), the Nosology and Classification of Genetic Skeletal Diseases opted to continue with the classification into five subtypes based predominantly on clinical features. These are largely based on the original Sillence classification, whilst recognizing that multiple genetic mutations now account for each subtype, and this list is likely to continue expanding [10]. These are summarized in Table 12.1.

Type 1 is the commonest and mildest form of OI, and is usually due to an autosomal dominant mutation in either *COL1A1 or COL1A2,* which encode procollagen type 1 α1 and α2 chains, respectively. This results in either a qualitative or quantitative reduction in collagen. Affected individuals have an increased risk of fracture with minimal trauma, but bone deformity is usually absent or minimal and near-normal height is achieved. Other common, but not universal, features of type 1 OI include blue-grey discolouration of the sclera and dentinogenesis imperfecta, which results in discolouration of the teeth with a translucent appearance and increased risk of tooth fracture and decay.

Type 2 OI results in severe deformity and intrauterine fractures with death occurring during fetal life or in the neonatal period due to pulmonary hypoplasia. Type 3 OI is the most severe form amongst those that survive the intrauterine and neonatal period. Fracture risk is very high, with most affected individuals having evidence of fractures at birth. Progressive deformities to the limbs occur and extreme short stature is usually present. Scoliosis, hearing loss and dentinogenesis imperfecta are also typically observed in this group and in later childhood basilar invagination, a skull base deformity, may rarely occur. Individuals with type 4 OI are moderate-severely affected, but can range extensively in severity from very few fractures to a frequent fracturing bone deforming phenotype. Type 4 OI is associated with short stature which distinguishes it from Type 1 OI, in which stature is typically within the expected range. Dentinogenesis imperfecta and hearing loss can occur, but are not

Table 12.1 Genetic causes of poor bone health in childhood

Condition	Clinical Features (in addition to osteoporosis/ low bone mass)	Inheritance	Genes involved	Protein
Osteogenesis imperfecta type 1	Blue-grey sclera, dentinogenesis imperfecta. Normal stature	AD	*COL1A1* *COL1A2*	Collagen 1 alpha-1 chain Collagen 1 alpha-2 chain
Osteogeneis imperfecta type 2	Lethal in perinatal period, pulmonary hypoplasia	AD, AR	*COL1A1* *COL1A2* *CRTAP* *LEPRE1* *PPIB*	Collagen 1 alpha-1 chain Collagen 1 alpha-2 chain Cartilage-associated protein Leucine proline-enriched proteoglycan (leprecan) 1 Peptidylprolyl isomerase B

(continued)

Table 12.1 (continued)

Condition	Clinical Features (in addition to osteoporosis/ low bone mass)	Inheritance	Genes involved	Protein
Osteogeneis imperfecta type 3	Limb deformities secondary to fractures, severe short stature, hearing loss, dentinogenesis imperfecta	AD, AR	*COL1A1* *COL1A2* *CRTAP* *LEPRE1* *PPIB* *SERPINH1* *BMP1* *FKBP10* *PLOD2* *SERPINF1* *SP7* *WNT1* *TMEM38B* *CREB3L1* *SEC24D*	Collagen 1 alpha-1 chain Collagen 1 alpha-2 chain Cartilage-associated protein Leucine proline-enriched proteoglycan (leprecan) 1 Peptidylprolyl isomerase B Seroin peptidase inhibitor, clade H, member 1 Bone morphogenetic protein 1 FK506 binding protein 10 Procollagen lysyl hydroxylase 2 Serpin peptidase inhibitor, clade F, member 1 SP7 transcription factor (Osterix) Wingless-type MMTV integration site family, member Transmembrane protein 38B OASIS SEC24-related gene family, member D

Table 12.1 (continued)

Condition	Clinical Features (in addition to osteoporosis/ low bone mass)	Inheritance	Genes involved	Protein
Osteogeneis imperfecta type 4	Short stature, dentinogenesis imperfecta may occur	AD, AR	*COL1A1* *COL1A2* *CRTAP* *PPIB* *FKBP10* *SERPINF1* *WNT1* *SP7*	Collagen 1 alpha-1 chain Collagen 1 alpha-2 chain Cartilage-associated protein Peptidylprolyl isomerase B FK506 binding protein 10 Serpin peptidase inhibitor, clade F, member 1 Wingless-type MMTV integration site family, member SP7 transcription factor (Osterix)
Osteogeneis imperfecta type 5	Short stature, hypertrophic callus formation	AD	*IFITM5*	BRIL
Bruck syndrome type 1 [11, 12]	Congenital joint contractures	AR	*FKBP10*	FK506 binding protein 10
Bruck syndrome type 2 [11, 13, 14]	Congenital joint contractures, grey-blue sclera may be present	AR	*PLOD2*	Procollagen lysyl hydroxylase 2
Osteoporosis-pseudoglioma syndrome	Severe visual impairment, short stature	AR	*LRP5*	LDL-receptor related protein 5
LRP5 primary osteoporosis [15, 16]		AD	*LRP5*	LDL-receptor related protein 5
Calvarial doughnut lesions with bone fragility [17]	Sclerotic doughnut shaped lesions in the cranial bones, short stature, cranial sclerosis, spondylometaphyseal dysplasia	AD	*SGMS2*	Sphingomyelin synthase 2 gene
Cole-Carpenter dysplasia [18]	Craniosynostosis, ocular proptosis, hydrocephalus, facial dysmorphism	AD	*P4HB*	Prolyl 4-hydroxylase, beta subunit

(continued)

Table 12.1 (continued)

Condition	Clinical Features (in addition to osteoporosis/ low bone mass)	Inheritance	Genes involved	Protein
Spondylo-ocular dysplasia [19, 20]	Ocular abnormalities (eg cataract, retinal detachment), facial hypotonia, facial dysmorphism, vertebral anomalies, scoliosis, short trunk, hearing impariment	AR	*XYLT2*	Xylosyltransferase 2
Gnathodiaphyseal dysplasia [21]	Cementoosseous lesions of the jawbones, cortical thickening and sclerosis of diaphyses of tubular bones leading to bowing	AD	*ANO5*	
Ehlers-Danlos syndrome, progeroid form [22]	Short stature, hypermobility, facial dysmorphism, radioulnar synostosis, hypermetropia	AR	*B4GALT7*	Xylosylprotein 4-beta-galactosyltransferase deficiency
Geroderma osteodysplasticum [23, 24]	Progeroid features, hypermobility, inelastic wrinkled skin, flat feet, hypotonia, congenital hip dislocation, maxillary hypoplasia	AR	*GORAB*	SCYL1-binding protein 1
Cutis laxa type 2B [24]	Progeroid features, hypermobility, inelastic wrinkled skin, flat feet, hypotonia, congenital hip dislocation, short stature, facial dysmorphism, intrauterine growth restriction, intellectual impairment	AR	*PYCR1*	Pyrroline-5-carboxylate reductase
Cutis laxa type 2A (wrinkly skin syndrome) [24]	Progeroid features, hypermobility, inelastic wrinkled skin, flat feet, hypotonia, congenital hip dislocation, short stature, facial dysmorphism, abnormal fat distribution, intellectual impairment	AR	*ATP6VDA2*	ATPase

Table 12.1 (continued)

Condition	Clinical Features (in addition to osteoporosis/ low bone mass)	Inheritance	Genes involved	Protein
Singleton-Merten syndrome	Dental dysplasia, vascular and cardiac calcification, hypotonia and muscular atrophy, short stature, delayed motor development, glaucoma,	AD		
Hajdu-Cheney Syndrome [25]	Acrolysis, craniofacial defects, short stature, polycystic kidneys, cardiac anomalies	AD	*NOTCH2*	NOTCH
X-lined osteoporosis [26]		X linked	*PLS3*	Plastin 3
Juvenile idiopathic osteoporosis		Spontaneous		

always present. Types 2, 3 and 4 OI, like type 1, can be caused my mutations in *COL1A1* and *COL1A2*, but have also been associated with genetic errors in proteins involved in the post-translational modification and folding of collagen. For example, cartilage associated protein (CRTAP) and P3H1encoded by *LEPRE1* both form part of a multi-protein complex located in the endoplasmic reticulum and are essential for proper folding of procollagen. Mutations in both *CRTAP* and *LEPRE1* are associated with severe forms of OI (type 2 and 3) resulting in neonatal fractures, rhizomelia, broad undertubulated bones and severe growth deficiency [27]. Mutations in genes associated with collagen stability (*FKBP10* and *SERPINH1*), collagen cleavage (*BMP1*) and osteoblast and osteocyte function (WNT1, SP7, PLS3, SERPINF1) have also been associated with OI types 2, 3 and 4 [10, 27].

Type 5 OI results from a dominantly inherited mutation in *IFITM5,* which encodes BRIL, a protein involved in mineralization by the osteoblast [28]. Presentation is similar to type 4, but additionally includes the distinctive features of hypertrophic callus formation at sites of fracture or surgical sites and ossification of the forearm interosseous membrane often resulting in radial head dislocation [29].

Other Genetic Causes of Low Bone Density

There are a number of other recognized rare genetic causes of primary osteoporosis leading to fracture in childhood, typically caused by monogenic defects in the bone metabolism pathway. Many are associated with distinct clinical features, for example osteoporosis-pseudoglioma syndrome (OPPG). This condition is characterized by severe osteoporosis and visual loss. It is caused by autosomal recessive inactivating mutations in the low-density lipoprotein receptor-related protein 5 (LRP5) gene

[30]. LRP5 is a membrane co-receptor in the canonical Wnt signaling pathway, which acts to regulate bone mass through stimulation of preosteoblast replication, induction of osteoblastogenesis and inhibition of osteoblast and osteocyte apoptosis. Loss of function of this pathway results in reduced bone mineralization, and conversely gain of function mutations result in a high bone mass phenotype. Autosomal dominant mutations in the coding-regions of LRP5 have also been associated with childhood-onset primary osteoporosis without features of OI or OPPG [15, 16]. A detailed discussion of all conditions associated with childhood-onset primary osteoporosis is outside of the remit of this article. These conditions are summarized in Table 12.1 [11–26].

Finally, juvenile idiopathic osteoporosis (JIO) is a primary osteoporosis of unknown aetiology, and a diagnosis of exclusion once OI and other causes of primary and secondary osteoporosis have been excluded. JIO typically presents in children age 8–13 years, before the onset of puberty, with long bone fractures, back pain associated with vertebral fractures and reduced mobility [31]. Spontaneous remission usually occurs coinciding with puberty, but supportive treatment is often required until that time.

Secondary Osteoporosis

Secondary osteoporosis occurs as a result of another pathological process and/or its treatments that leads to alterations in bone metabolism and/or bone mineral accrual. At birth, whole body bone mineral content (BMC) of an infant with a weight of 3.0–3.5 kg is approximately 66 g [32]. Thereafter bone mass increases throughout childhood and adolescence to reach a peak in the third decade when whole body BMC averages 2.5 kg in females and 3.5 kg in males [33]. Puberty is a critical period for bone mass accrual. Whole body bone mass approximately doubles during the period of pubertal growth. However, the rate of gain in bone mass temporally lags behind peak growth velocity by approximately 6 months, resulting in a period of relative under-mineralisation [34]. This coincides with the increase in fracture rates observed in adolescence, even in otherwise healthy individuals [1]. Chronic medical conditions can impact on bone strength and mineral accrual through malnutrition, chronic inflammation, impaired bone-muscle interactions or disruption to endocrine pathways. In many chronic conditions, osteoporosis results from a combination of these detrimental effects. Inflicted injury should also be considered in cases of unexplained fracture.

Malnutrition is associated with poor bone accrual. Anorexia nervosa is an example of an extreme form of nutritional deprivation and is associated with loss of muscle mass and bone mass, particularly in the trabecular compartment [35]. Hypogonadotrophic hypogonadism resulting in delayed puberty and/or amenorrhoea, and growth hormone resistance will also contribute to bone loss in adolescents with eating disorders. Although some recovery of BMD can occur after restoration of normal weight and menses [36, 37], it is possible that lifetime fracture risk remains elevated in both men and women [38]. Poor nutrition and low body mass index is also implicated in impaired bone mineral accrual in adolescents with cystic fibrosis [39].

Low BMD has been demonstrated in a number of paediatric inflammatory medical conditions, including inflammatory bowel disease, coeliac disease, systemic lupus erythematosus, inflammatory arthritides, and nephrotic syndrome [40–42]. The underlying inflammatory process may contribute directly to detrimental bone outcomes and indeed vertebral fractures have been identified at diagnosis in children with systemic inflammatory conditions [43, 44]. In inflammatory bowel disease, interactions between IL-6, TNF-alpha and RANK-ligand on osteoblasts and osteoclasts lead to increased bone resorption [45]. Malabsorption effects, particularly impaired absorption of calcium and vitamin D in inflammatory bowel disease and coeliac disease also contribute to reduced BMD [46]. In coeliac disease, adherence to a gluten free diet, plus calcium and vitamin D supplementation has been shown to improve bone health significantly, but in adults BMD often continues to be lower than in healthy controls [47]. Coeliac disease has also been associated with autoantibodies, which neutralise the action of osteoprotegerin (OPG), an inhibitor of bone resorption [48, 49]. These antibodies would be expected to result in increased bone resorption, and thus might further contribute to osteoporosis in individuals with coeliac disease.

Fractures can be a presenting feature of acute lymphoblastic leukaemia (ALL), and in particular vertebral fractures at diagnosis are well recognised. In the Canadian Steroid-Associated Osteoporosis in the Paediatric Population (STOPP) study, 16% of children had at least one vertebral fracture on spinal radiographs at diagnosis of ALL. Many participants had multiple vertebral fractures [50]. In the same study, just over one third of children had a fracture within the first 6 years after ALL diagnosis [51]. The exact pathophysiological process resulting in bone fragility is poorly understood. Whilst osteotoxic chemotherapy agents, including high dose steroids, are likely to contribute, the high prevalence of fractures prior to treatment initiation suggest an alternative process is also responsible. It has been suggested that cytokines produced by the malignant cells result in increased osteoclast activation and subsequent osteolysis [52].

The importance of muscular function to bone mineral accrual is well recognised. Reduced physical activity as part of the treatment of an eating disorder or as a result of a chronic medical condition (eg due to pain, poor lung function, hospitalisation, reduced energy levels) will contribute to secondary osteoporosis risk. Conditions directly affecting neuro-muscular function are often associated with an increased incidence of fragility fracture. For example, boys with Duchenne muscular dystrophy (DMD) are at high risk of fractures due to impaired immobility in addition to chronic inflammation, delayed puberty and high-dose glucocorticoid exposure. Similarly, children with cerebral palsy have a number of risk factors for osteoporosis including reduced ambulation and low muscle mass, poor nutrition, and exposure to osteotoxic medications eg anti-epileptic agents.

Many medications impact negatively on bone, of which glucocorticoids are the most commonly described. In adults, dose-dependent bone loss occurs rapidly on drug introduction, and is associated with increased fracture risk [53]. In children requiring recurrent courses of glucocorticoids an increased fracture risk has also been reported [54]. In one large study children who had received 4 or more prescriptions for oral steroids in a 12-month period had just over 30% increased risk of fracture compared to children who had never been prescribed steroids. Fracture incidence was not increased in children who had taken oral steroids more than 12 months previously, suggesting recovery of detrimental bony effects [54]. The use of inhaled steroids for childhood asthma has not been associated with increased fracture risk [55]. Importantly, achieving a balance between the bone loss associated with glucocorticoids use, and minimizing the underlying disease/inflammatory process, which impacts negatively on growth, puberty, skeletal mineralisation, nutrition and muscular function, is important. One such example is boys with DMD, in whom oral corticosteroids have been shown to preserve ambulation and therefore discontinuation of these is not feasible, but modification of treatment regimens might be important to minimise bone demineralisation. In a recent study comparing the use of daily to intermittent (10 days on-10 days off) steroid dosing over a 2-year period in a non-randomised convenience sample, a greater proportion of boys on daily dosing remained ambulant, but at a cost of more vertebral fractures than observed in boys receiving intermittent steroid dosing [56]. Further studies to establish the optimal dosing schedule for preservation of ambulation with minimal bone loss are needed.

Other medications associated with increased fracture incidence or reduced BMD in childhood include acid suppression therapy [57], selective serotonin reuptake inhibitors (SSRI) [58], heparin, low-molecular weight heparins, warfarin, stimulant medication for attention deficit hyperactivity disorder (ADHD) [59], anti-epileptic agents [60] and anti-retroviral therapy [61].

Investigation of Suspected Bone Fragility in Children

A diagnosis of osteoporosis should be considered in children presenting with frequent low to moderate trauma fractures or vertebral fractures, or in children at risk of osteoporosis due to a medical condition associated with osteoporosis, a family history of primary osteoporosis or other clinical signs suspicious of a syndrome associated with osteoporosis.

History and Examination

A detailed fracture history should be obtained, and importantly, attempts made to confirm that a bony injury was sustained. In a recent study, 16% of previous injuries reported by parents to have included a fracture did not have evidence of a radiographically detectable fracture. In that study 11% of children who would have had a clinically significant fracture history on parental report alone, did not have a clinically significant fracture history on review of radiological reports [62].

The history and examination in a child with suspected osteoporosis should aim to elucidate signs and symptoms of conditions associated with secondary osteoporosis and the family history of fractures, joint dislocation, osteoporosis and intrauterine deaths. Assessment of growth and pubertal stage is vital, and examination should include observation of dysmorphic features, hypermobility, scleral colour, presence/absence of dentinogenesis imperfecta, vertebral tenderness, scoliosis, limb deformity, herniae and abnormal scarring. Signs of conditions associated with secondary osteoporosis eg apthous ulceration, abdominal tenderness in inflammatory bowel disease, clubbing, chest signs in cystic fibrosis should be noted.

Blood Investigations

Baseline investigations should include blood sampling for full blood count, renal profile, PTH, calcium, phosphate, alkaline phosphatase, inflammatory markers, 25-hydroxyvitamin D status, thyroid function and coeliac screen. If a primary osteoporosis is considered likely, then a genetic panel for OI should be considered.

Vertebral Imaging

Many vertebral fractures in children are asymptomatic [43, 50]. Imaging is therefore required to determine their presence or absence if a diagnosis of osteoporosis is considered clinically likely. In children who are high risk of osteoporosis, regular screening for vertebral fractures is often advised even if bone mineral density is within the normal range. For example, screening for vertebral fractures is recommended in boys with DMD every 1–2 years in those taking steroids, and every 2–3 years in boys not treated with steroids [63].

Lateral thoracolumbar spinal radiographs are considered the gold standard to identify vertebral fractures, and are the most commonly used imaging modality due to widespread availability and low radiation exposure. The Genant scoring system can be used to provide a semi-quantitative score for the degree of spinal deformity. Vertebral fracture assessment (VFA) using dual energy X-ray absorptiometry (DXA) is also increasingly used. The main benefit of this approach is the lower radiation exposure, but the accuracy of automated morphometric vertebral fracture analysis software in children remains debatable [64].

Dual Energy X-ray Absorptiometry

As discussed in Chap. 2, measurement of BMD is performed by DXA. Algorithms are used for bone edge detections, and the reported BMD is the mean BMD measured within the pixels identified as bone. Importantly in children, bone edge detection is more difficult than in adults due to the relatively lower BMD. This can lead to underestimation of the bone area and false identification of bone as soft tissue. The use of paediatric software is important to overcome this issue. DXA reports an areal BMD in g/cm^2 as during the acquisition of the scan a three dimensional structure is converted into a two dimensional image. As such, a thick low density bone and a thin high density bone might have the same aBMD. aBMD will overestimate true volumetric BMD in larger bones and underestimate in small bones and this needs to be considered in children. A number of mathematical models and approaches have been developed to adjust for this, including bone mineral apparent density (BMAD) [65] and bone mineral content (BMC) for height [66]. The typical sites for assessment of BMD in children are total body less head (TBLH) and lumbar spine (LS) due to the reproducibility at these sites [4].

The main limitation of DXA in young children is movement artefact reducing scan interpretation. Acquisition time for a TBLH DXA scan in approximately 5 min, during which the child needs to remain still. LS, proximal femur (PF), lateral distal femur (LDF) and distal radial scans are considerably quicker to obtain, however the latter scanning sites should only be used when TBLH and/or LS cannot be obtained, for example, due to non-removable artifacts (e.g. orthopaedic hardware, feeding tubes) or positioning difficulties (e.g. severe scoliosis, contractures) [4]. Radiation exposure for a DXA scan is low; a TBLH and LS scan exposes a preschool child and an adult to an effective radiation dose of approximately 21 and 16 microsieverts, respectively. In comparison, a transatlantic flight exposes an individual to roughly 80 microsieverts of radiation [67].

Management

Bone modeling and remodeling during growth has the potential to restore bone strength if risk factors contributing to poor bone mineralization can be reversed. Vertebral fractures can also reshape in the growing skeleton. Approaches to minimizing risk factors, for example discontinuing unnecessary medications, optimizing mobility, steroid-sparing/minimizing strategies, addressing underlying inflammation should be undertaken in all cases.

Multidisciplinary Management

The management of osteoporosis in childhood requires a multidisciplinary team approach. Occupational therapists, physiotherapists and orthotists should be involved to improve physical function and provide necessary aids to overcome limitations due to contractures, short stature and limited mobility. Surgical involvement is likely to be necessary for management of fractures, long bone deformities and scoliosis. Audiological review is necessary for children with OI.

Lifestyle Advice

Children with osteoporosis should be counselled on minimizing fracture risk whilst promoting a normal healthy lifestyle. Participation in contact sports should be advised against, and high impact repetitive sports which place excessive forces on the vertebral column, for example trampolining, gymnastics, horse-riding should be avoided. Similarly, participation in activities which are associated with an increased falls risk eg ice-skating, skiing, should be recommended against.

Further advice should aim to optimize bone health by promoting nutrition and physical activity. Calcium and vitamin D are well recognized as necessary for bone health, but other dietary factors including protein, vitamins A, C and K, magnesium and phosphate are also important to bone metabolism. Maintenance of a body mass index (BMI) within the normal range is important as both undernutrition and obesity have been linked to increased fracture propensity [68]. Poor nutrition can delay initiation and progression through puberty, which is an important period for bone mass accrual and bone remodeling. Similarly, restoration of menses in amenorrhoeic adolescents will have a positive effect on bone mineral accrual during late adolescence and early adulthood prior to attainment of peak bone mass. Multidisciplinary input from dietetics should be sought in children at risk of dietary deficiencies or with an abnormal BMI due to malabsorption, increased caloric demands or eating disorders to ensure this is achieved.

The importance of muscular strain on bone modelling and remodeling is well recognized and therefore physical activity, within the limits of the underlying diagnosis, should be encouraged. In otherwise healthy children [69], physical activity has been shown to increase BMD in randomized controlled trials. There are fewer studies on the effects of physical activity in children with a diagnosis of osteoporosis. One recent randomised controlled trial of whole body vibration (WBV) in children with OI in an attempt to improve muscle strength and subsequently bone mass showed no increase in BMD over a 5 month period despite an increase in total body lean mass [70].

Dental Care

OI type 1 is commonly associated with dentinogenesis imperfecta, an abnormality at the dentinoenamel junction, which increases the likelihood of dental fracture, attrition and decay. Regular dental review and good dental hygiene should be encouraged. Children with OI are also at increased risk of dental malocclusion and orthodontic review may be necessary.

Pharmacological Therapy

Bisphosphonates

Bisphosphonates inhibit bone resorption by binding to calcium crystals in hydroxyapatite and inhibiting osteoclastic action. In children, bisphosphonates increase bone mass and strength by reducing bone resorption, but have no effect on bone growth, periosteal bone formation or trabecular bone formation. Histomorphometric studies have shown that children with OI treated with pamidronate had an increase in cortical thickness and trabecular number [71]. When increased, both of these parameters, when measured by high-resolution peripheral quantitative computed tomography (HR-pQCT), have been associated with lower fracture risk in healthy children and adults [72–74].

The decision whether to initiate bisphosphosphate treatment is often individualised following a discussion with the patient and/or carer. This involves consideration of the underlying cause of osteoporosis, the benefit/risks of therapy and discussion of the side effect profile, reversibility and likelihood of spontaneous resolution of osteoporosis. In children with primary osteoporosis, resolution is less likely than those with secondary osteoporosis in whom the underlying cause for poor bone health can be managed. As such, in children with primary osteoporosis with vertebral compression fractures or frequent (>2 per year) long bone fractures, then intravenous bisphosphonate therapy would be recommended [75]. In children with OI, a recent Cochrane systematic review of 14 trials of bisphosphonate treatment showed, bisphosphonates resulted in an increase in BMD, although the effects on vertebral remodeling and fracture incidence remain uncertain [76]. Currently there are no trials on the use of bisphosphonates to prevent primary fracture in children with secondary osteoporosis, and therefore initiation of therapy based solely on a low BMD measurement cannot be recommended at the current time. Some groups of children with secondary osteoporosis are more likely to have persistence of risk factors, for example boys with DMD who are likely to remain on long term steroids until ambulation is lost and children with CP or spinal injuries in whom neuromuscular function is unlikely to improve. In contrast, children with IBD or rheumatological conditions are more likely to achieve control of the underlying inflammatory disorder and/or reduce steroid exposure. The opportunity for vertebral reshaping and bone remodeling is also lower in peripubertal children, and therefore earlier initiation of bisphosphonates might be warranted. Similarly to studies in OI, the use of bisphosphonates in secondary osteoporosis has been associated with an increased BMD, but typically have limited power to assess the effect on fracture incidence [75].

The most commonly studied and used bisphosphonates in children are intravenous pamidronate and zoledronate. The main benefit of zoledronate over pamidronate is the dosing schedule: zoledronate is administered as a single dose every 6 months, whereas pamidronate is given over 2 days every 3 months. A recent study in children with OI showed that the clinical efficacy of the two drug regimens were similar in terms of fracture rate and lumbar spine BMD, but zoledronate was significantly cheaper, mostly due to the reduced administration costs [77]. Clearly, the benefits for the patient and their family in terms of hospital visits, missed school and employment and fewer painful procedures (intravenous cannulation) are also important.

The most frequent side effect of bisphosphonate therapy is an "acute phase reaction". Symptoms include fever, malaise, bone pain, headache, nausea and vomiting, and typically occur within 48 hours of the infusion. This reaction is more commonly seen in bisphosphate-naïve patients, with one recent study reporting it to occur in 27% of children following their first treatment [78]. Interestingly, in the same study, acute phase reactions in subsequent infusions were more common in children with secondary osteoporosis than those with primary osteoporosis, but no difference was seen between pamidronate and zoledronic acid [78]. Treatment is with symptom management.

Hypocalcaemia is also commonly seen after bisphosphonate therapy, with one recent report suggesting 7% of infusions were complicated by this. As with acute phase reactions, hypocalcaemia was more commonly observed in children with secondary and glucocorticoid induced osteoporosis compared to primary osteoporosis [78]. Routine calcium supplementation and attention to ensuring vitamin D sufficiency prior to administration are strategies to reduce symptomatic hypocalcaemia.

In adults, osteonecrosis of the jaw (ONJ) and atypical femoral fractures (AFF) are recognized rare complications of bisphosphonate therapy [79, 80]. In a recently published systematic review of the literature up to August 2018, there were no published cases of ONJ in children and young adults under 24 years of age [81]. Nonetheless, awareness of the condition by medical professionals treating children with bisphosphonates and counselling of parents and children as to the very small potential risk is needed. AFF are a recognized complication of adult long term bisphosphonate therapy. They are a form of stress fracture thought to result from the presence of overmineralized older bone, repetitive loading and microcrack formation. AFF are defined according to an American Society of Bone Mineral Research (ASBMR) task force definition [82]. There are case reports of children undergoing BP therapy for OI and with fractures suggestive of AFF [83, 84], although the unique nature of bone morphology and fractures in this group of patients it is difficult to determine causality to BPs.

Denosumab

Denosumab is a humanized monoclonal antibody that binds with high affinity and specificity to RANK ligand (RANKL), resulting in rapid suppression of bone resorption. It is licensed for use in postmenopausal osteoporosis, but there have been few studies of its use in paediatric osteoporosis. One study in 4 boys with OI type 4 demonstrated an increase in areal BMD and stabilization or improvement in vertebral morphology following treatment with denosumab for 2 years [85]. A second study by the same research group involving ten children with OI due to genetically confirmed mutations in *COL1A1* or *COL1A2* similarly showed an increased in lumbar spine aBMD and BMD z-score from baseline following 48 weeks of denosumab treatment. No control group was included [86]. In adults with osteoporosis a rebound of vertebral fractures is observed following discontinuation of denosumab. Severe rebound hypercalcaemia following discontinuation of denosumab in children with other conditions has been observed. Further studies in children are therefore needed prior to routine use in clinical practice.

Teriparatide

Teriparatide, a synthetic form of parathyroid hormone, significantly reduces the risk of vertebral fractures in post-menopausal osteoporosis, but the effect on long bone fractures is less well documented [87]. However, its use in the paediatric population has not been explored as a study in rats found a high incidence of osteosarcoma following recombinant PTH administration [88].

Romosozumab

Romosozumab, an anti-sclerotin monoclonal antibody, is the newest treatment available for postmenopausal osteoporosis. A 2020 Endocrine Society guideline has suggested romosozumab should be used as first line therapy in patients with multiple vertebral fractures, or hip fracture and BMD in the osteoporotic range [89]. Its use has not yet been investigated in children with osteoporosis.

Summary

Whilst poor bone health in children has a broad range of causes including genetic, pharmacologically induced and secondary to other health conditions, the increased propensity to fracture defines the condition. Importantly, the investigation and treatment of childhood osteoporosis is unique to this age group and diagnostic and management guidelines for adults cannot be used.

References

1. Moon RJ, Harvey NC, Curtis EM, de Vries F, van Staa T, Cooper C. Ethnic and geographic variations in the epidemiology of childhood fractures in the United Kingdom. Bone. 2016;85:9–14. https://doi.org/10.1016/j.bone.2016.01.015.
2. Consensus Development Conference. Consensus development conference: diagnosis, prophylaxis, and treatment of osteoporosis. Am J Med. 1993;94(6):646–50.

3. Bishop N, Arundel P, Clark E, Dimitri P, Farr J, Jones G, et al. Fracture prediction and the definition of osteoporosis in children and adolescents: the ISCD 2013 pediatric official positions. J Clin Densitom. 2014;17(2):275–80. https://doi.org/10.1016/j.jocd.2014.01.004.
4. Shuhart CR, Yeap SS, Anderson PA, Jankowski LG, Lewiecki EM, Morse LR, et al. Executive summary of the 2019 ISCD position development conference on monitoring treatment, DXA cross-calibration and least significant change, spinal cord injury, peri-prosthetic and orthopedic bone health, transgender medicine, and pediatrics. J Clin Densitom. 2019;22(4):453–71. https://doi.org/10.1016/j.jocd.2019.07.001.
5. Ma J, Siminoski K, Alos N, Halton J, Ho J, Lentle B, et al. The choice of normative pediatric reference database changes spine bone mineral density Z-scores but not the relationship between bone mineral density and prevalent vertebral fractures. J Clin Endocrinol Metab. 2015;100(3):1018–27. https://doi.org/10.1210/jc.2014-3096.
6. Ward LM, Weber DR, Munns CF, Högler W, Zemel BS. A contemporary view of the definition and diagnosis of osteoporosis in children and adolescents. J Clin Endocrinol Metabol. 2020;105(5):e2088–97. https://doi.org/10.1210/clinem/dgz294.
7. Folkestad L, Hald JD, Ersboll AK, Gram J, Hermann AP, Langdahl B, et al. Fracture rates and fracture sites in patients with osteogenesis imperfecta: a nationwide register-based cohort study. J Bone Miner Res. 2017;32(1):125–34. https://doi.org/10.1002/jbmr.2920.
8. Sillence DO, Senn A, Danks DM. Genetic heterogeneity in osteogenesis imperfecta. J Med Genet. 1979;16(2):101–16. https://doi.org/10.1136/jmg.16.2.101.
9. Van Dijk FS, Sillence DO. Osteogenesis imperfecta: clinical diagnosis, nomenclature and severity assessment. Am J Med Genet A. 2014;164A(6):1470–81. https://doi.org/10.1002/ajmg.a.36545.
10. Bonafe L, Cormier-Daire V, Hall C, Lachman R, Mortier G, Mundlos S, et al. Nosology and classification of genetic skeletal disorders: 2015 revision. Am J Med Genet A. 2015;167(12):2869–92. https://doi.org/10.1002/ajmg.a.37365.
11. Viljoen D, Versfeld G, Beighton P. Osteogenesis imperfecta with congenital joint contractures (Bruck syndrome). Clin Genet. 1989;36(2):122–6. https://doi.org/10.1111/j.1399-0004.1989.tb03174.x.
12. Alanay Y, Avaygan H, Camacho N, Utine GE, Boduroglu K, Aktas D, et al. Mutations in the gene encoding the RER protein FKBP65 cause autosomal-recessive osteogenesis imperfecta. Am J Hum Genet. 2010;86(4):551–9. https://doi.org/10.1016/j.ajhg.2010.02.022.
13. van der Slot AJ, Zuurmond AM, Bardoel AF, Wijmenga C, Pruijs HE, Sillence DO, et al. Identification of PLOD2 as telopeptide lysyl hydroxylase, an important enzyme in fibrosis. J Biol Chem. 2003;278(42):40967–72. https://doi.org/10.1074/jbc.M307380200.
14. Lv F, Xu X, Song Y, Li L, Asan, Wang J, et al. Novel mutations in PLOD2 cause rare Bruck syndrome. Calcif Tissue Int. 2018;102(3):296–309. https://doi.org/10.1007/s00223-017-0360-6.
15. Korvala J, Juppner H, Makitie O, Sochett E, Schnabel D, Mora S, et al. Mutations in LRP5 cause primary osteoporosis without features of OI by reducing Wnt signaling activity. BMC Med Genet. 2012;13:26. https://doi.org/10.1186/1471-2350-13-26.
16. Hartikka H, Makitie O, Mannikko M, Doria AS, Daneman A, Cole WG, et al. Heterozygous mutations in the LDL receptor-related protein 5 (LRP5) gene are associated with primary osteoporosis in children. J Bone Miner Res. 2005;20(5):783–9. https://doi.org/10.1359/jbmr.050101.
17. Pekkinen M, Terhal PA, Botto LD, Henning P, Mäkitie RE, Roschger P, et al. Osteoporosis and skeletal dysplasia caused by pathogenic variants in SGMS2. JCI Insight. 2019;4(7):e126180. https://doi.org/10.1172/jci.insight.126180.
18. Rauch F, Fahiminiya S, Majewski J, Carrot-Zhang J, Boudko S, Glorieux F, et al. Cole-carpenter syndrome is caused by a heterozygous missense mutation in P4HB. Am J Hum Genet. 2015;96(3):425–31. https://doi.org/10.1016/j.ajhg.2014.12.027.
19. Schmidt H, Rudolph G, Hergersberg M, Schneider K, Moradi S, Meitinger T. Retinal detachment and cataract, facial dysmorphism, generalized osteoporosis, immobile spine

and platyspondyly in a consanguinous kindred—a possible new syndrome. Clin Genet. 2001;59(2):99–105. https://doi.org/10.1034/j.1399-0004.2001.590206.x.
20. Munns CF, Fahiminiya S, Poudel N, Munteanu MC, Majewski J, Sillence DO, et al. Homozygosity for frameshift mutations in XYLT2 result in a spondylo-ocular syndrome with bone fragility, cataracts, and hearing defects. Am J Hum Genet. 2015;96(6):971–8. https://doi.org/10.1016/j.ajhg.2015.04.017.
21. Jin L, Liu Y, Sun F, Collins MT, Blackwell K, Woo AS, et al. Three novel ANO5 missense mutations in Caucasian and Chinese families and sporadic cases with gnathodiaphyseal dysplasia. Sci Rep. 2017;7:40935. https://doi.org/10.1038/srep40935.
22. Salter CG, Davies JH, Moon RJ, Fairhurst J, Bunyan D, Foulds N. Further defining the phenotypic spectrum of B4GALT7 mutations. Am J Med Genet A. 2016;170(6):1556–63. https://doi.org/10.1002/ajmg.a.37604.
23. Takeda R, Takagi M, Shinohara H, Futagawa H, Narumi S, Hasegawa T, et al. Novel compound heterozygous mutations identified by whole exome sequencing in a Japanese patient with geroderma osteodysplastica. Eur J Med Genet. 2017;60(12):635–8. https://doi.org/10.1016/j.ejmg.2017.08.002.
24. Kariminejad A, Afroozan F, Bozorgmehr B, Ghanadan A, Akbaroghli S, Khorram Khorshid HR, et al. Discriminative features in three autosomal recessive Cutis Laxa syndromes: Cutis Laxa IIA, Cutis Laxa IIB, and Geroderma Osteoplastica. Int J Mol Sci. 2017;18(3):635. https://doi.org/10.3390/ijms18030635.
25. Canalis E, Zanotti S. Hajdu-Cheney syndrome: a review. Orphanet J Rare Dis. 2014;9(1):200. https://doi.org/10.1186/s13023-014-0200-y.
26. Kampe AJ, Makitie RE, Makitie O. New genetic forms of childhood-onset primary osteoporosis. Horm Res Paediatr. 2015;84(6):361–9. https://doi.org/10.1159/000439566.
27. Forlino A, Marini JC. Osteogenesis imperfecta. Lancet. 2016;387(10028):1657–71. https://doi.org/10.1016/S0140-6736(15)00728-X.
28. Moffatt P, Gaumond MH, Salois P, Sellin K, Bessette MC, Godin E, et al. Bril: a novel bone-specific modulator of mineralization. J Bone Miner Res. 2008;23(9):1497–508. https://doi.org/10.1359/jbmr.080412.
29. Glorieux FH, Rauch F, Plotkin H, Ward L, Travers R, Roughley P, et al. Type V osteogenesis imperfecta: a new form of brittle bone disease. J Bone Miner Res. 2000;15(9):1650–8. https://doi.org/10.1359/jbmr.2000.15.9.1650.
30. Streeten EA, McBride D, Puffenberger E, Hoffman ME, Pollin TI, Donnelly P, et al. Osteoporosis-pseudoglioma syndrome: description of 9 new cases and beneficial response to bisphosphonates. Bone. 2008;43(3):584–90. https://doi.org/10.1016/j.bone.2008.04.020.
31. Smith R. Idiopathic juvenile osteoporosis: experience of twenty-one patients. Br J Rheumatol. 1995;34(1):68–77. https://doi.org/10.1093/rheumatology/34.1.68.
32. Koo WW, Walters J, Bush AJ, Chesney RW, Carlson SE. Dual-energy X-ray absorptiometry studies of bone mineral status in newborn infants. J Bone Miner Res. 1996;11(7):997–102. https://doi.org/10.1002/jbmr.5650110717.
33. Alwis G, Rosengren B, Stenevi-Lundgren S, Duppe H, Sernbo I, Karlsson MK. Normative dual energy X-ray absorptiometry data in Swedish children and adolescents. Acta Paediatr. 2010;99(7):1091–9. https://doi.org/10.1111/j.1651-2227.2010.01713.x.
34. Kirmani S, Christen D, van Lenthe GH, Fischer PR, Bouxsein ML, McCready LK, et al. Bone structure at the distal radius during adolescent growth. J Bone Miner Res. 2009;24(6):1033–42. https://doi.org/10.1359/jbmr.081255.
35. DiVasta AD, Feldman HA, O'Donnell JM, Long J, Leonard MB, Gordon CM. Skeletal outcomes by peripheral quantitative computed tomography and dual-energy X-ray absorptiometry in adolescent girls with anorexia nervosa. Osteoporos Int. 2016;27(12):3549–58. https://doi.org/10.1007/s00198-016-3685-5.
36. El Ghoch M, Gatti D, Calugi S, Viapiana O, Bazzani PV, Dalle Grave R. The association between weight gain/restoration and bone mineral density in adolescents with anorexia nervosa: a systematic review. Nutrients. 2016;8(12):769. https://doi.org/10.3390/nu8120769.

37. Miller KK, Lee EE, Lawson EA, Misra M, Minihan J, Grinspoon SK, et al. Determinants of skeletal loss and recovery in anorexia nervosa. J Clin Endocrinol Metab. 2006;91(8):2931–7. https://doi.org/10.1210/jc.2005-2818.
38. Lucas AR, Melton LJ 3rd, Crowson CS, O'Fallon WM. Long-term fracture risk among women with anorexia nervosa: a population-based cohort study. Mayo Clin Proc. 1999;74(10):972–7. https://doi.org/10.4065/74.10.972.
39. Sharma S, Jaksic M, Fenwick S, Byrnes C, Cundy T. Accrual of bone mass in children and adolescents with cystic fibrosis. J Clin Endocrinol Metab. 2017;102(5):1734–9. https://doi.org/10.1210/jc.2016-3459.
40. Dubner SE, Shults J, Baldassano RN, Zemel BS, Thayu M, Burnham JM, et al. Longitudinal assessment of bone density and structure in an incident cohort of children with Crohn's disease. Gastroenterology. 2009;136(1):123–30. https://doi.org/10.1053/j.gastro.2008.09.072.
41. Kohler JA, Moon RJ, Sands R, Doherty LJ, Taylor PA, Cooper C, et al. Selective reduction in trabecular volumetric bone mineral density during treatment for childhood acute lymphoblastic leukemia. Bone. 2012;51(4):765–70. https://doi.org/10.1016/j.bone.2012.06.025.
42. Viswanathan A, Sylvester FA. Chronic pediatric inflammatory diseases: effects on bone. Rev Endocr Metab Disord. 2008;9(2):107–22. https://doi.org/10.1007/s11154-007-9070-0.
43. Huber AM, Gaboury I, Cabral DA, Lang B, Ni A, Stephure D, et al. Prevalent vertebral fractures among children initiating glucocorticoid therapy for the treatment of rheumatic disorders. Arthritis Care Res. 2010;62(4):516–26. https://doi.org/10.1002/acr.20171.
44. Dias Costa F, Maia C, Almeida S, Ferreira R. Child with multiple fractures: a rare presentation of a common disease. BMJ Case Rep. 2017;2017:bcr2016218477. https://doi.org/10.1136/bcr-2016-218477.
45. Laakso S, Valta H, Verkasalo M, Toiviainen-Salo S, Viljakainen H, Makitie O. Impaired bone health in inflammatory bowel disease: a case-control study in 80 pediatric patients. Calcif Tissue Int. 2012;91(2):121–30. https://doi.org/10.1007/s00223-012-9617-2.
46. Fouda MA, Khan AA, Sultan MS, Rios LP, McAssey K, Armstrong D. Evaluation and management of skeletal health in celiac disease: position statement. Can J Gastroenterol. 2012;26(11):819–29.
47. Zanchetta MB, Longobardi V, Costa F, Longarini G, Mazure RM, Moreno ML, et al. Impaired bone microarchitecture improves after one year on gluten-free diet: a prospective longitudinal HRpQCT study in women with celiac disease. J Bone Miner Res. 2017;32(1):135–42. https://doi.org/10.1002/jbmr.2922.
48. Riches PL, McRorie E, Fraser WD, Determann C, van't Hof R, Ralston SH. Osteoporosis associated with neutralizing autoantibodies against osteoprotegerin. N Engl J Med. 2009;361(15):1459–65. https://doi.org/10.1056/NEJMoa0810925.
49. Real A, Gilbert N, Hauser B, Kennedy N, Shand A, Gillett H, et al. Characterisation of osteoprotegerin autoantibodies in coeliac disease. Calcif Tissue Int. 2015;97(2):125–33. https://doi.org/10.1007/s00223-015-0023-4.
50. Halton J, Gaboury I, Grant R, Alos N, Cummings EA, Matzinger M, et al. Advanced vertebral fracture among newly diagnosed children with acute lymphoblastic leukemia: results of the Canadian Steroid-Associated Osteoporosis in the Pediatric Population (STOPP) research program. J Bone Miner Res. 2009;24(7):1326–34. https://doi.org/10.1359/jbmr.090202.
51. Ward LM, Ma J, Lang B, Ho J, Alos N, Matzinger MA, et al. Bone morbidity and recovery in children with acute lymphoblastic leukemia: results of a six-year prospective cohort study. J Bone Miner Res. 2018;33(8):1435–43. https://doi.org/10.1002/jbmr.3447.
52. Jayanthan A, Miettunen PM, Incoronato A, Ortiz-Neira CL, Lewis VA, Anderson R, et al. Childhood acute lymphoblastic leukemia (ALL) presenting with severe osteolysis: a model to study leukemia-bone interactions and potential targeted therapeutics. Pediatr Hematol Oncol. 2010;27(3):212–27. https://doi.org/10.3109/08880011003663382.
53. Van Staa TP, Leufkens HG, Abenhaim L, Zhang B, Cooper C. Use of oral corticosteroids and risk of fractures. J Bone Miner Res. 2000;15(6):993–1000. https://doi.org/10.1359/jbmr.2000.15.6.993.

54. van Staa TP, Cooper C, Leufkens HG, Bishop N. Children and the risk of fractures caused by oral corticosteroids. J Bone Miner Res. 2003;18(5):913–8. https://doi.org/10.1359/jbmr.2003.18.5.913.
55. Gray N, Howard A, Zhu J, Feldman LY, To T. Association between inhaled corticosteroid use and bone fracture in children with asthma. JAMA Pediatr. 2018;172(1):57–64. https://doi.org/10.1001/jamapediatrics.2017.3579.
56. Crabtree NJ, Adams JE, Padidela R, Shaw NJ, Hogler W, Roper H, et al. Growth, bone health & ambulatory status of boys with DMD treated with daily vs. intermittent oral glucocorticoid regimen. Bone. 2018;116:181–6. https://doi.org/10.1016/j.bone.2018.07.019.
57. Malchodi L, Wagner K, Susi A, Gorman G, Hisle-Gorman E. Early acid suppression therapy exposure and fracture in young children. Pediatrics. 2019;144(1):e20182625. https://doi.org/10.1542/peds.2018-2625.
58. Wadhwa R, Kumar M, Talegaonkar S, Vohora D. Serotonin reuptake inhibitors and bone health: a review of clinical studies and plausible mechanisms. Osteoporos Sarcopenia. 2017;3(2):75–81. https://doi.org/10.1016/j.afos.2017.05.002.
59. Howard JT, Walick KS, Rivera JC. Preliminary evidence of an association between ADHD medications and diminished bone health in children and adolescents. J Pediatr Orthop. 2017;37(5):348–54. https://doi.org/10.1097/bpo.0000000000000651.
60. Petty SJ, Wilding H, Wark JD. Osteoporosis associated with epilepsy and the use of anti-epileptics—a review. Curr Osteoporos Rep. 2016;14(2):54–65. https://doi.org/10.1007/s11914-016-0302-7.
61. Shiau S, Arpadi SM, Yin MT. Bone update: is it still an issue without Tenofovir Disoproxil fumarate? Curr HIV/AIDS Rep. 2020;17(1):1–5. https://doi.org/10.1007/s11904-019-00474-1.
62. Moon RJ, Lim A, Farmer M, Segaran A, Clarke NM, Harvey NC, et al. Validity of parental recall of children's fracture: implications for investigation of childhood osteoporosis. Osteoporos Int. 2016;27(2):809–13. https://doi.org/10.1007/s00198-015-3287-7.
63. Birnkrant DJ, Bushby K, Bann CM, Alman BA, Apkon SD, Blackwell A, et al. Diagnosis and management of Duchenne muscular dystrophy, part 2: respiratory, cardiac, bone health, and orthopaedic management. Lancet Neurol. 2018;17(4):347–61. https://doi.org/10.1016/S1474-4422(18)30025-5.
64. Alqahtani FF, Offiah AC. Diagnosis of osteoporotic vertebral fractures in children. Pediatr Radiol. 2019;49(3):283–96. https://doi.org/10.1007/s00247-018-4279-5.
65. Carter DR, Bouxsein ML, Marcus R. New approaches for interpreting projected bone densitometry data. J Bone Miner Res. 1992;7(2):137–45. https://doi.org/10.1002/jbmr.5650070204.
66. Zemel BS, Leonard MB, Kelly A, Lappe JM, Gilsanz V, Oberfield S, et al. Height adjustment in assessing dual energy x-ray absorptiometry measurements of bone mass and density in children. J Clin Endocrinol Metab. 2010;95(3):1265–73. https://doi.org/10.1210/jc.2009-2057.
67. Public Health England. Ionising radiation: dose comparisons. 2011. https://www.gov.uk/government/publications/ionising-radiation-dose-comparisons/ionising-radiation-dose-comparisons. Accessed 29 Mar 2017.
68. Dimitri P, Bishop N, Walsh JS, Eastell R. Obesity is a risk factor for fracture in children but is protective against fracture in adults: a paradox. Bone. 2012;50(2):457–66. S8756-3282(11)00985-9 [pii]. https://doi.org/10.1016/j.bone.2011.05.011.
69. Yang X, Zhai Y, Zhang J, Chen J-Y, Liu D, Zhao W-H. Combined effects of physical activity and calcium on bone health in children and adolescents: a systematic review of randomized controlled trials. World J Pediatr. 2020;16(4):356–65. https://doi.org/10.1007/s12519-019-00330-7.
70. Högler W, Scott J, Bishop N, Arundel P, Nightingale P, Mughal MZ, et al. The effect of whole body vibration training on bone and muscle function in children with osteogenesis imperfecta. J Clin Endocrinol Metabol. 2017;102(8):2734–43. https://doi.org/10.1210/jc.2017-00275.
71. Rauch F, Travers R, Plotkin H, Glorieux FH. The effects of intravenous pamidronate on the bone tissue of children and adolescents with osteogenesis imperfecta. J Clin Invest. 2002;110(9):1293–9. https://doi.org/10.1172/JCI15952.

72. Stein EM, Liu XS, Nickolas TL, Cohen A, Thomas V, McMahon DJ, et al. Abnormal microarchitecture and reduced stiffness at the radius and tibia in postmenopausal women with fractures. J Bone Miner Res. 2010;25(12):2572–81. https://doi.org/10.1002/jbmr.152.
73. Farr JN, Amin S, Melton LJ, Kirmani S, McCready LK, Atkinson EJ, et al. Bone strength and structural deficits in children and adolescents with a distal forearm fracture resulting from mild trauma. J Bone Miner Res. 2014;29(3):590–9. https://doi.org/10.1002/jbmr.2071.
74. Chevalley T, Bonjour JP, van Rietbergen B, Ferrari S, Rizzoli R. Fractures during childhood and adolescence in healthy boys: relation with bone mass, microstructure, and strength. J Clin Endocrinol Metab. 2011;96(10):3134–42. jc.2011-1445 [pii]. https://doi.org/10.1210/jc.2011-1445.
75. Simm PJ, Biggin A, Zacharin MR, Rodda CP, Tham E, Siafarikas A, et al. Consensus guidelines on the use of bisphosphonate therapy in children and adolescents. J Paediatr Child Health. 2018;54(3):223–33. https://doi.org/10.1111/jpc.13768.
76. Dwan K, Phillipi CA, Steiner RD, Basel D. Bisphosphonate therapy for osteogenesis imperfecta. Cochrane Database Syst Rev. 2016;10(10):CD005088. https://doi.org/10.1002/14651858.CD005088.pub4.
77. Saraff V, Sahota J, Crabtree N, Sakka S, Shaw NJ, Högler W. Efficacy and treatment costs of zoledronate versus pamidronate in paediatric osteoporosis. Arch Dis Child. 2018;103(1):92–4. https://doi.org/10.1136/archdischild-2017-313234.
78. Nasomyont N, Hornung LN, Gordon CM, Wasserman H. Outcomes following intravenous bisphosphonate infusion in pediatric patients: a 7-year retrospective chart review. Bone. 2019;121:60–7. https://doi.org/10.1016/j.bone.2019.01.003.
79. Zervas K, Verrou E, Teleioudis Z, Vahtsevanos K, Banti A, Mihou D, et al. Incidence, risk factors and management of osteonecrosis of the jaw in patients with multiple myeloma: a single-centre experience in 303 patients. Br J Haematol. 2006;134(6):620–3. https://doi.org/10.1111/j.1365-2141.2006.06230.x.
80. Wotton CJ, Green J, Brown A, Armstrong MEG, Floud S, Beral V, et al. Use of oral bisphosphonates and risk of hospital admission with osteonecrosis of the jaw: large prospective cohort study in UK women. Bone. 2019;124:69–74. https://doi.org/10.1016/j.bone.2019.04.003.
81. Duarte NT, Rech BO, Martins IG, Franco JB, Ortega KL. Can children be affected by bisphosphonate-related osteonecrosis of the jaw? A systematic review. Int J Oral Maxillofac Surg. 2020;49(2):183–91. https://doi.org/10.1016/j.ijom.2019.08.004.
82. Shane E, Burr D, Abrahamsen B, Adler RA, Brown TD, Cheung AM, et al. Atypical subtrochanteric and diaphyseal femoral fractures: second report of a task force of the American Society for Bone and Mineral Research. J Bone Miner Res. 2014;29(1):1–23. https://doi.org/10.1002/jbmr.1998.
83. Vasanwala RF, Sanghrajka A, Bishop NJ, Högler W. Recurrent proximal femur fractures in a teenager with osteogenesis imperfecta on continuous bisphosphonate therapy: are we overtreating? J Bone Miner Res. 2016;31(7):1449–54. https://doi.org/10.1002/jbmr.2805.
84. Trejo P, Fassier F, Glorieux FH, Rauch F. Diaphyseal femur fractures in osteogenesis imperfecta: characteristics and relationship with bisphosphonate treatment. J Bone Miner Res. 2017;32(5):1034–9. https://doi.org/10.1002/jbmr.3071.
85. Hoyer-Kuhn H, Netzer C, Koerber F, Schoenau E, Semler O. Two years' experience with denosumab for children with osteogenesis imperfecta type VI. Orphanet J Rare Dis. 2014;9:145. https://doi.org/10.1186/s13023-014-0145-1.
86. Hoyer-Kuhn H, Franklin J, Allo G, Kron M, Netzer C, Eysel P, et al. Safety and efficacy of denosumab in children with osteogenesis imperfect—a first prospective trial. J Musculoskelet Neuronal Interact. 2016;16(1):24–32.
87. Kanis JA, Cooper C, Rizzoli R, Reginster JY, Scientific Advisory Board of the European Society for Clinical and Economic Aspects of Osteoporosis (ESCEO) and the Committees of Scientific Advisors and National Societies of the International Osteoporosis Foundation (IOF). European guidance for the diagnosis and management of osteoporosis in postmenopausal women. Osteoporos Int. 2019;30(1):3–44. https://doi.org/10.1007/s00198-018-4704-5.

88. Vahle JL, Sato M, Long GG, Young JK, Francis PC, Engelhardt JA, et al. Skeletal changes in rats given daily subcutaneous injections of recombinant human parathyroid hormone (1-34) for 2 years and relevance to human safety. Toxicol Pathol. 2002;30(3):312–21. https://doi.org/10.1080/01926230252929882.
89. Shoback D, Rosen CJ, Black DM, Cheung AM, Murad MH, Eastell R. Pharmacological management of osteoporosis in postmenopausal women: an endocrine society guideline update. J Clin Endocrinol Metab. 2020;105(3):dgaa048. https://doi.org/10.1210/clinem/dgaa048.

Index

E. Dennison (ed.), *Osteoporosis Treatment*, https://doi.org/10.1007/978-3-030-78128-6

GPSR Compliance

The European Union's (EU) General Product Safety Regulation (GPSR) is a set of rules that requires consumer products to be safe and our obligations to ensure this.

If you have any concerns about our products, you can contact us on ProductSafety@springernature.com

In case Publisher is established outside the EU, the EU authorized representative is:

Springer Nature Customer Service Center GmbH
Europaplatz 3
69115 Heidelberg, Germany

Batch number: 10732090

Printed by Printforce, the Netherlands